KU-200-635

THE INTERNATIONAL
HAIRSTYLE INDEX

THE PEPIN PRESS
AMSTERDAM & SINGAPORE

646 724 INT
151080

All rights reserved.
Copyright © 2003 The Pepin Press BV, Amsterdam

The Pepin Press BV
P.O. Box 10349
1001 EH Amsterdam
The Netherlands

Tel +31 20 4202021
Fax +31 20 4201152
mail@pepinpress.com
www.pepinpress.com

ISBN 90 5496 104 x

Concept & book design: Pepin van Roojen
Editor and picture researcher: Femke van Eijk

10 9 8 7 6 5 4 3 2 1
2008 07 06 05 04 03

Manufactured in China

WITHDRAWN

page 2

INTERCOIFFURE SOUTH AFRICA
ISJON, P.O. Box 4921, Halfway House 1685, Johannesburg, South Africa
Hair: Johan Nortje, Isjon, Intercoiffure South Africa

page 3

THE LOUNGE HAIR STUDIO
100-1039 Richards Street, Vancouver, British Columbia V6B 3E4, Canada
www.loungehairstudio.com
Hair: Martin Hillier
Salon: The Lounge Hair Studio
Make-up: Sharon Fisher
Photography: Lance Blanchette

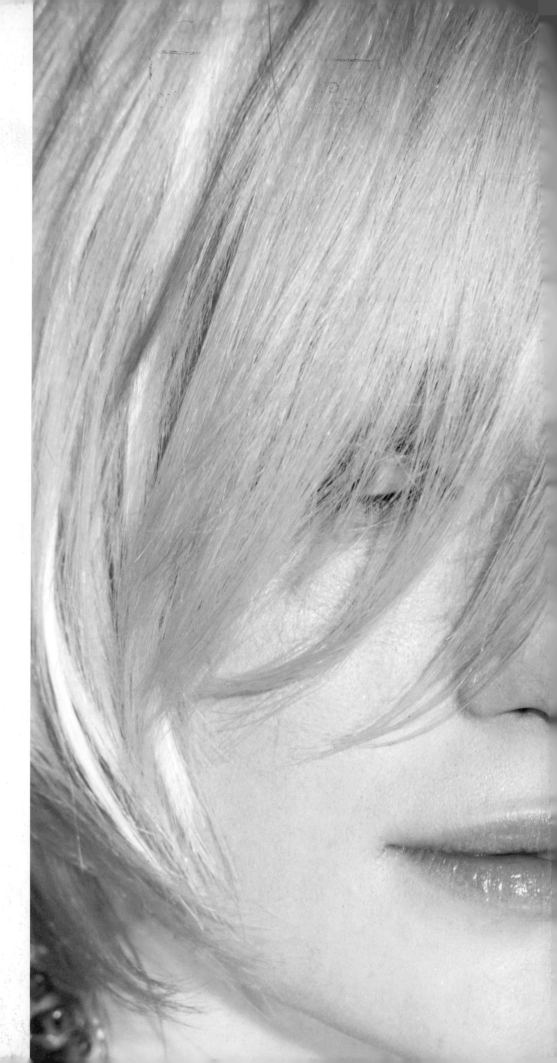

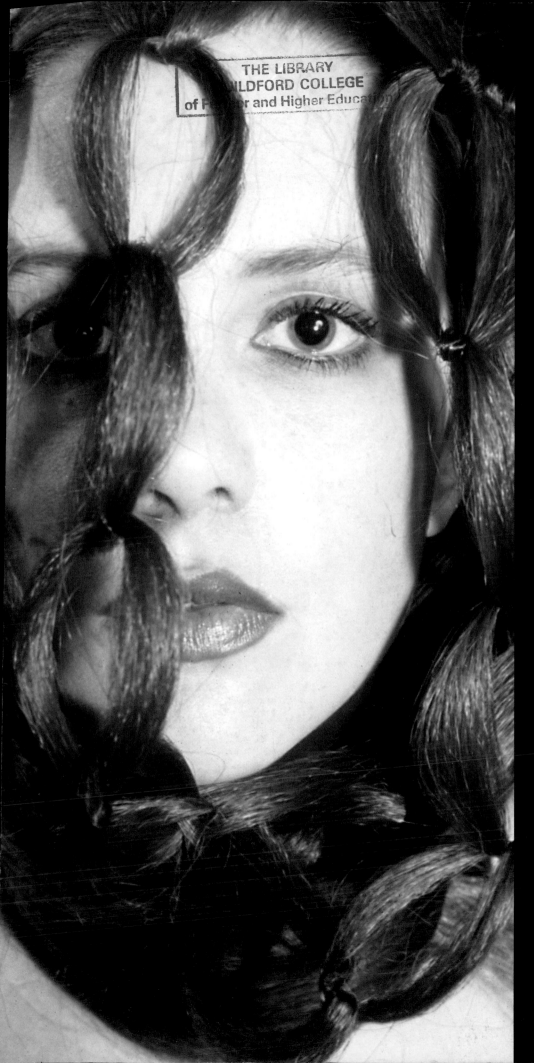

THE LIBRARY
ILDFORD COLLEGE
of F   er and Higher Education

Introduction en français
Introduzione in Italiano
Einführung auf deutsch
Introduction in English
緒言繁體中文版
日本語での紹介
Introdução em Português
Introducción en Español

380 Hairstyles

Country Index
Alphabetical Index

INTRODUCTION

L'objectif de l'*Index international de la coiffure* est de présenter un choix de photographies de grande qualité représentant le travail passionnant et innovant de coiffeurs du monde entier. Cet ouvrage se veut avant tout une source d'inspiration et de communication pour tous ceux qui s'intéressent à la coiffure et à la photographie.
Le premier volume présente une centaine de coiffeurs. Outre leurs noms et adresses, les photographes, maquilleurs, mannequins et agences sont également mentionnés ainsi que, lorsqu'ils sont connus, les produits coiffants utilisés.

PRESENTEZ-NOUS VOTRE TRAVAIL
Index international de la coiffure
L'*Index international de la coiffure* paraît chaque année. La sélection des coiffures prend en compte leur qualité et celle de la photographie. L'intégration à l'index est gratuite. Si vous souhaitez proposer votre travail pour la prochaine édition, remplissez le formulaire de candidature disponible à l'adresse www.hairstyleindex.com ou contactez notre directeur des publications consacrées à la mode à l'adresse : fashion-editor@pepinpress.com.

Maquillage, mode et photographie de mode
Outre l'*Index international de la coiffure*, The Pepin Press travaille à une collection d'ouvrages dans les domaines du maquillage, de la coiffure, des accessoires, de la mode et de la photographie de mode. Si vous souhaitez figurer dans l'un de ces ouvrages, vous pouvez contacter notre directeur des publications consacrées à la mode à l'adresse : fashion-editor@pepinpress.com.

ÉDITIONS PEPIN PRESS / AGILE RABBIT
Les éditions Pepin Press / Agile Rabbit publient un vaste choix de livres et de CD-ROM proposant des documents visuels de référence et des images prêtes à l'emploi pour les stylistes, les créateurs de textiles, les graphistes et tous ceux qui s'intéressent aux arts appliqués. Pour en savoir plus, visitez la page Web www.pepinpress.com.

INTRODUZIONE

L'*indice internazionale delle acconciature* offre una rassegna di eccellenti fotografie che mostrano le acconciature più interessanti e innovative di professionisti di tutto il mondo. Il libro rappresenta una fonte d'ispirazione e di comunicazione per chiunque sia interessato all'acconciatura e alla fotografia.
Questo primo volume raccoglie le creazioni di circa cento stilisti. Oltre al loro nome e indirizzo, compaiono quelli di fotografi, truccatori, modelli, agenzie e, quando è stato possibile, anche i dettagli dei prodotti utilizzati.

PRESENTATE LE VOSTRE CREAZIONI
L'indice internazionale delle acconciature
L'*indice internazionale delle acconciature* è una pubblicazione annuale. Le creazioni presenti nel libro vengono scelte a seconda della qualità delle acconciature e delle fotografie. La partecipazione è gratuita. Se volete candidarvi alla selezione per la prossima pubblicazione, troverete il modulo di iscrizione al sito www.hairstyleindex.com o potete mettervi in contatto con la redazione tramite l'indirizzo e-mail: fashion-editor@pepinpress.com

Make-up, Design e Fotografia di Moda
Oltre a *L'indice internazionale delle acconciature*, The Pepin Press sta elaborando una serie di libri su make-up, acconciature, accessori, design e fotografia di moda. Se volete veder pubblicate le vostre creazioni, potete mettervi in contatto con la redazione tramite l'indirizzo e-mail: fashion-editor@pepinpress.com

THE PEPIN PRESS / AGILE RABBIT EDITIONS
The Pepin Press / Agile Rabbit Editions pubblica una vasta gamma di libri e CD-ROM con materiale informativo ed immagini indirizzate ai professionisti del mondo della moda, del settore dell'abbigliamento, del disegno grafico e a tutti coloro che hanno uno speciale interesse nelle arti applicate in generale. Per ulteriori informazioni potete visitare il sito www.pepinpress.com

EINLEITUNG

Der internationale Frisuren-Index bietet eine Übersicht exzellenter Fotos von sensationellen und innovativen Kreationen von Hairstylisten aus aller Welt. Das vorliegende Buch soll all jenen, die sich für Hairstyling und Fotografie interessieren, als Anregung und Kommunikationsplattform dienen.
In diesem ersten Band sind rund 100 Stylisten vertreten. Neben den Namen und Adressen der Stylisten finden Sie auch Angaben zu den Fotografen, Make-up Artists, Models und Agenturen. Sofern bekannt, sind auch die verwendeten Styling-Produkte verzeichnet.

SENDEN SIE UNS IHRE KREATIONEN
Der internationale Frisuren-Index
Der internationale Frisuren-Index ist eine jährliche Publikation. Die Auswahl der Abbildungen basiert auf der Qualität des Hairstylings (oder Stylings) und des Fotos. Die Veröffentlichung ist kostenlos. Wenn Sie Ihre Arbeit für die nächste Ausgabe einreichen möchten, verwenden Sie bitte das Teilnahmeformular auf www.hairstyleindex.com oder kontaktieren Sie unseren Fashion-Editor unter fashion-editor@pepinpress.com.

Make-up, Mode-Design und Modefotografie
Neben dem *Internationalen Frisuren-Index* arbeitet The Pepin Press auch an einer Reihe von Büchern im Bereich Make-up, Frisuren, Accessoires, Mode-Design und Modefotografie. Wenn Sie sich für eine Veröffentlichung in einem dieser Bücher interessieren, kontaktieren Sie bitte unseren Fashion-Editor unter fashion-editor@pepinpress.com.

THE PEPIN PRESS / AGILE RABBIT EDITIONS
The Pepin Press / Agile Rabbit Editions veröffentlicht eine breite Palette an Büchern und CD-ROMs mit visuellem Referenzmaterial und sofort verwendbaren Bildern für Mode-, Textil- und Grafik-Designer und alle Personen, die sich für angewandte Kunst interessieren. Weitere Informationen entnehmen Sie bitte der Website www.pepinpress.com.

INTRODUCTION

The objective of *The International Hairstyle Index* is to provide an overview of excellent photographs of exciting and innovative work by hairstylists from all over the world. This book is meant as a source of inspiration and communication for anyone with an interest in hairstyles and photography.
In this first volume, about a hundred stylists are featured. In addition to the stylists' names and addresses, the photographers, make-up artists, models and agencies have also been credited. When known, the styling products that have been used are mentioned as well.

SUBMIT YOUR WORK
The International Hairstyle Index
The International Hairstyle Index will be published annually and selection is based on the quality of (hair) styling and photography. Inclusion is free of charge. Should you wish to submit your work for consideration for the next edition, please access the submission form at www.hairstyleindex.com or contact our fashion editor at: fashion-editor@pepinpress.com

Make-up, Fashion Design and Fashion Photography
In addition to *The International Hairstyle Index*, The Pepin Press is working on a series of books in the fields of make-up, coiffures, accessories, fashion design and fashion photography. Should you wish to be considered for publication in books in these fields, please contact our fashion editor at: fashion-editor@pepinpress.com

THE PEPIN PRESS / AGILE RABBIT EDITIONS
The Pepin Press / Agile Rabbit Editions publishes a wide range of books and CD-ROMs with visual reference material and ready-to-use images for fashion, textile and graphic designers, and anyone with an interest in the applied arts. For more information, please visit www.pepinpress.com

はじめに

この国際ヘアースタイル年鑑は、世界中のヘアースタイリストの手になる見事な作品を、美しい写真でお目にかけるために刊行された本です。ヘアースタイルや写真に興味のある方ならどなたでも、この本をインスピレーションやコミュニケーションのベースとしてご利用いただけます。
この第1巻には約100人のスタイリストがフィーチャーされています。各スタイリストの氏名と住所に加えて、フォトグラファー、メーキャップアーティスト、モデル、エージェントの名称も記載いたしました。分かる限りで、使用されているスタイリング製品の名称も含めました。

応募について

国際ヘアースタイル年鑑

国際ヘアースタイル年鑑は年次刊行されます。掲載作品を選ぶ基準は、(ヘアー)スタイリングと写真の質の高さです。次回の年鑑にご自身の作品を応募なさりたい方は、www.hairstyleindex.com からダウンロードできる応募用紙でお申し込み頂くか、fashion-editor@pepinpress.com あてに E-メールで弊社のファッション部門編集者にご連絡下さい。

メーキャップ、ファッションデザイン、ファッション写真

ペピン・プレスでは、国際ヘアースタイル年鑑の他にもメーキャップ、ヘアーファッション、アクセサリー、ファッションデザイン、ファッション写真の分野で数多くの書籍を出版しています。この分野の本を出版したいとお考えの方は、fashion-editor@pepinpress.com あてに E-メールで弊社のファッション部門編集者にご相談下さい。

ペピン・プレス/アジール・ラビット・エディションについて

ペピン・プレス/アジール・ラビット・エディションは、ファッション、テキスタイル、グラフィック分野のデザイナーや応用美術に興味を持たれる全ての方に向けたビジュアル資料やレディーメード素材付きの書籍及び CD-ROM を幅広く手がけています。
詳細については www.pepinpress.com でご覧下さい。

緒言

《國際髮型檢索》（International Hairstyle Index）彙萃了全球頂尖髮型設計師的優秀作品圖片。本書旨在?髮型設計和攝影技術發燒友提供一個交流的空間並激發其創作靈感。
在本書第一卷中，對約 100 位設計師進行了專門介紹。除列出他們的姓名和地址外，還列出了相關的攝影師、化妝師、模特及代理商的名稱。也對已經使用的著名髮型作品進行了介紹。

提交你的作品

《國際髮型檢索》

《國際髮型檢索》每年出版一次，內容根據（髮式）造型和圖片進行篩選。入選作品是沒有稿酬的。如果你希望?下一輯出版物提交你的作品，請訪問 www.hairstyleindex.com 或聯絡我們的時尚編輯： fashion-editor@pepinpress.com ，以索取提交表格。

化妝、時裝設計及時尚攝影

除了《國際髮型檢索》外，Pepin 出版社現正致力於有關化妝、頭飾、飾配物、時裝設計和時尚攝影等方面的系列書目。如果你希望對這些書目投稿，請與我們時尚編輯聯絡：
fashion-editor@pepinpress.com

THE PEPIN PRESS / AGILE RABBIT EDITIONS 出版社

The Pepin Press/Agile Rabbit Editions 出版了大量的書籍和 CD-ROM ，?時裝、織物和圖案設計師以及對實用藝術感興趣的所有讀者，提供直觀的參考材料和現成的圖片素材。
欲獲得更多資訊，請訪問 www.pepinpress.com 。

INTRODUÇÃO

O objectivo do *Índice internacional de estilos de penteado* é proporcionar, através de fotografias excelentes, uma visão global do trabalho inovador de cabeleireiros de todo o mundo. A intenção deste livro é ser uma fonte de inspiração e comunicação para todas as pessoas que se interessam por penteados e fotografia.
Neste primeiro volume, encontram-se apresentados cerca de cem cabeleireiros.
Para além dos nomes e endereços dos cabeleireiros, os fotógrafos, maquilhadores, manequins e agências encontram-se igualmente incluídos na lista de créditos.
Quando conhecidos, os produtos utilizados são igualmente referidos.

ENVIE O SEU TRABALHO
Índice internacional de estilos de penteado
O *Índice internacional de estilos de penteado* será publicado anualmente e a selecção é feita com base na qualidade do penteado e da fotografia. A inclusão na obra é grátis. Caso pretenda submeter o seu trabalho a consideração para a próxima edição, aceda ao respectivo formulário em www.hairstyleindex.com ou contacte o nosso editor de moda através do endereço fashion-editor@pepinpress.com

Fotografia de Moda, Maquilhagem e Design de Moda
Para além do *Índice internacional de estilos de penteado*, a Pepin Press encontra-se a trabalhar numa série de livros nas áreas de fotografia de design de moda, maquilhagem, penteados e acessórios. Caso deseje ser considerado para publicação nos livros destas áreas, contacte o nosso editor de moda através do endereço fashion-editor@pepinpress.com

PEPIN PRESS / AGILE RABBIT EDITIONS
A Pepin Press / Agile Rabbit Editions publica um vasto leque de livros e CD-ROMs com material de consulta visual e imagens prontas-a-utilizar para designers de moda, gráficos e da indústria têxtil, bem como todas as pessoas interessadas nas artes aplicadas. Para obter informações adicionais, visite o endereço www.pepinpress.com

INTRODUCCIÓN

El *Índice internacional de peluquería* tiene como objetivo presentar una amplia selección de excelentes fotografías que muestran trabajos atrevidos e innovadores de peluqueros de todo el mundo.
Este libro ha sido concebido como fuente de inspiración y comunicación para todos aquellos interesados en el mundo de la peluquería y la fotografía.
En este primer volumen se incluyen alrededor de cien estilistas. Además de sus nombres y direcciones, aparecen los de los fotógrafos, maquilladores, modelos y agencias. Asimismo, se mencionan los productos de peluquería utilizados, en el caso de que se conozcan.

ENVÍENOS SUS TRABAJOS
Índice internacional de peluquería
El *Índice internacional de peluquería* se publicará de forma anual. Los criterios de selección se basan en la calidad de los diseños de peluquería o estilismo y de las fotografías. La aparición en el índice no supone coste alguno. Si desea enviarnos sus trabajos para que los tengamos en cuenta para la próxima edición, rellene el formulario de solicitud en www.hairstyleindex.com o póngase en contacto con nuestro editor de moda en: fashion-editor@pepinpress.com.

Maquillaje, diseño de moda y fotografía de moda
Además del *Índice internacional de peluquería*, la editorial The Pepin Press está trabajando en una serie de libros dedicada a los ámbitos del maquillaje, la peluquería, los accesorios, el diseño de moda y la fotografía de moda. Si desea enviarnos su candidatura para aparecer en alguno de ellos, contacte con nuestro editor de moda en: fashion-editor@pepinpress.com.

THE PEPIN PRESS / AGILE RABBIT EDITIONS
La editorial The Pepin Press / Agile Rabbit Editions publica una amplia variedad de libros y CD-ROM con material de referencia visual e imágenes destinados a diseñadores de moda, textiles o gráficos, o a cualquiera que esté interesado en las artes aplicadas. Si desea obtener más información, visite www.pepinpress.com.

ANITA COX pages 8–13

62 Britton Street, Clerkwell, London EC1M 5UY, United Kingdom

Hair: Anita Cox
Salon: Anita Cox
Make-up: Janet Dunford
Styling: Angela Barnard
Photography: Martin Evening

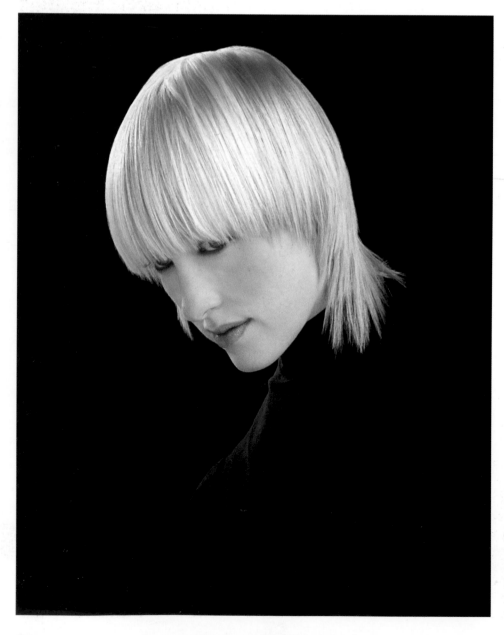 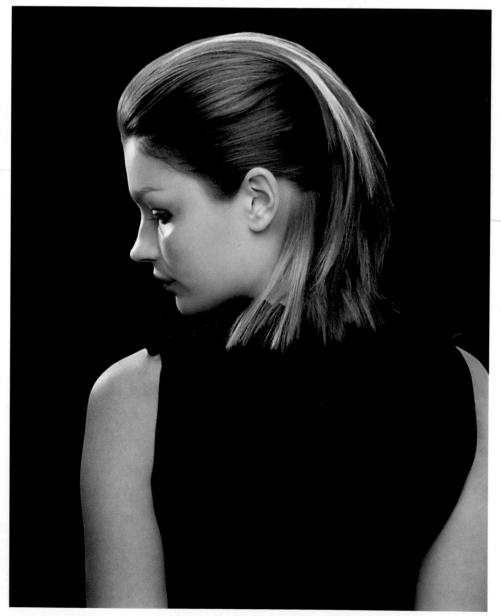

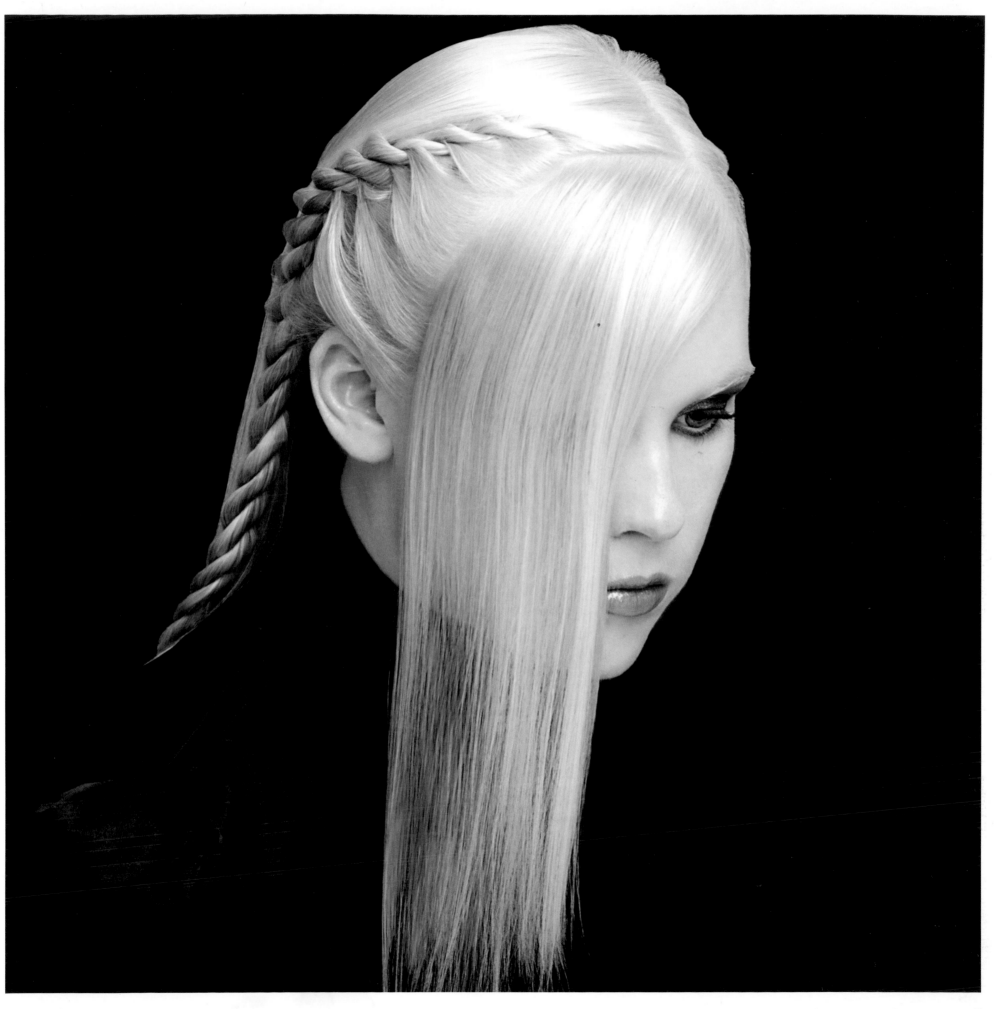

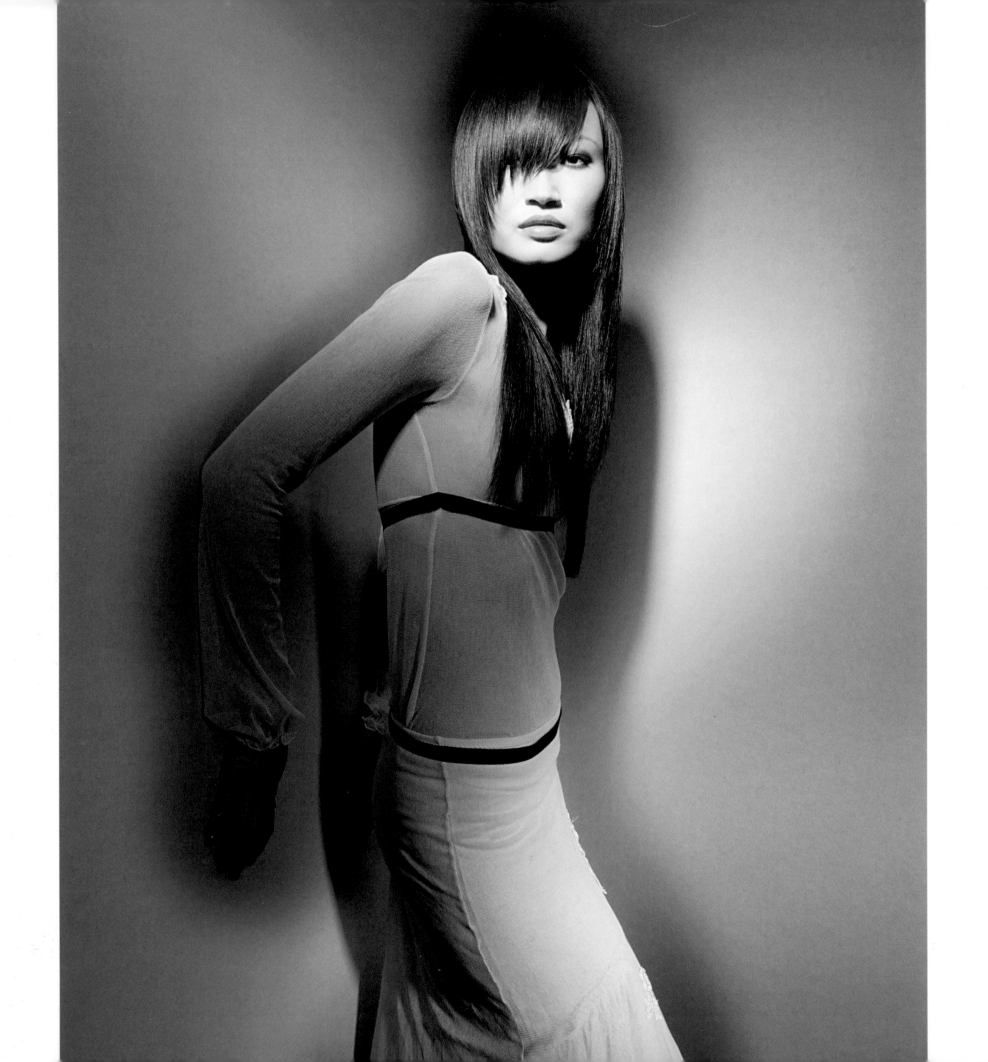

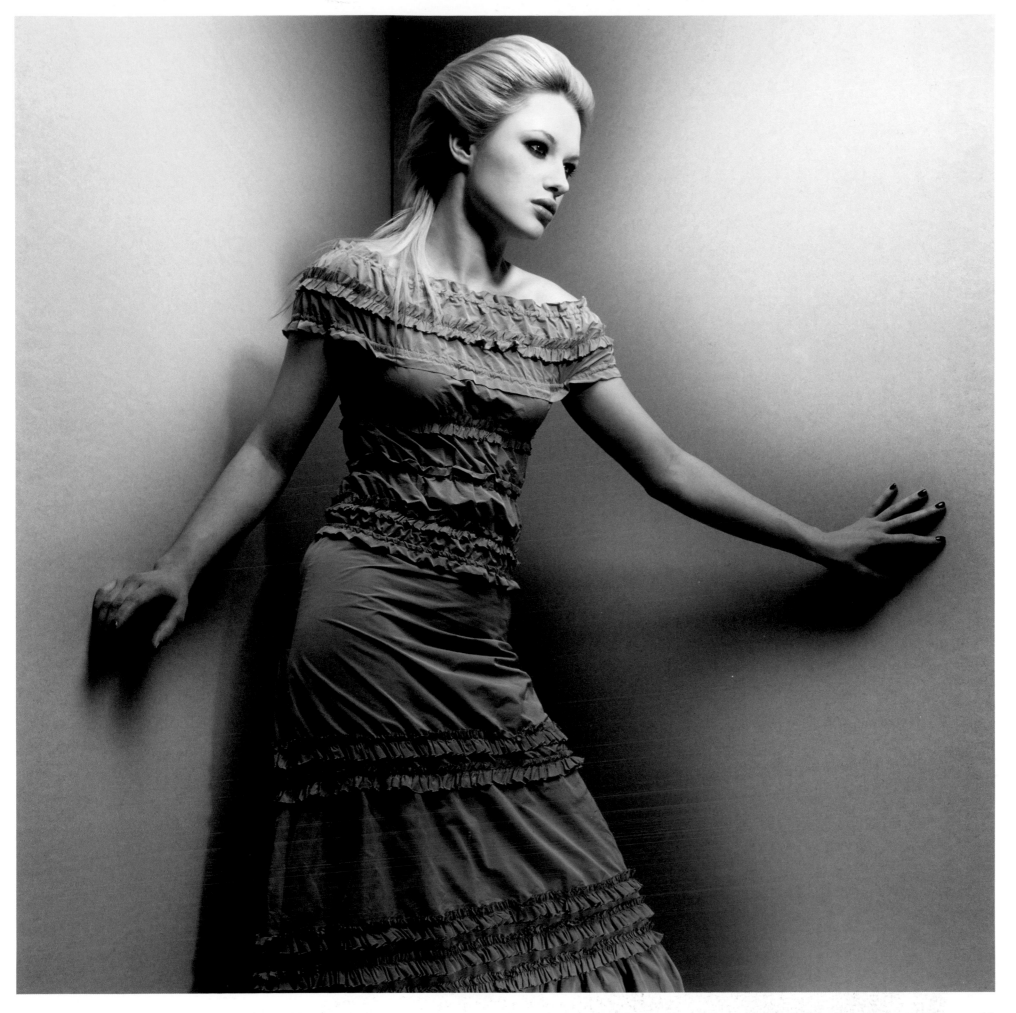

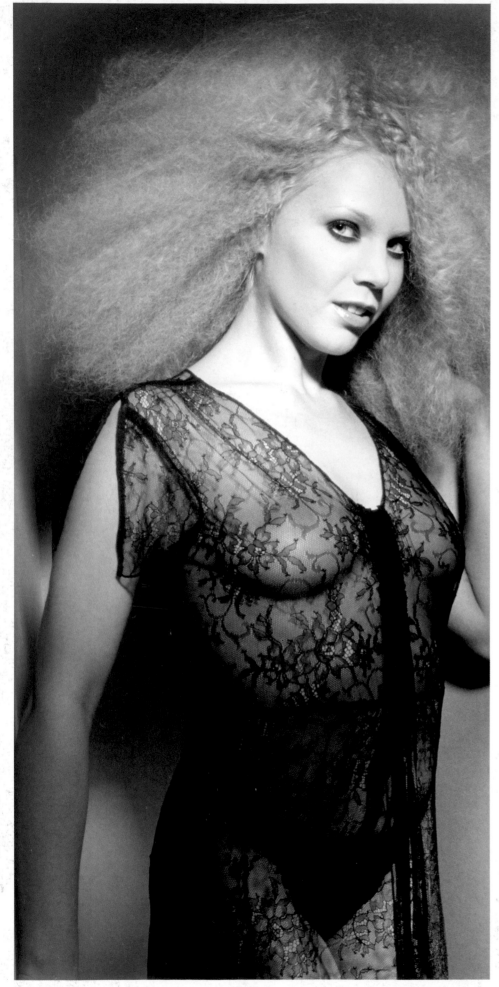
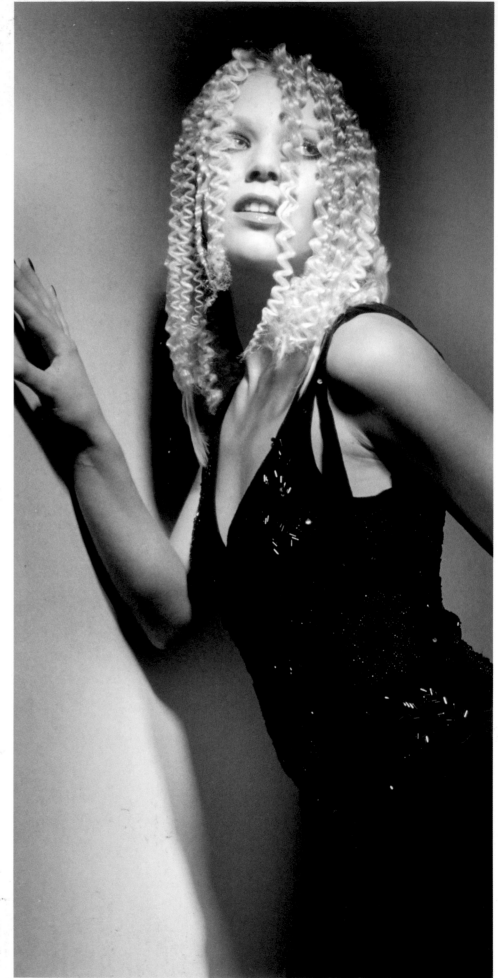

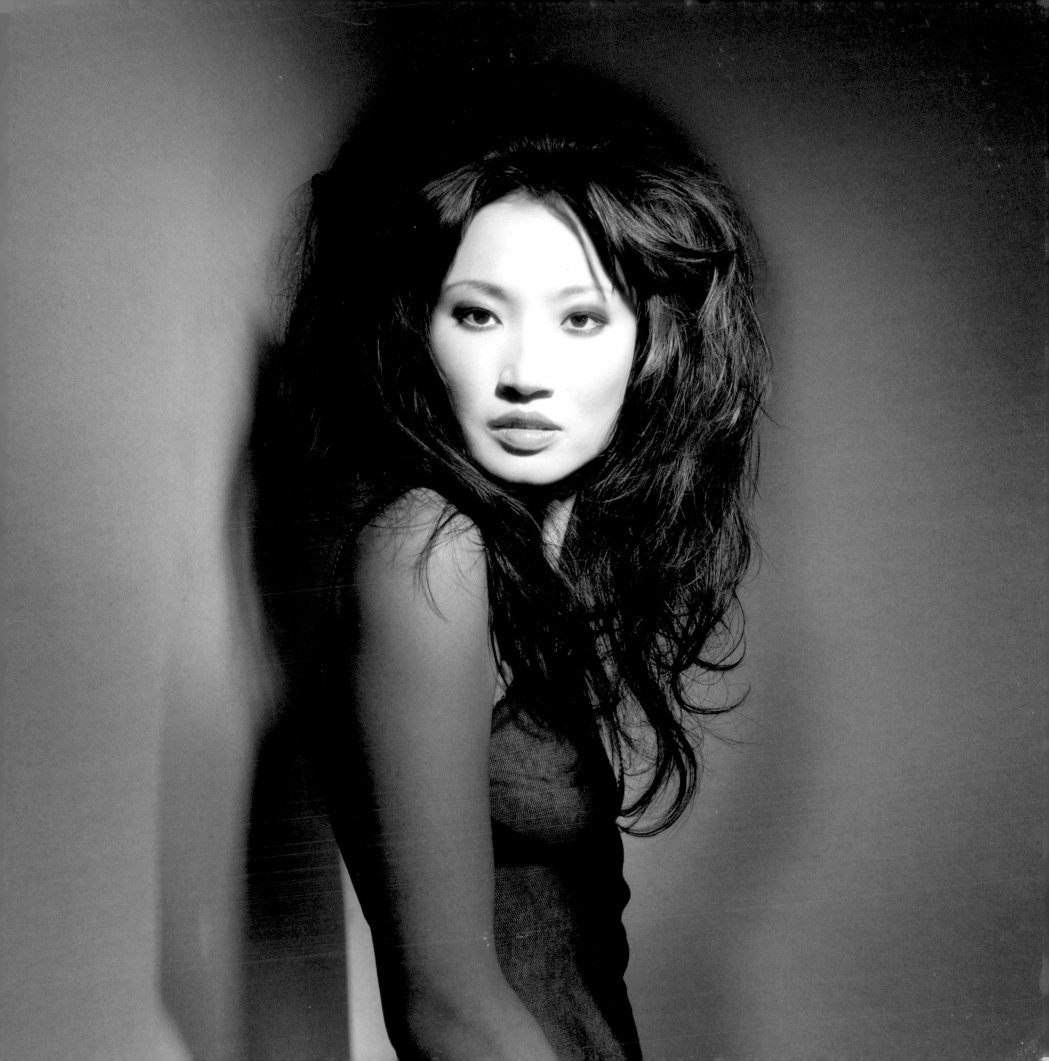

ATELIER KAZU pages 14–15

1-48-19-404 Sasazuka, Shibuya-ku, Tokyo, Japan, www.atelier-kazu.co.jp

Hair: Teru for Atelier KAZU
Salon: Atelier KAZU
Make-up: Ebara (p. 14, 15) Mina for Bridge (p. 15)
Styling: Maki Murata for Bridge
Photography: Rory Dennis (p. 14, 15) Mike Diver (p. 14)
Model: Satomi (p. 14) Aya (p. 14) Irving Cheung for Bridge

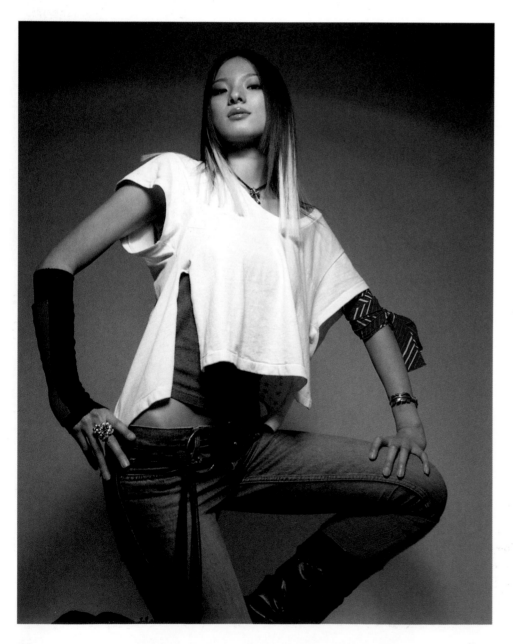

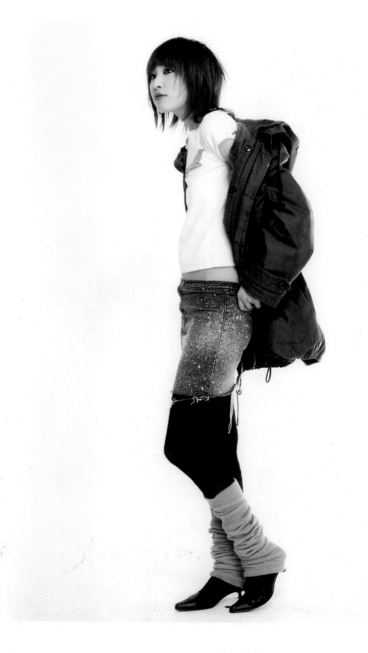

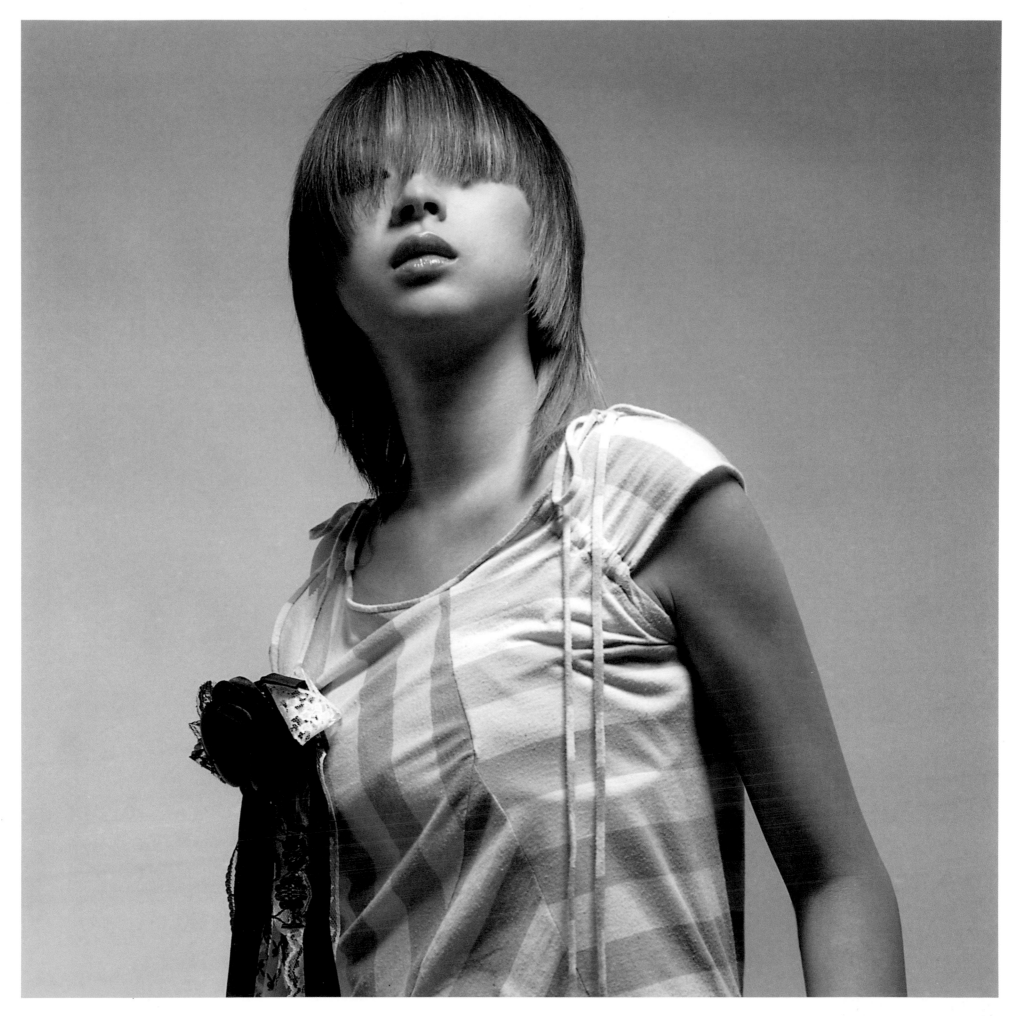

LLONGUERAS pages 16–17

Berlin 39, 08014 Barcelona, Spain, www.llongueras.com

Hair: Llongueras International
Make-up: Llongueras International
Photography: Yoye
Co-ordination: Lolita Llongueras

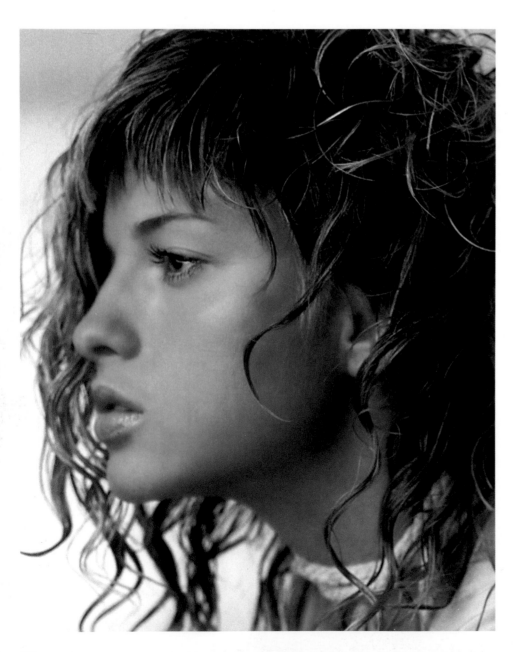

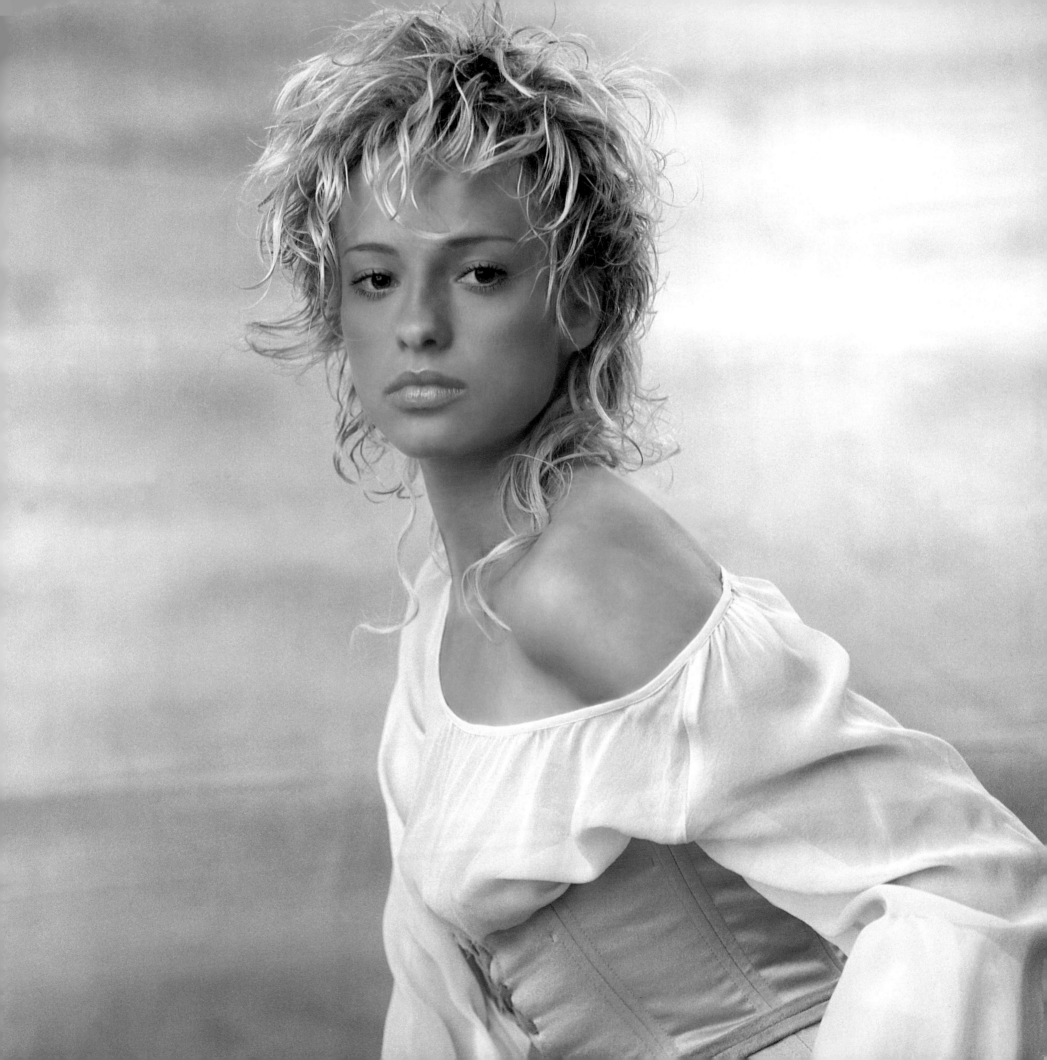

ENTRENOUS pages 18–23

579 Richmond Street, London Ontario N6A 3G2, Canada, www.salonentrenous.com

Hair: Heather Wenman
Salon: Entrenous
Make-up: April Maloney (p. 18, 19) and Lesley Balch (p. 21)
Photography: Paula Tizzard (p. 18, 19) David Raposo (p. 20) Babak (p. 21) and Benjamin Jordan (p. 22, 23)
Model: Marla Weaver (p. 20, 21)

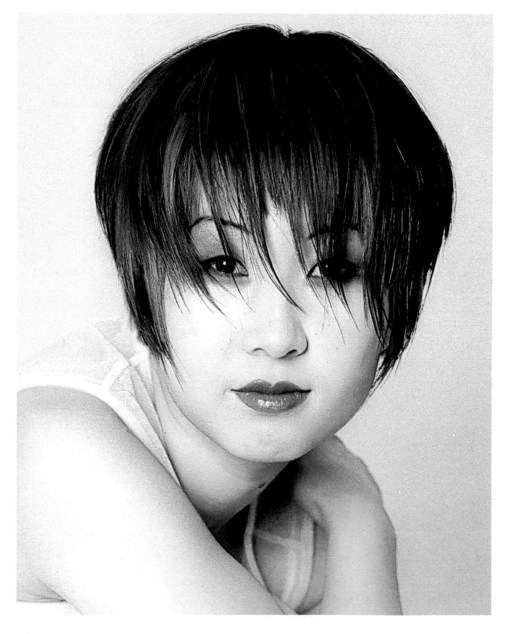

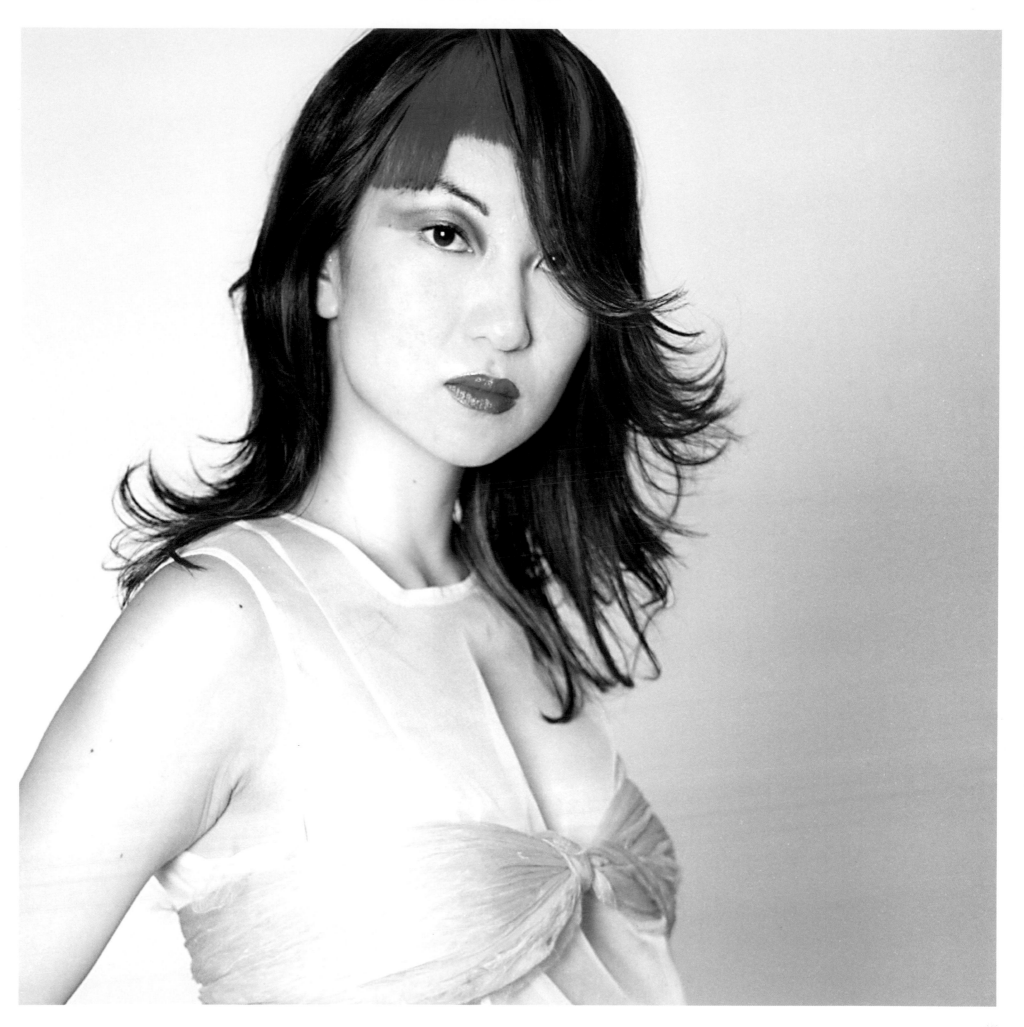

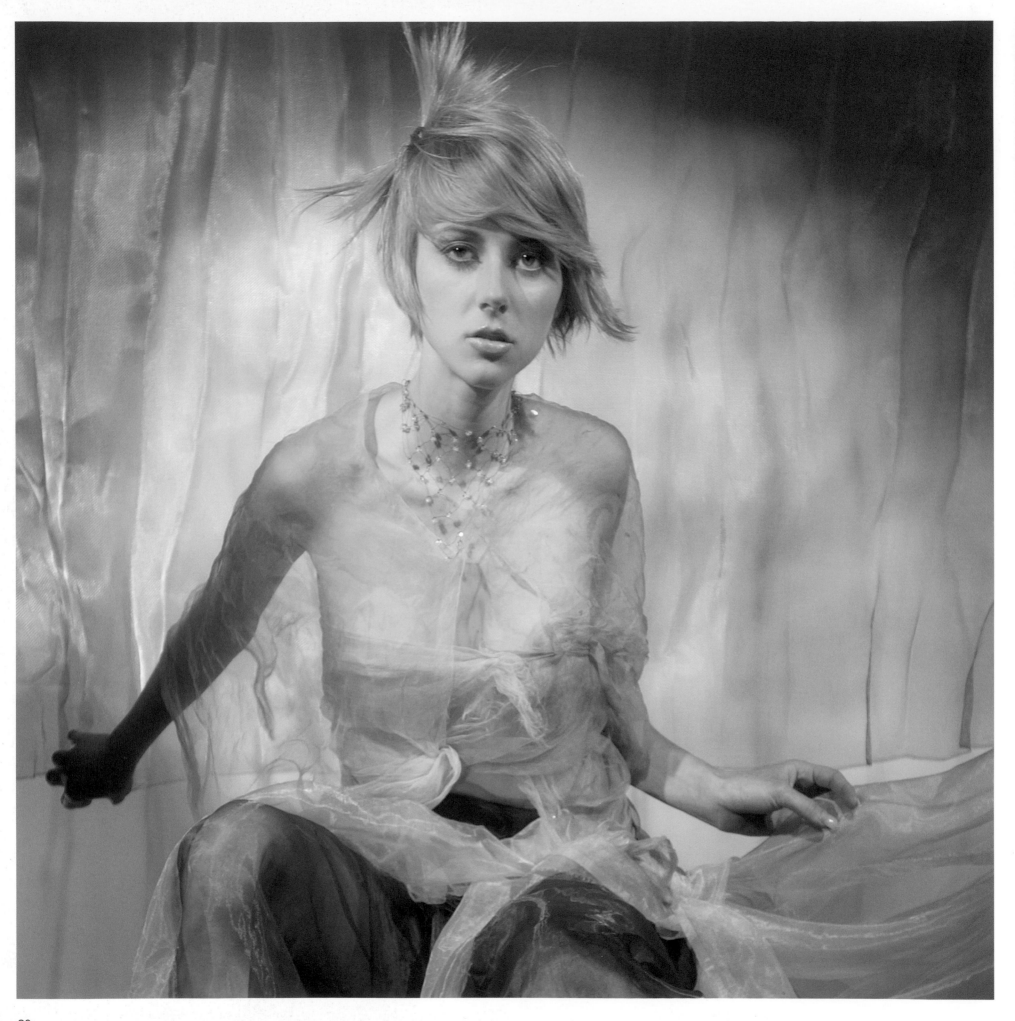

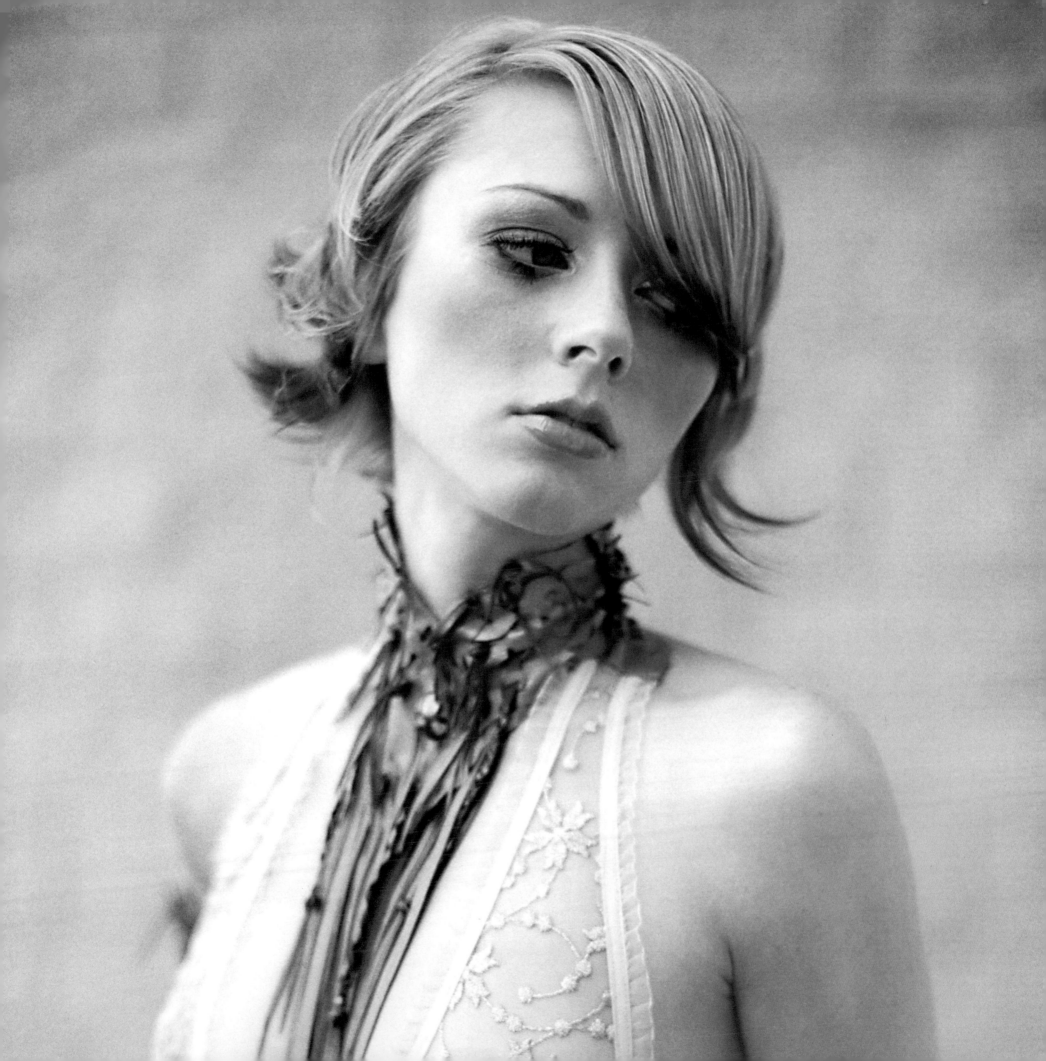

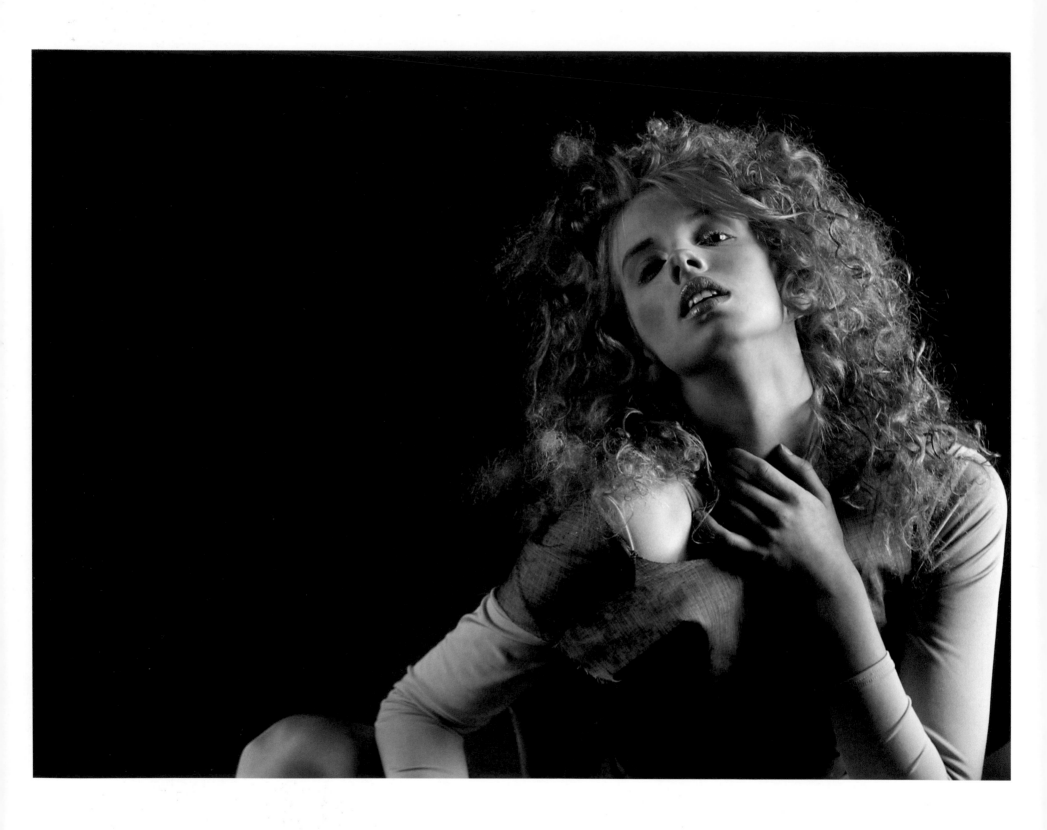

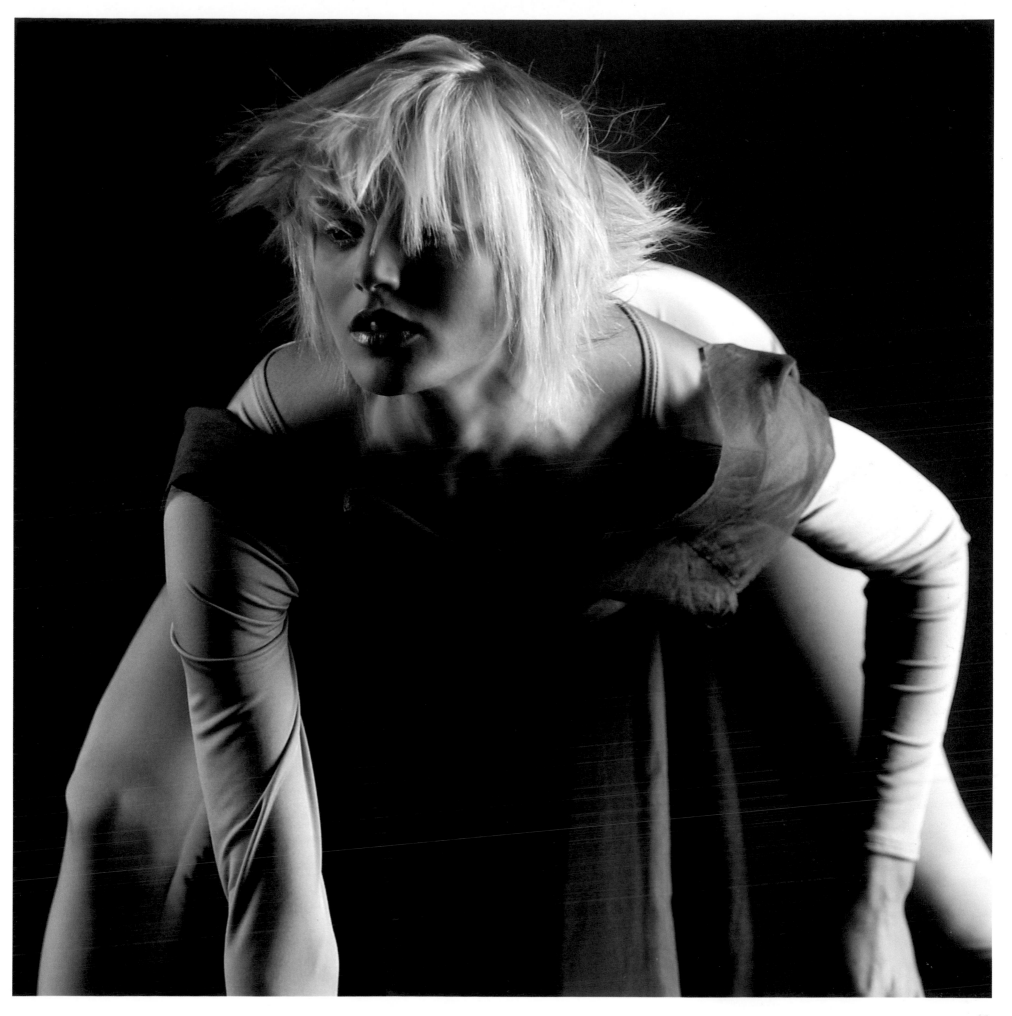

GUY KREMER pages 24–25

Stonemasons Court 67, Parchment Street, Winchester SO23 8AT, United Kingdom

Hair: Guy Kremer International
Make-up: Pascal Marin
Styling: Tracey-Lea Sayer
Photography: Carolo Lumiere
Products: L'Oréal Professionnel

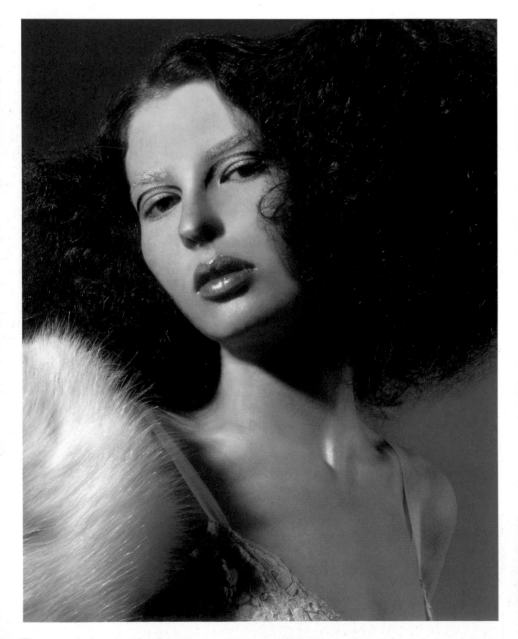

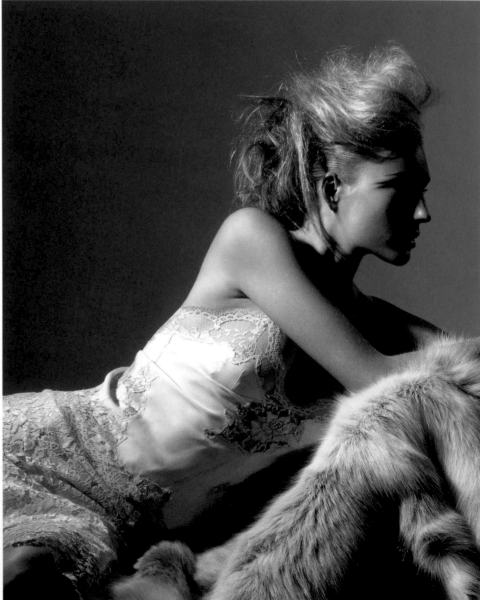

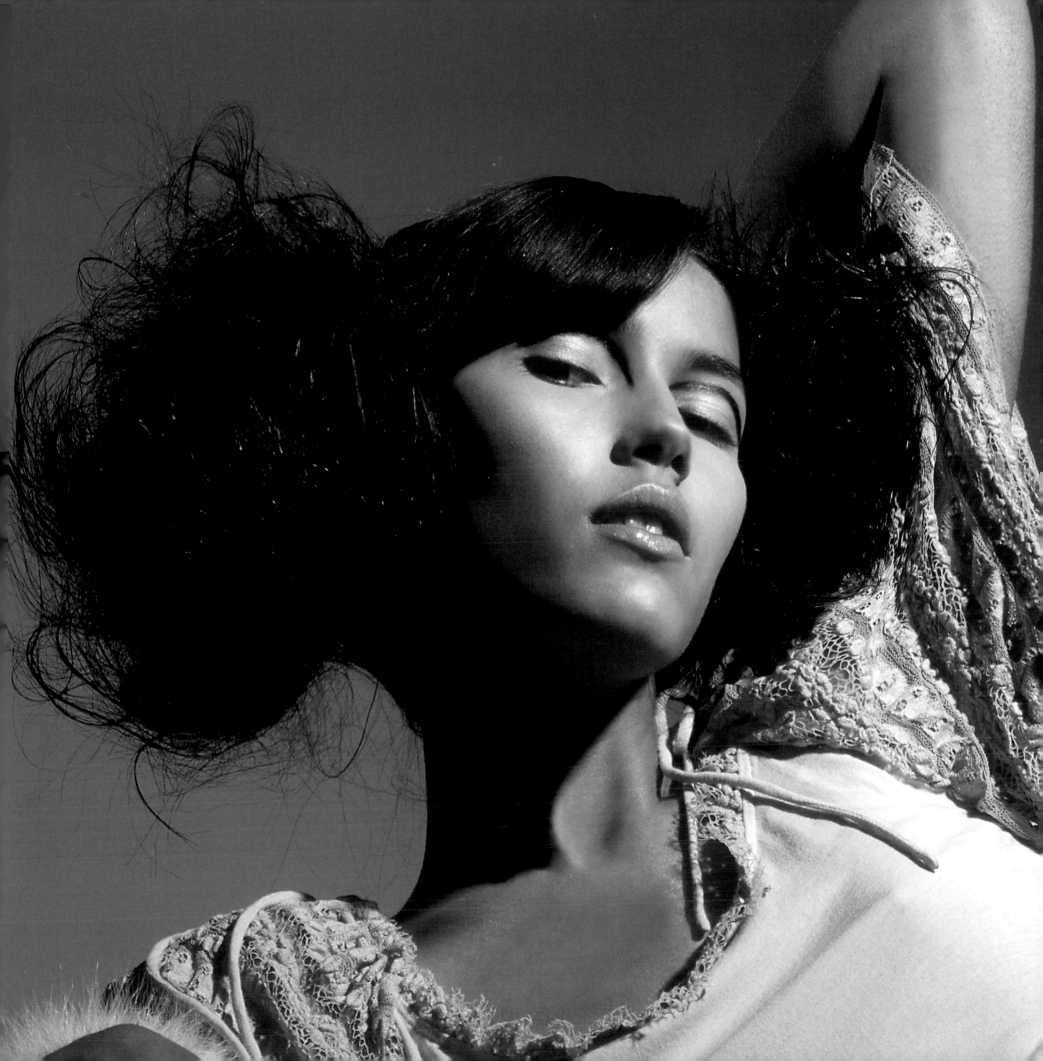

CARLO BAY HAIR DIFFUSION pages 26–27

Via Marsuppini 18 rosso, Firenze, Italy, www.carlobay.it

Hair: Carlo Bay Hair Diffusion

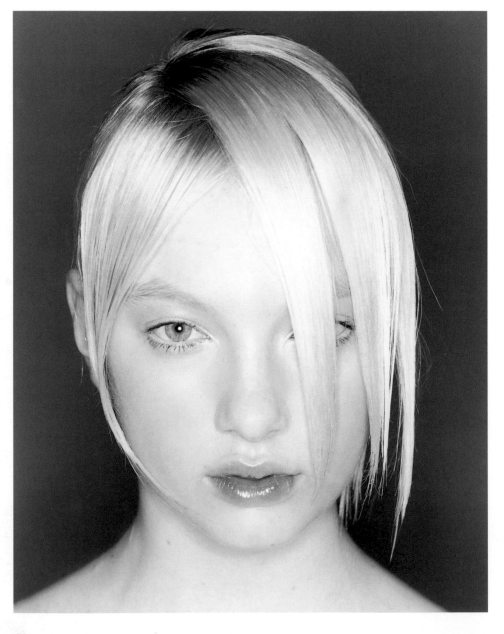 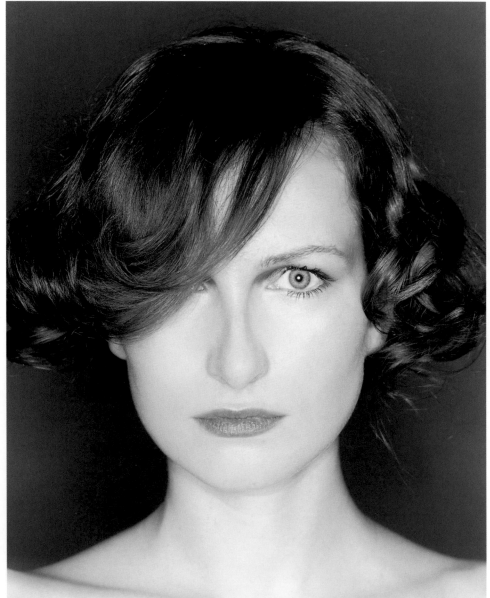

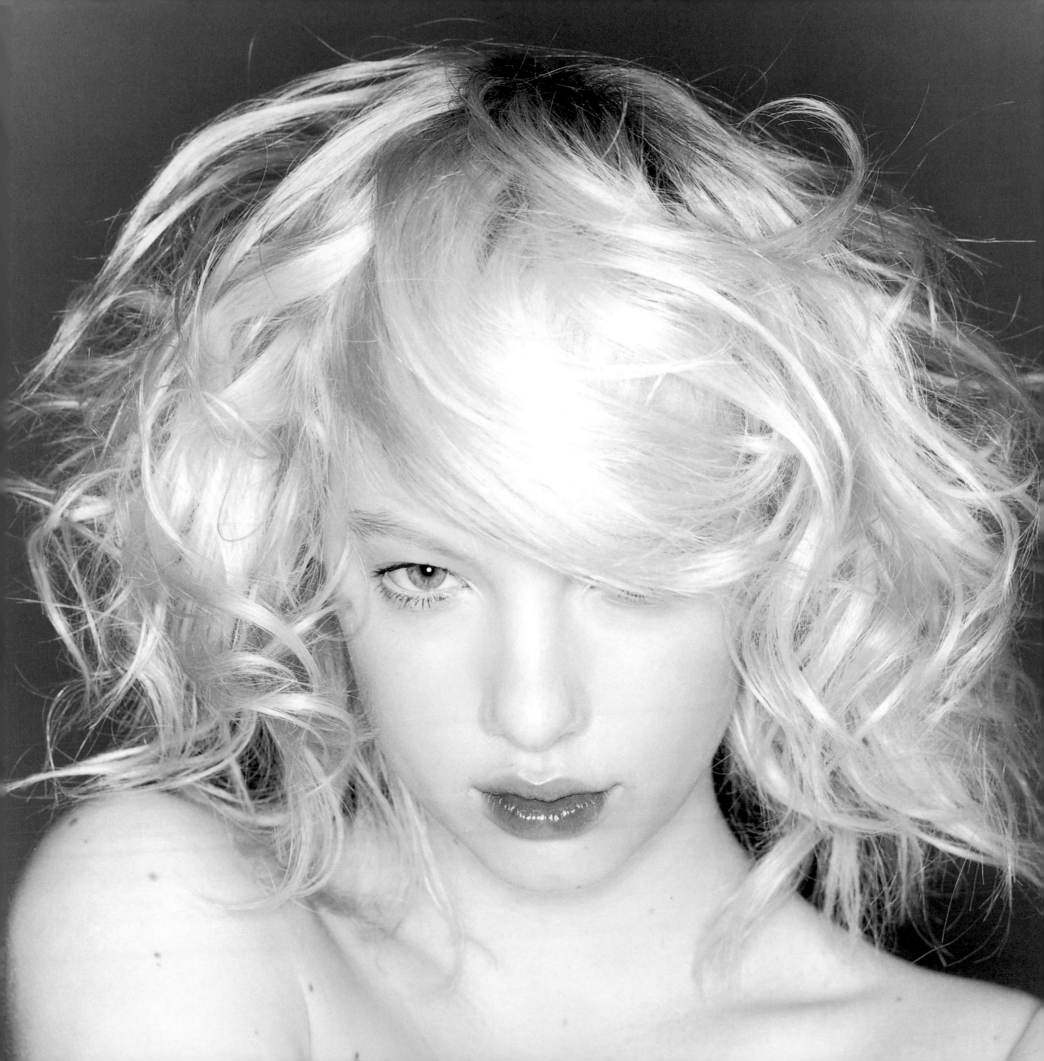

A CUT ABOVE pages 28–33

Bangsar Shopping Center 285, Jalan Maarof, 59000 Kuala Lumpur, Malaysia

Hair: Winnie Loo (p. 28, 29, 30, 31, 33) Jo T'ng and James Wong (p. 32)
Salon: A Cut Above
Make-up: Winnie Loo (p. 28, 29, 30) Jo T'ng and James Wong (p. 32) Faevien Yee and Jo T'ng (p. 33)
Styling: Jonathan Cheng (p. 28, 29) Syeba Yip (p. 30, 31) Khoon Hooi (p. 32) Lim Jimmy (p. 33)
Photography: Fai, IFL Studio (p. 28, 29, 30, 31, 33) Alvin Loh, New Looks Studio (p. 32)
Products: Schwarzkopf

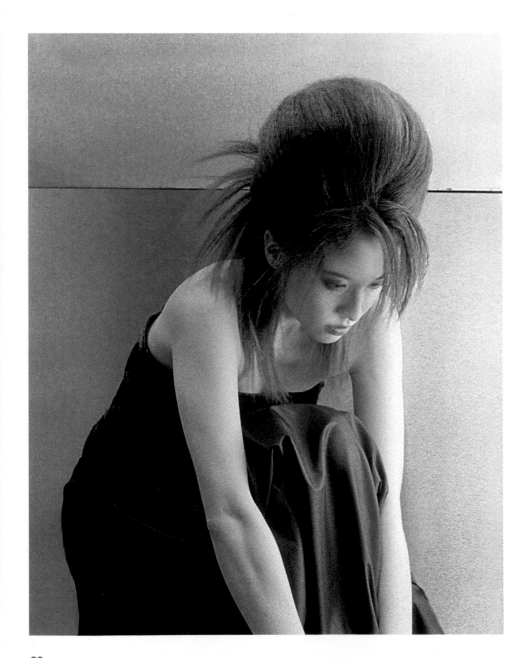

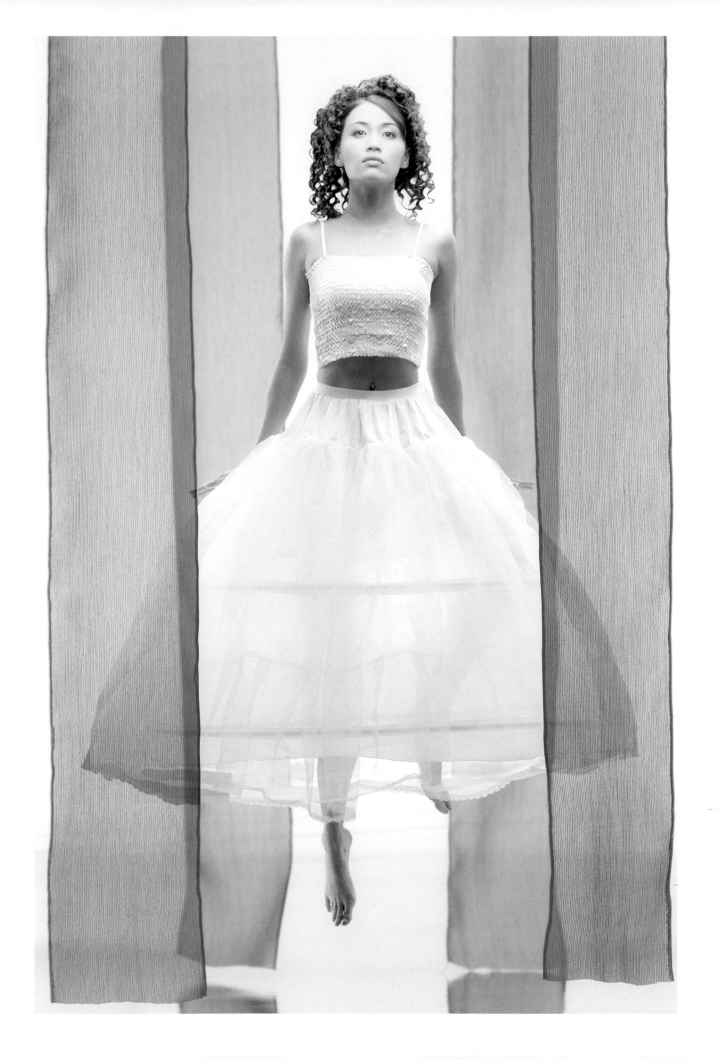

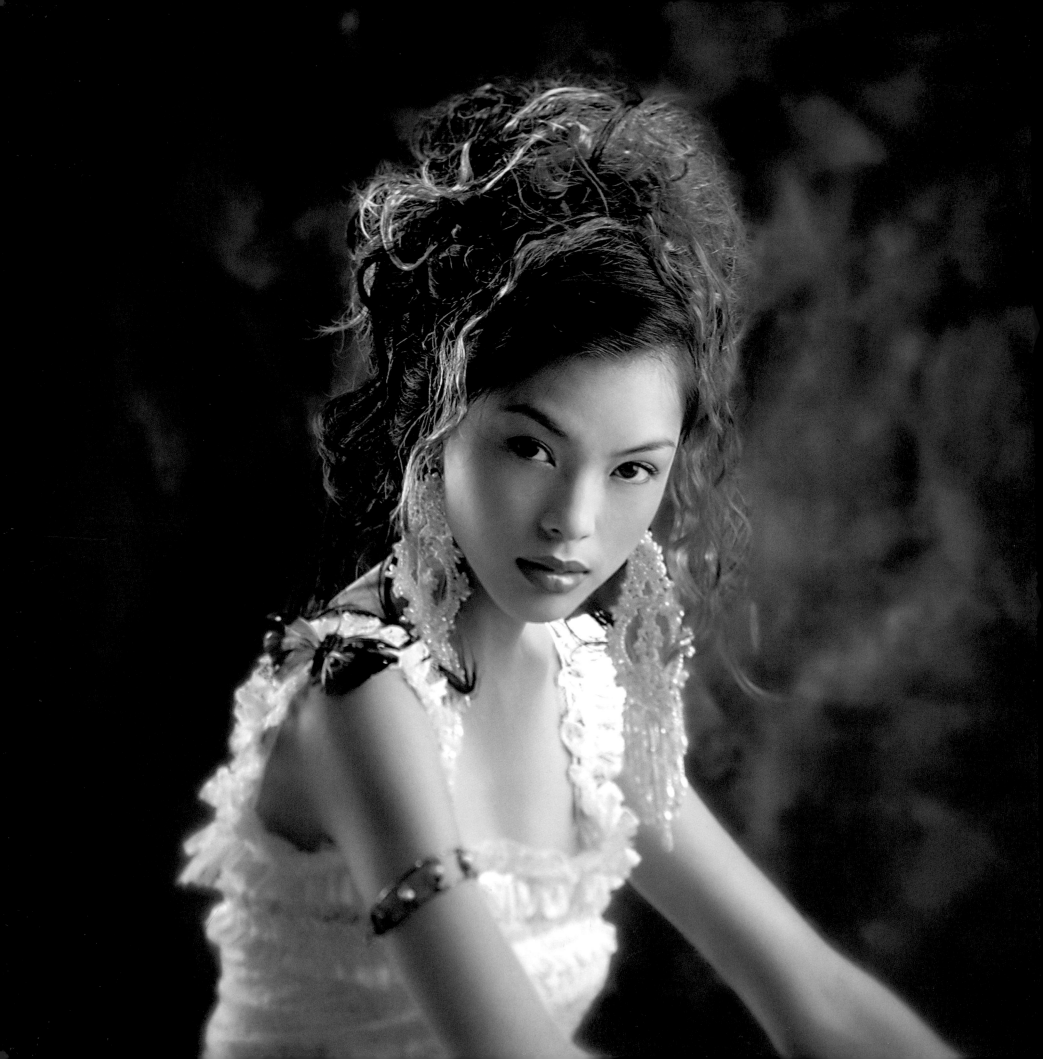

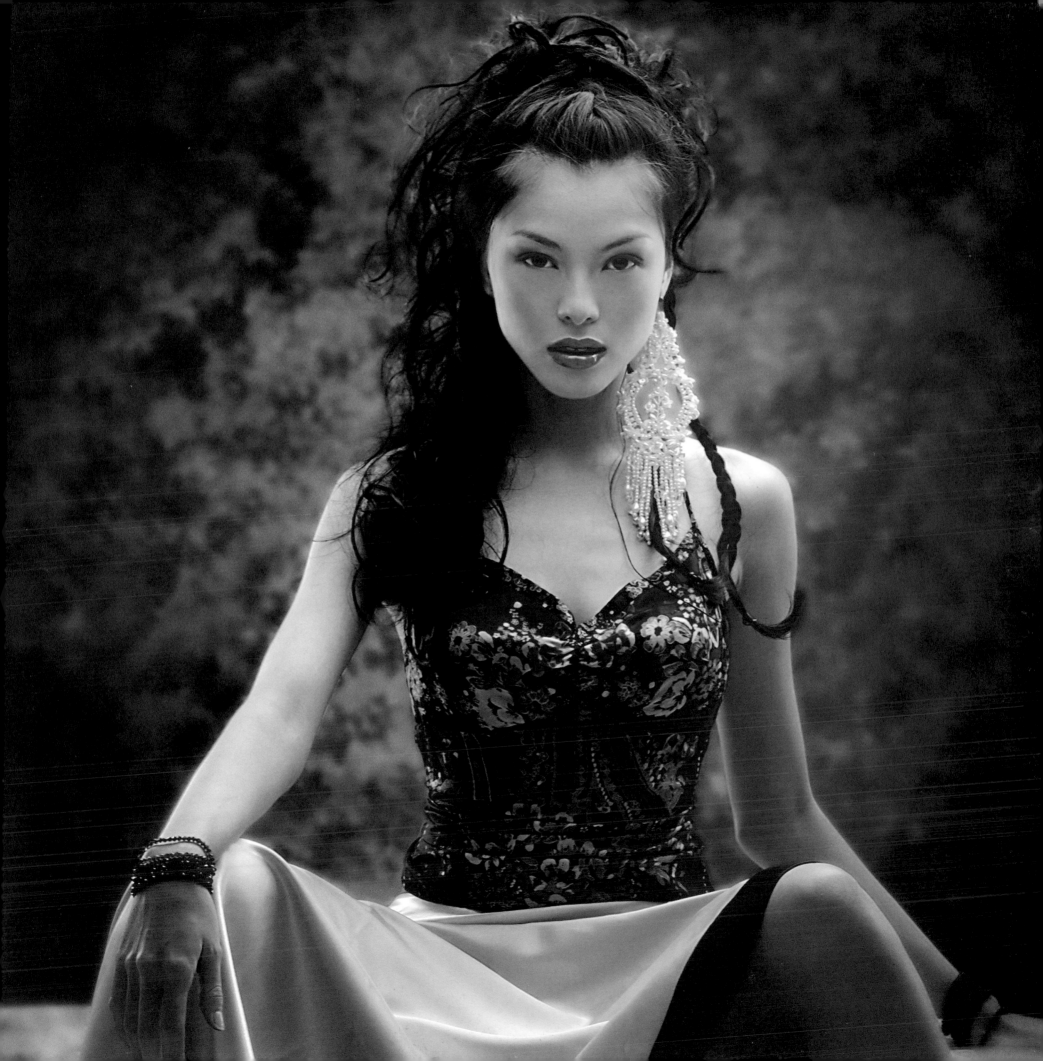

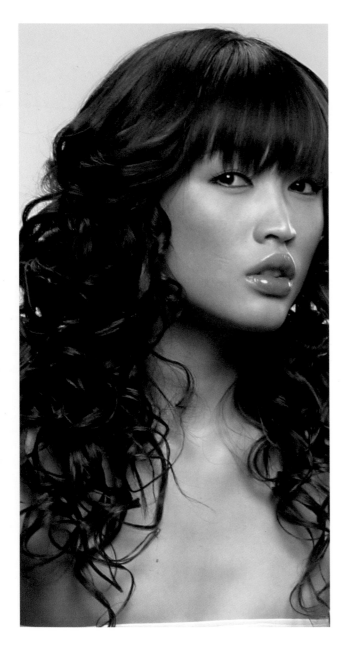
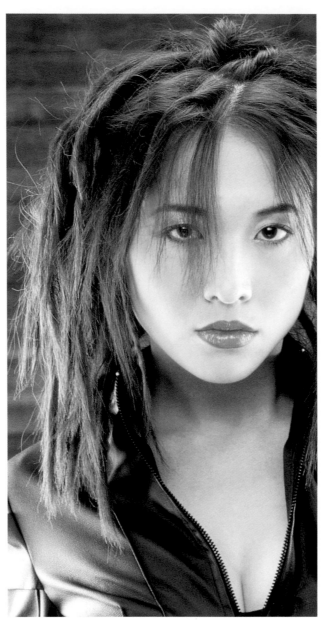
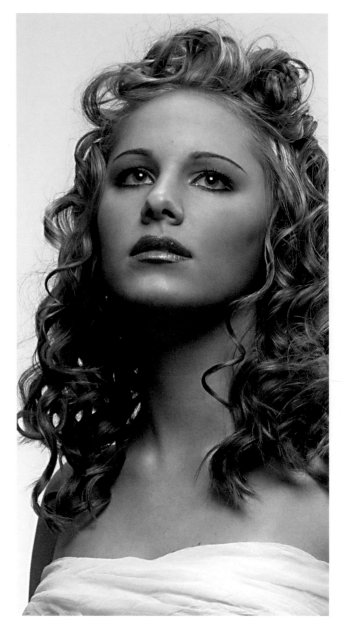

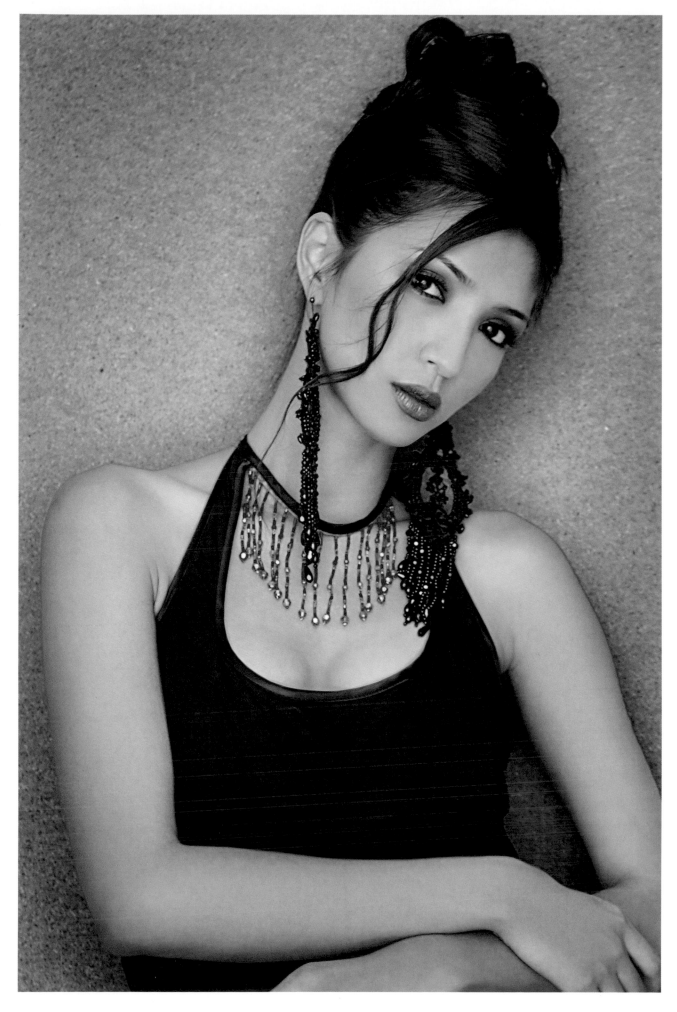
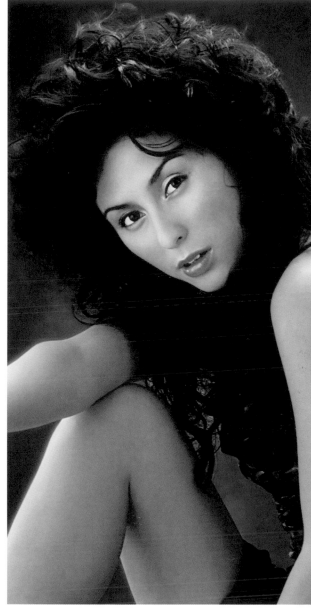

A-SQUARE pages 34–37

61 Lane, 233 TunHua S. Rd. Sec. 1, Taipei 106, Taiwan, www.a-square.com.tw

Hair: Michael Kwok (p. 34 - 37) Bron Hui (p. 36) Anne Hsieh (p. 36)
Salon: A-Square
Make-up: Laura Lan
Styling: Laura Lan
Photography: Arthur Chou and Amber

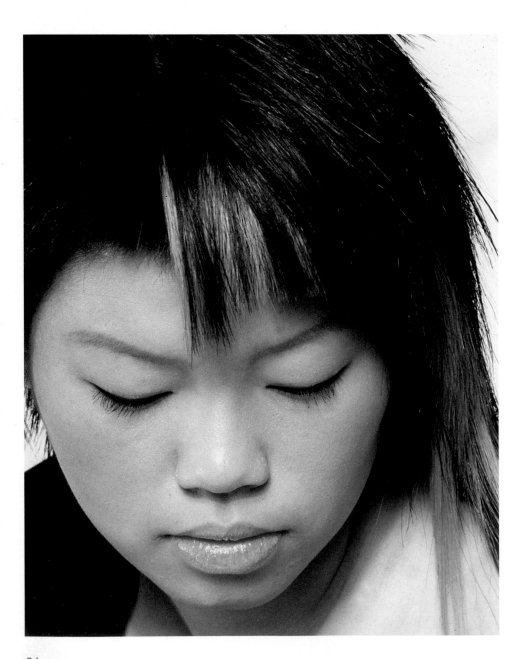

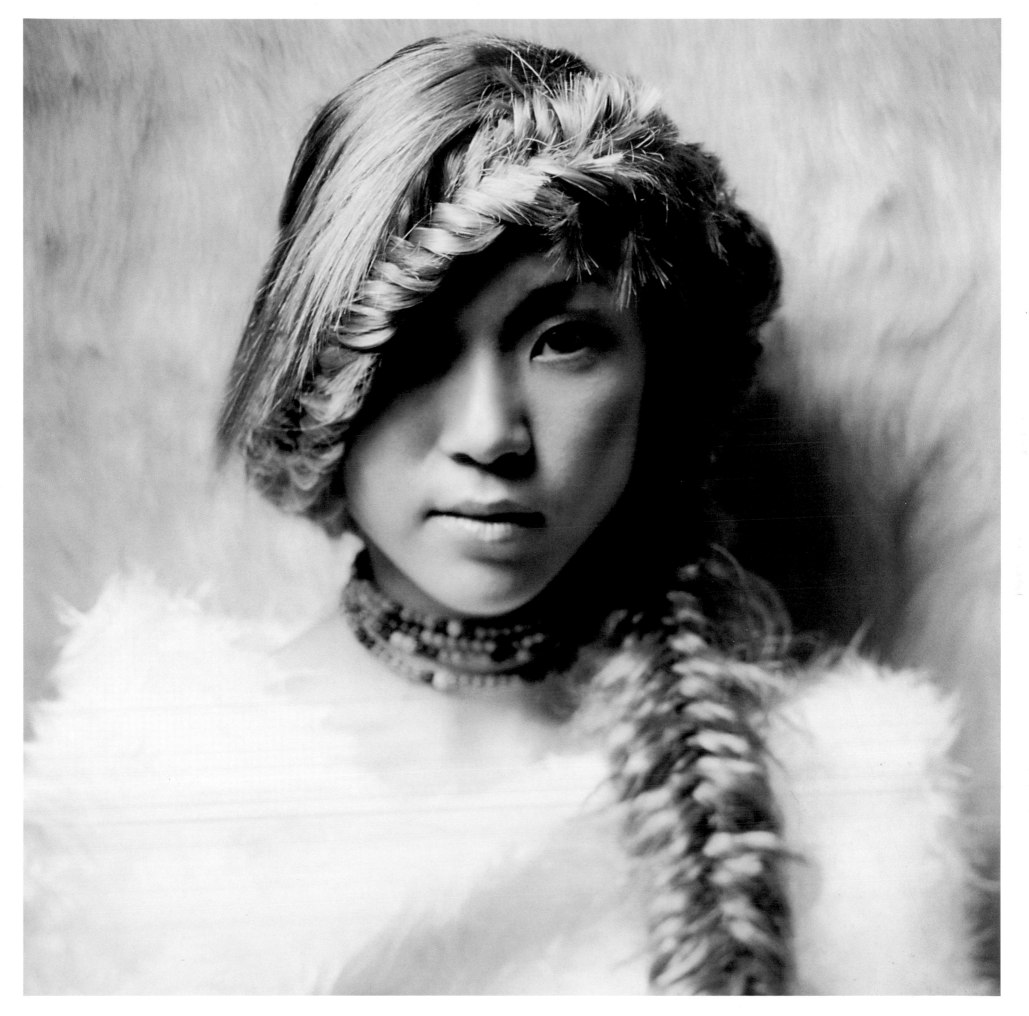

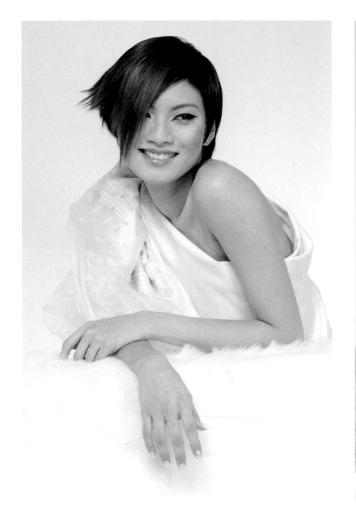
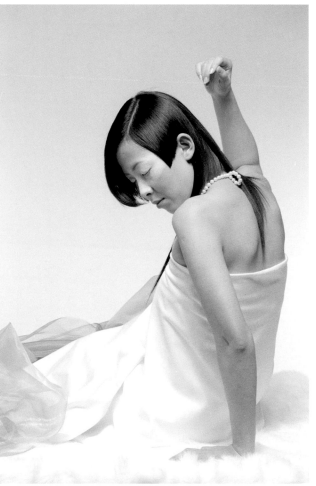
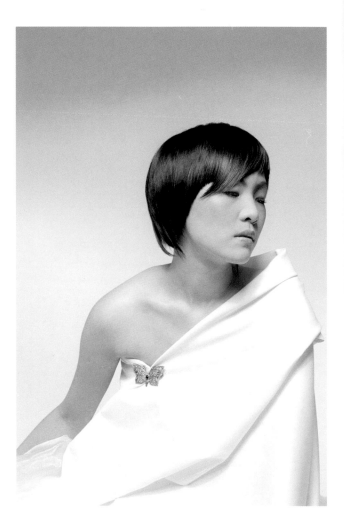

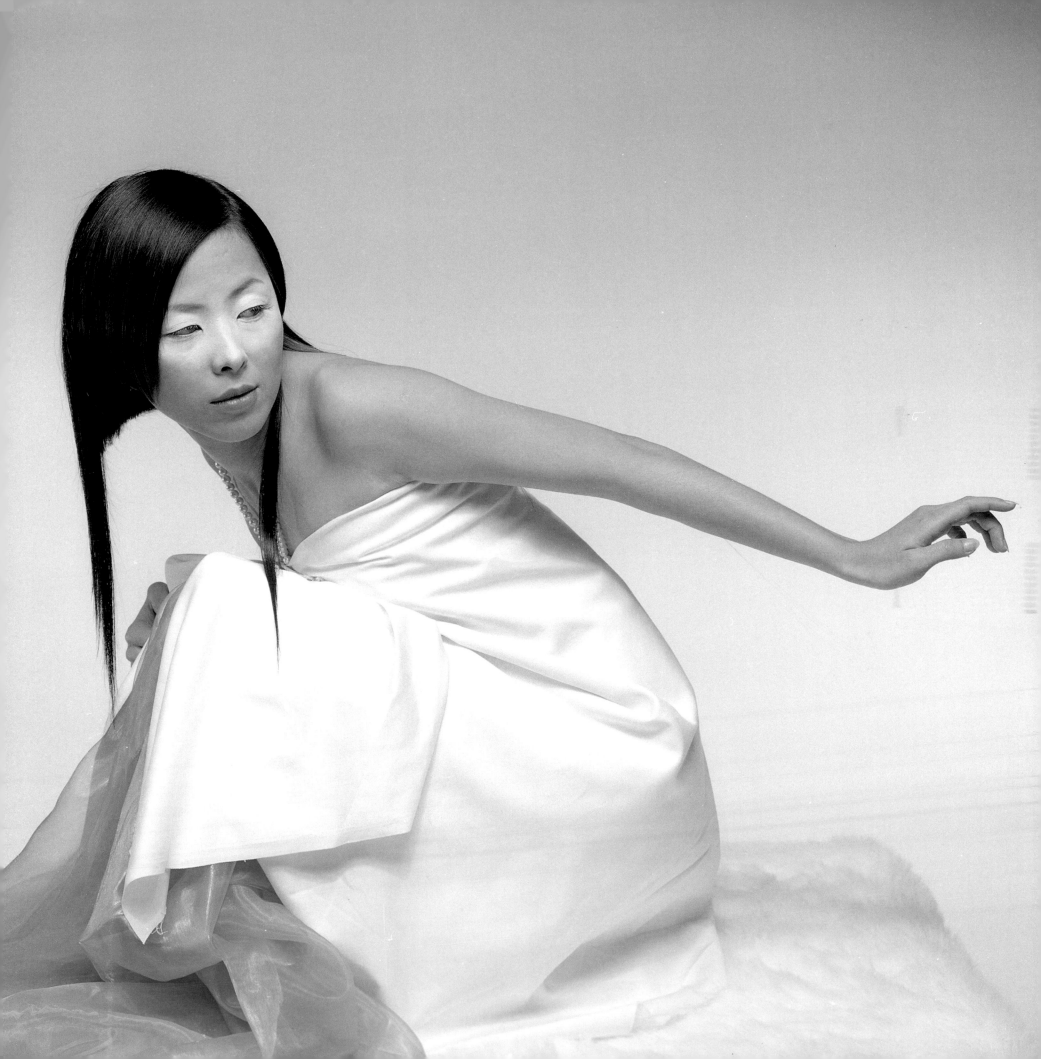

CATALDO'S SALON pages 38–41

55 Northbourne Avenue, Canberra City ACT 2601, Australia, www.cataldo's.com.au

Hair: Emilio Cataldo
Salon: Cataldo's
Make-up: Kylie O'Toole
Styling: Emma Cotterill
Photography: Andrew O'Toole

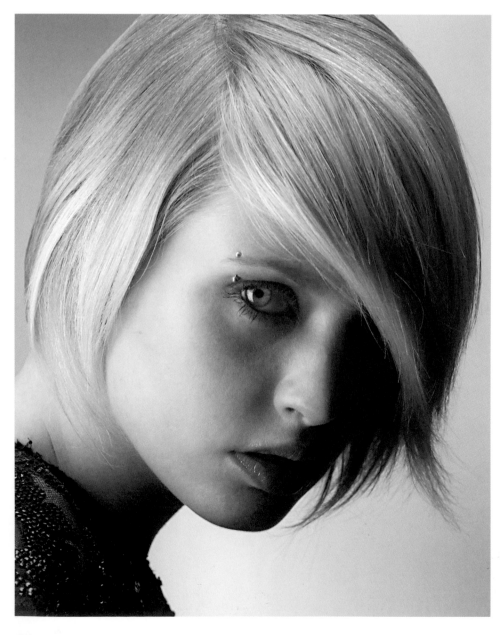
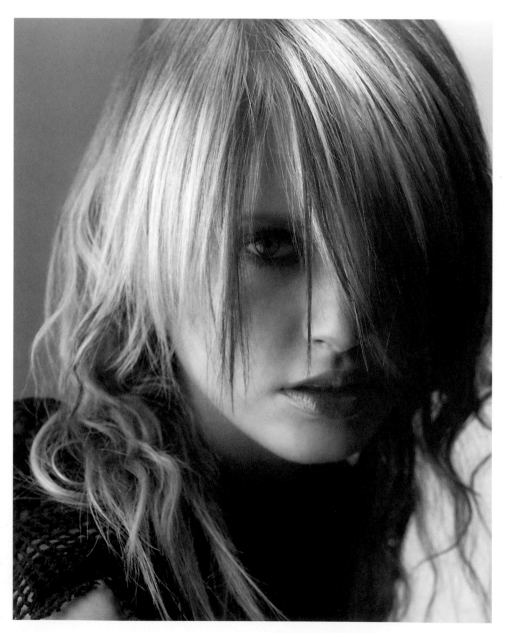

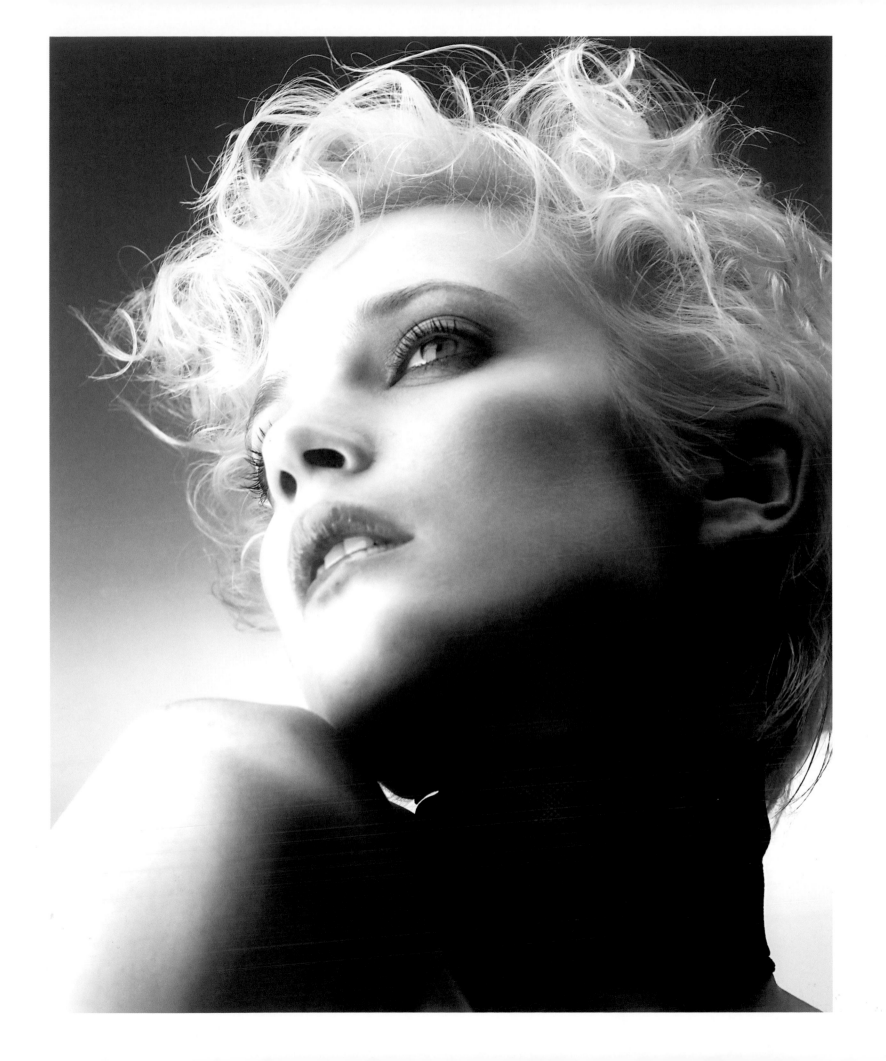

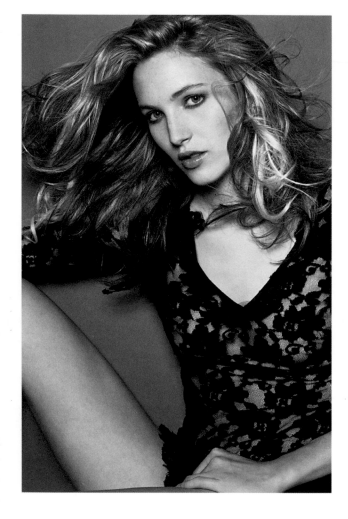
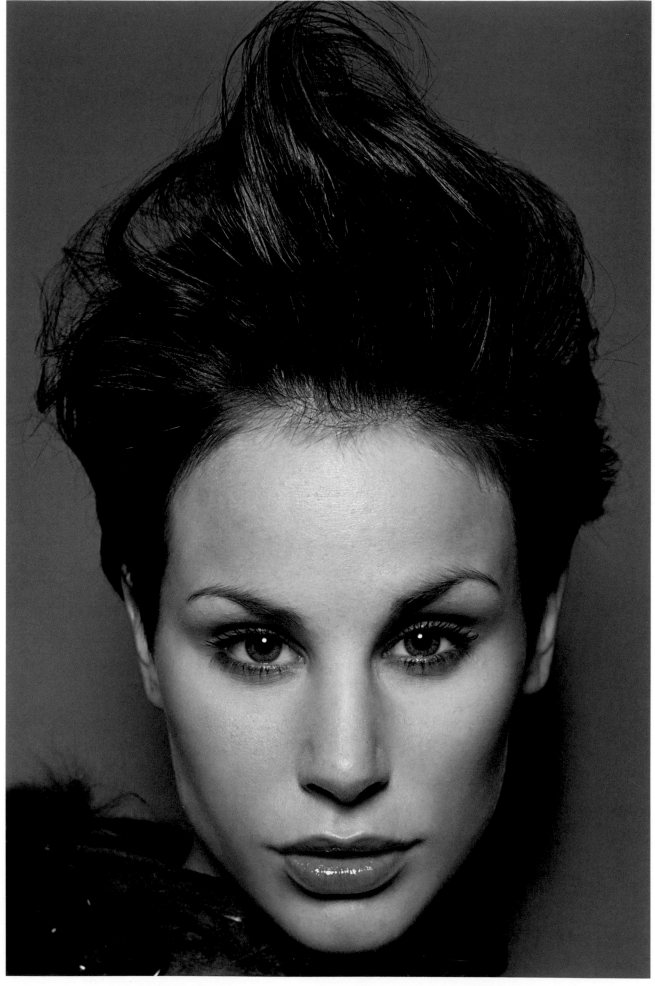

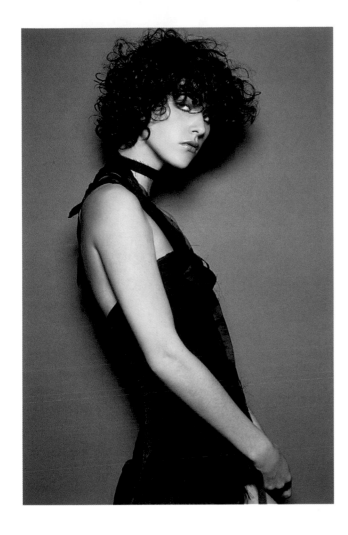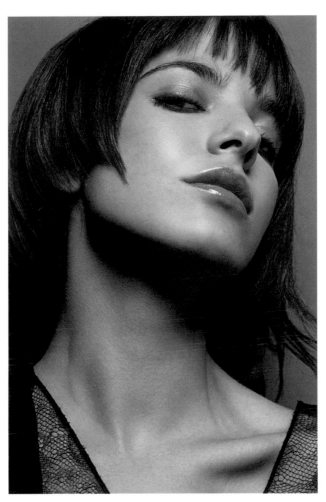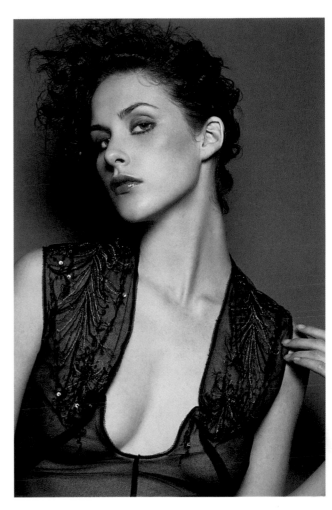

BEVERLY COBELLA pages 42–45

Cobella House, 5 Kensington High Street, London W8 5NP, United Kingdom

Hair: Beverly Cobella
Make-up: Cheryl Phelps Gardiner
Styling: Marcella Martinelli
Photography: Clive Arrowsmith

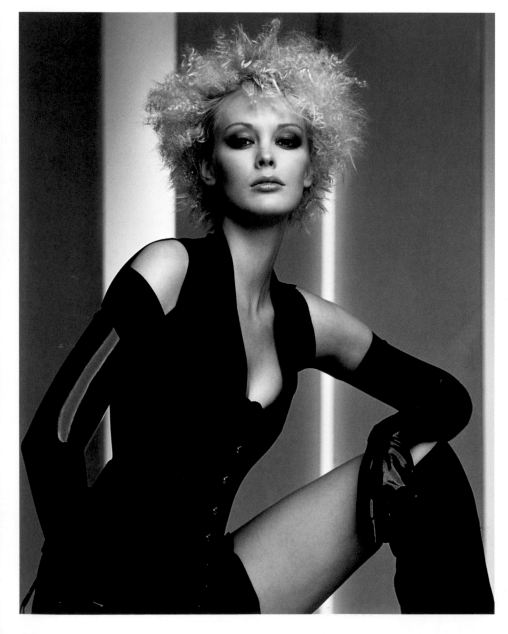
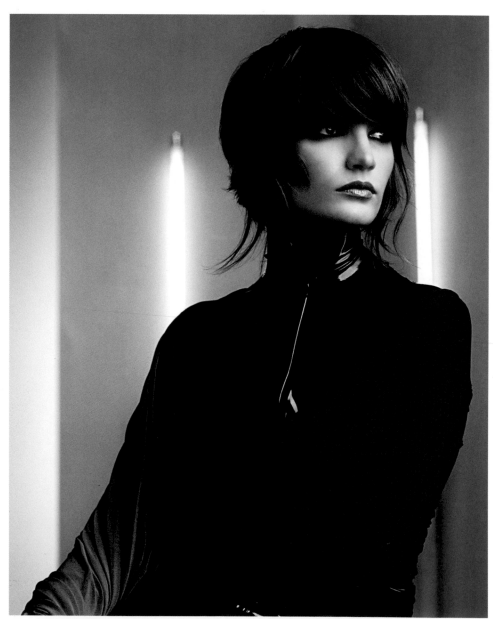

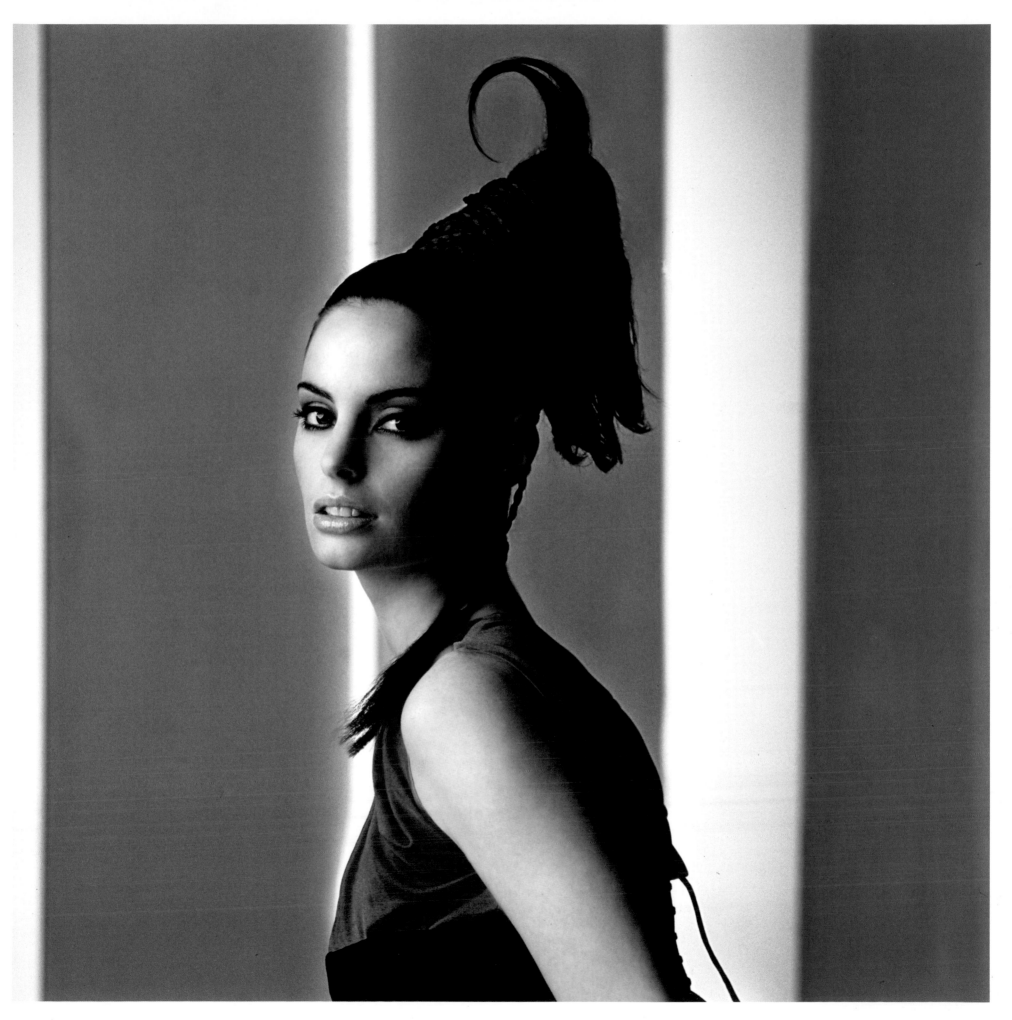

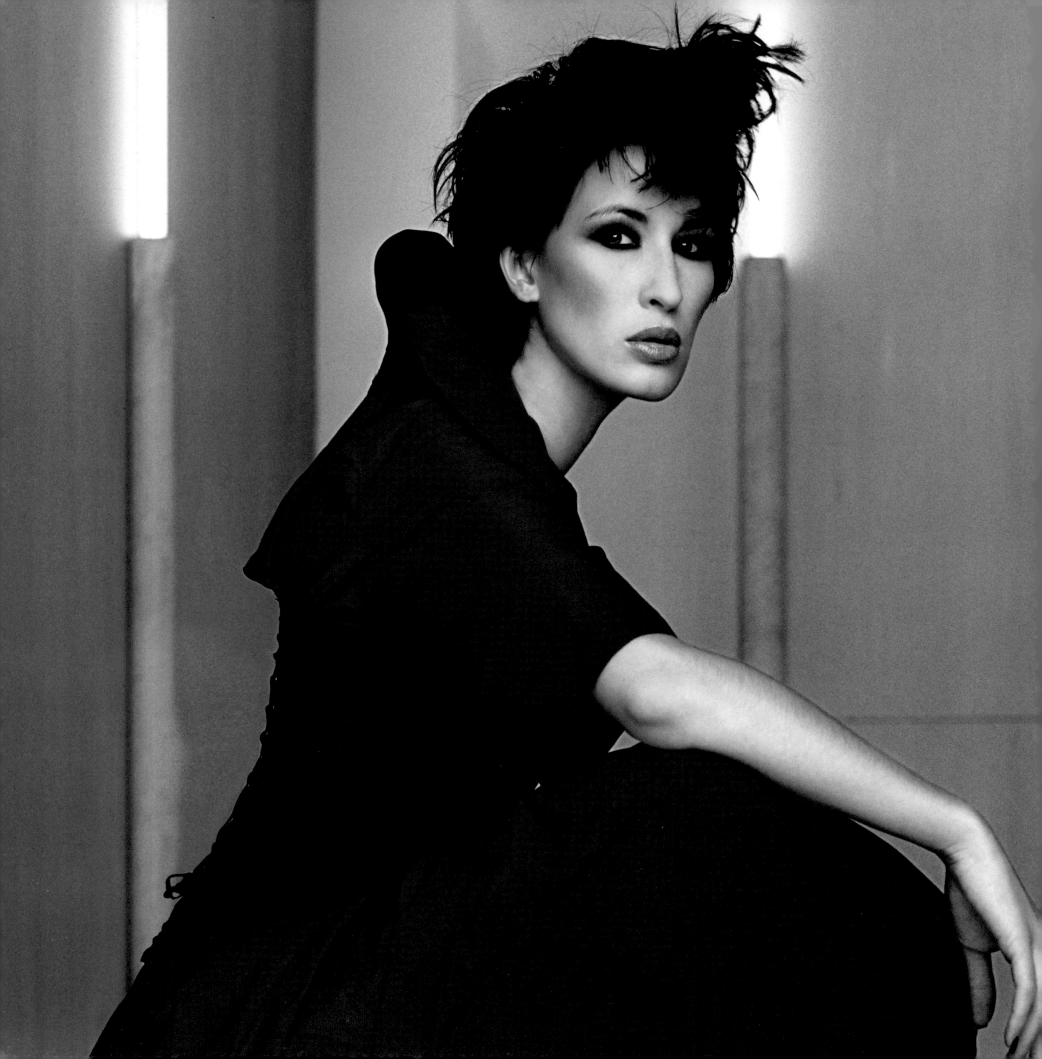

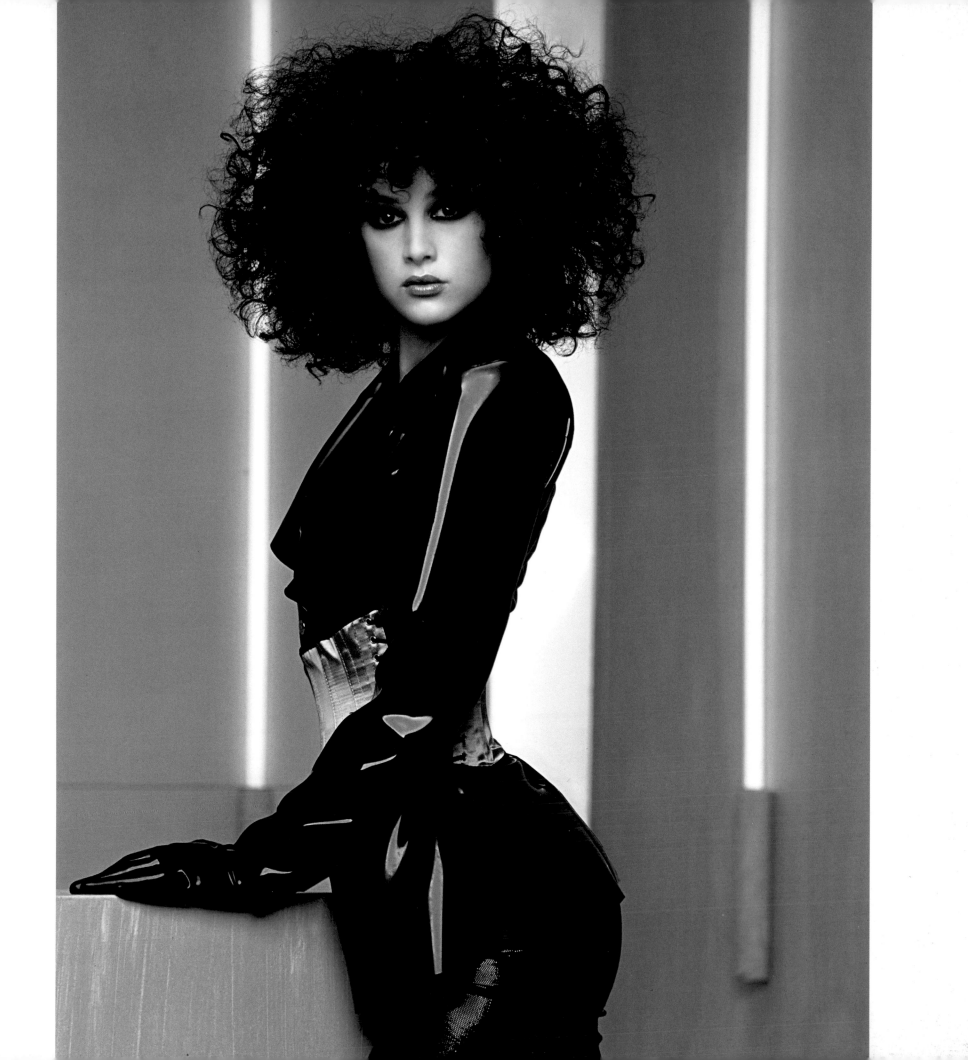

I SARGASSI pages 46–47

I Sargassi Training Centre, Via Ottaviano 6, (San Pietro), 00192 Roma, Italy

Hair: I Sargassi Roma Creative Team
Make-up: Daniela Pannella
Styling: Loredana Servadio
Photography: Andrea Camandona
Concept: Franco Romano
Model Agency: Talent's
Products: L'Oréal

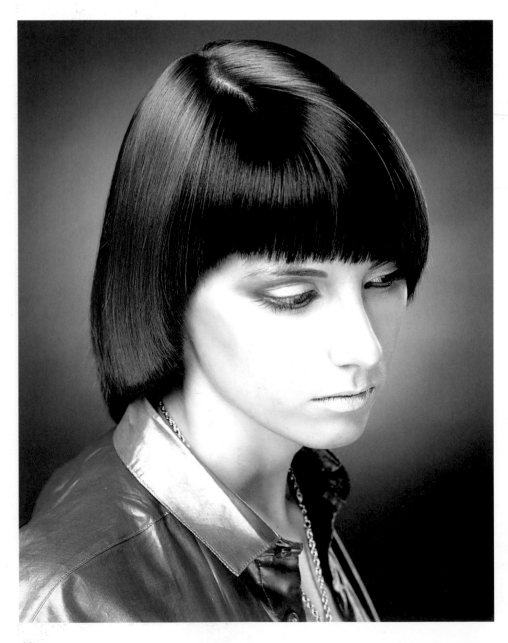 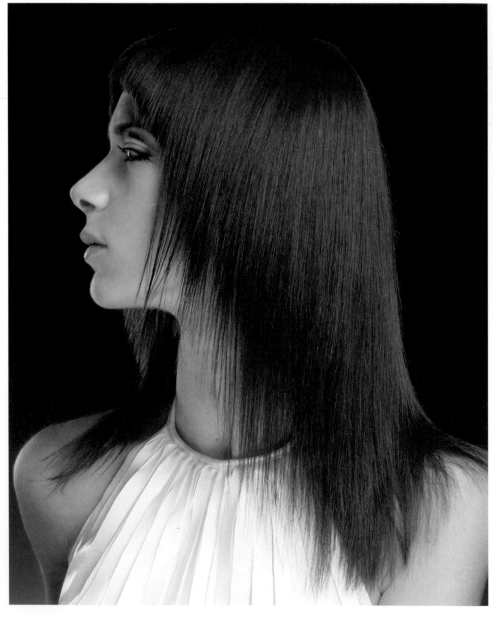

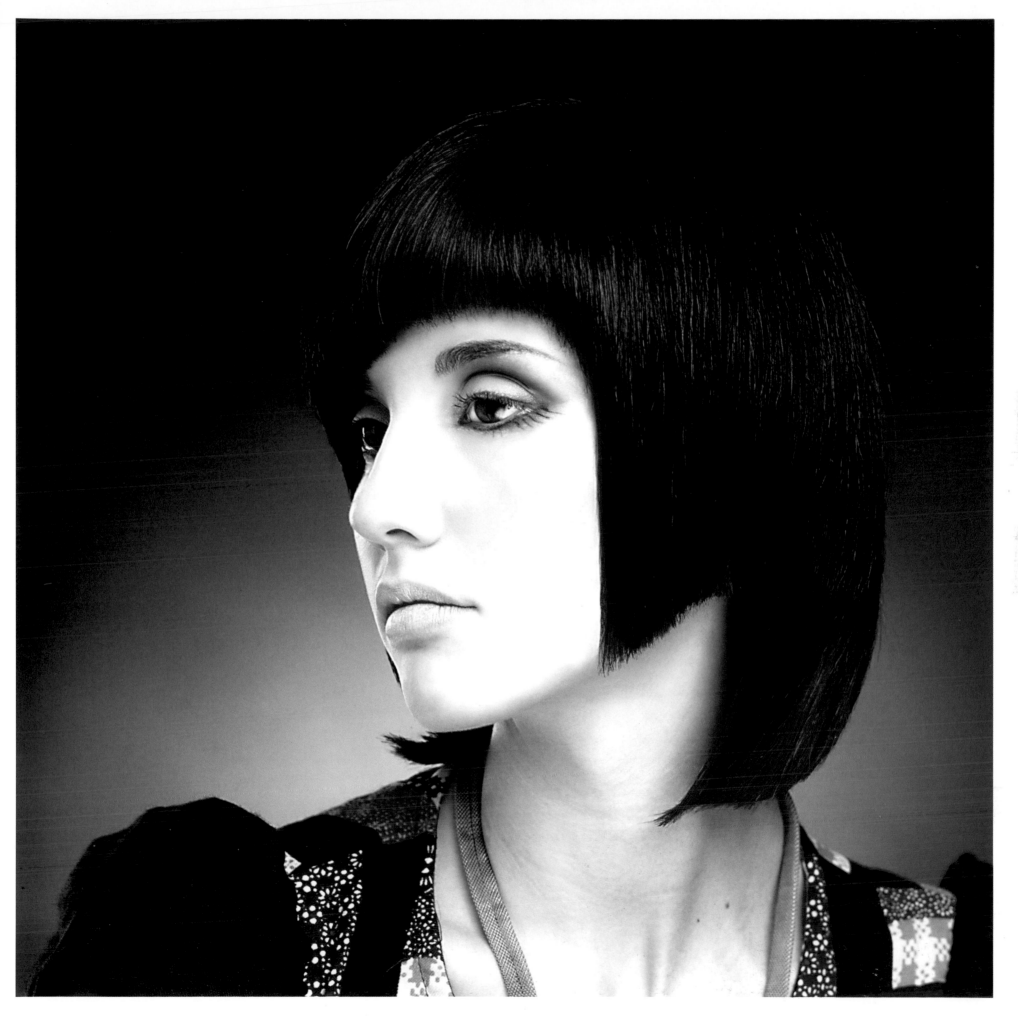

MICHAEL JUNG pages 48–49

Gärtnerstrasse 30, 20253 Hamburg, Germany

Hair: Michael Jung
Make-up: Diana Schairer
Photography: Adele Marschner

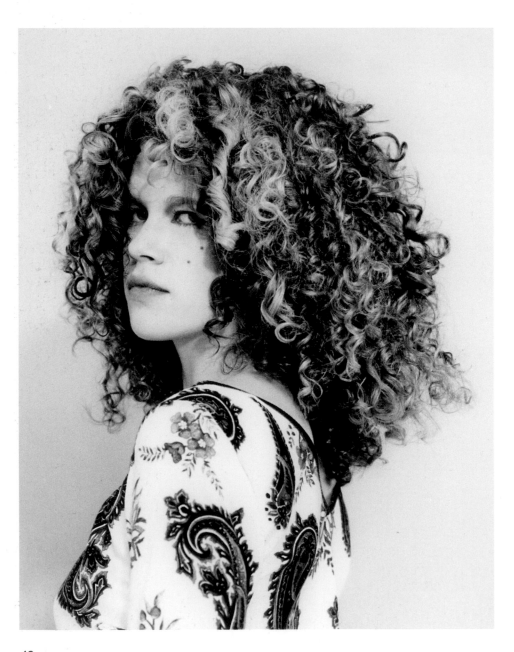

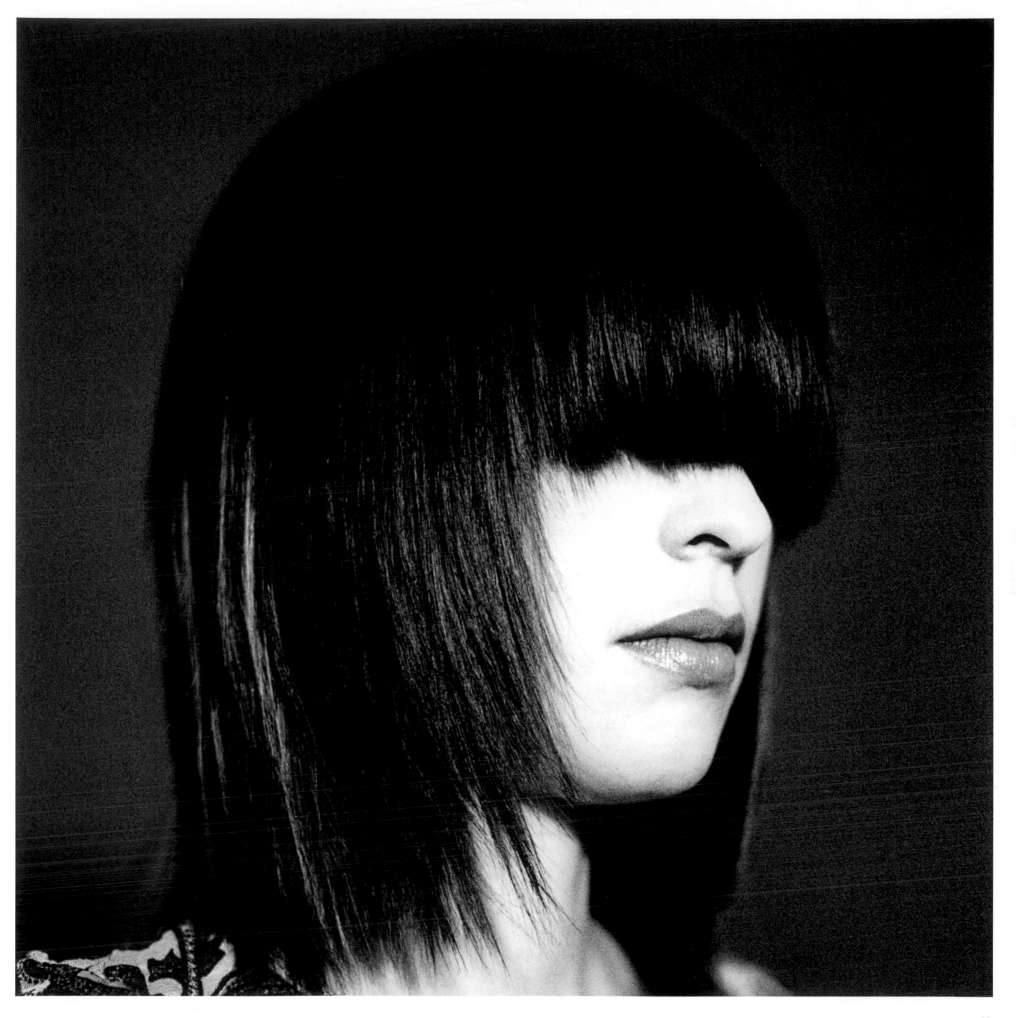

CARITÉ INTERNATIONAL pages 50–51

65 Tomas Montañana, 46021 Valencia, Spain, www.newcarite.com

Hair: Carité International

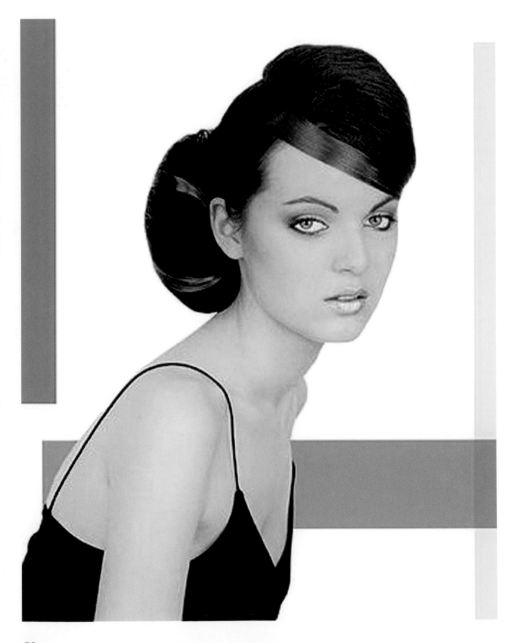

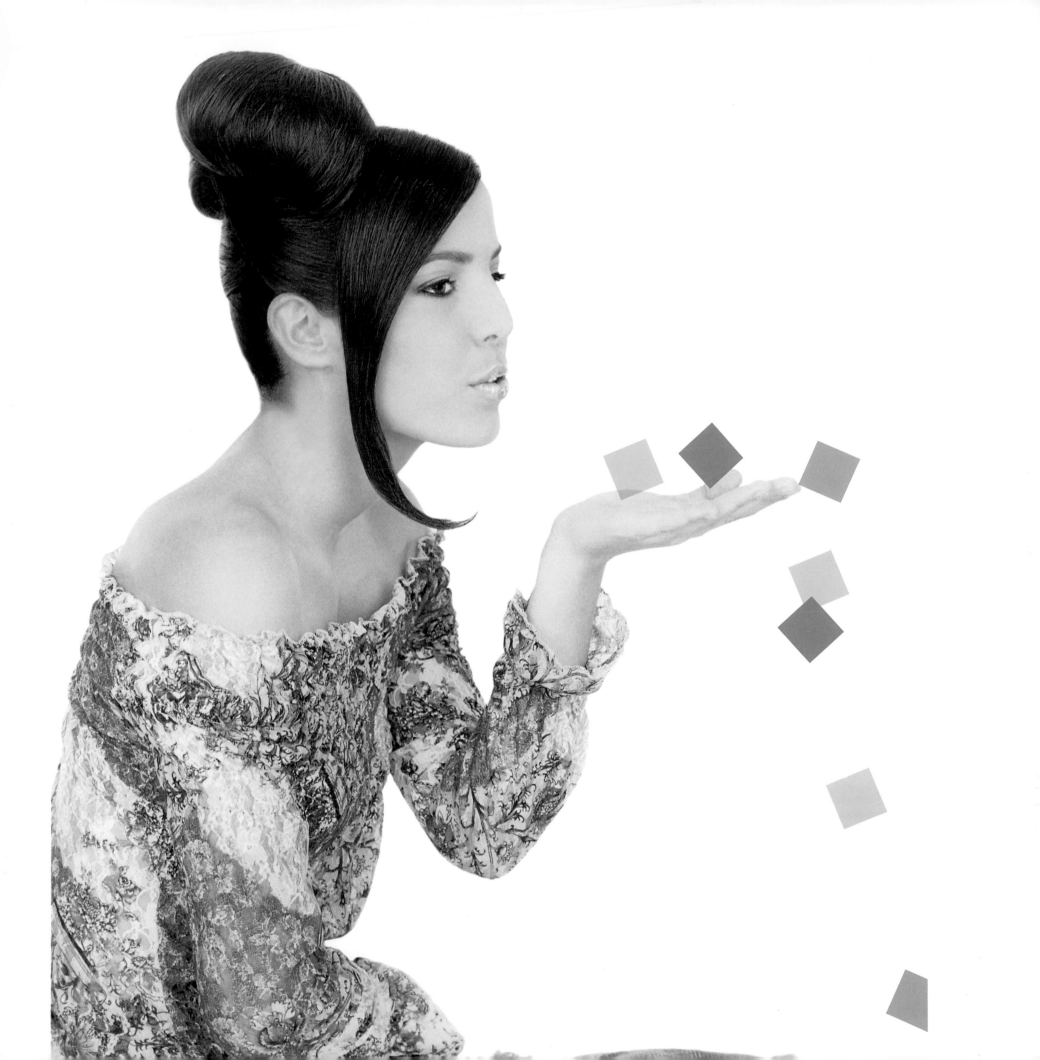

JAGA HUPALO & THOMAS WOLFF pages 52–55
Ul. Burakowska 5/7, 01-066 Warszawa, Poland, www.jagahairdesign.com

Hair: Jaga Hupalo & Thomas Wollf Hair Design
Make-up: Jerry Keszka (p. 52) Wiorika Zagorowska (p. 53, 55) Slawek Oszjaca (p. 54)
Photography: Thomas Wollf
Models: Weronika Iwaniuk D'Vision (p. 52) Karolina Raczynska D'Vision (p. 53)
Mira (p. 54) Wiorika Zagorowska Eastern Models (p. 55)

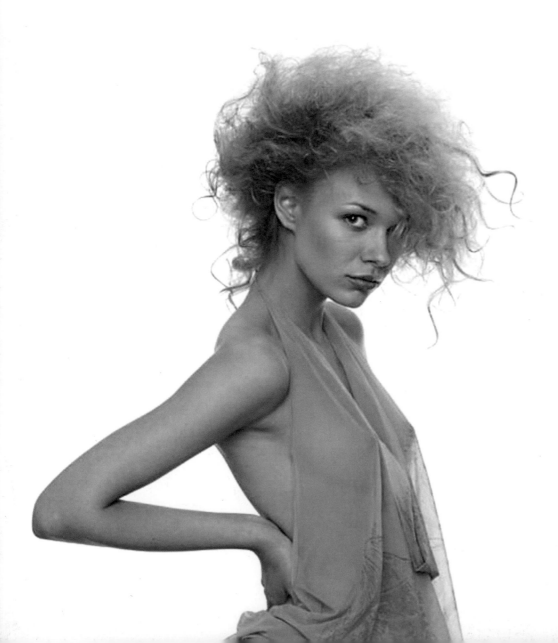

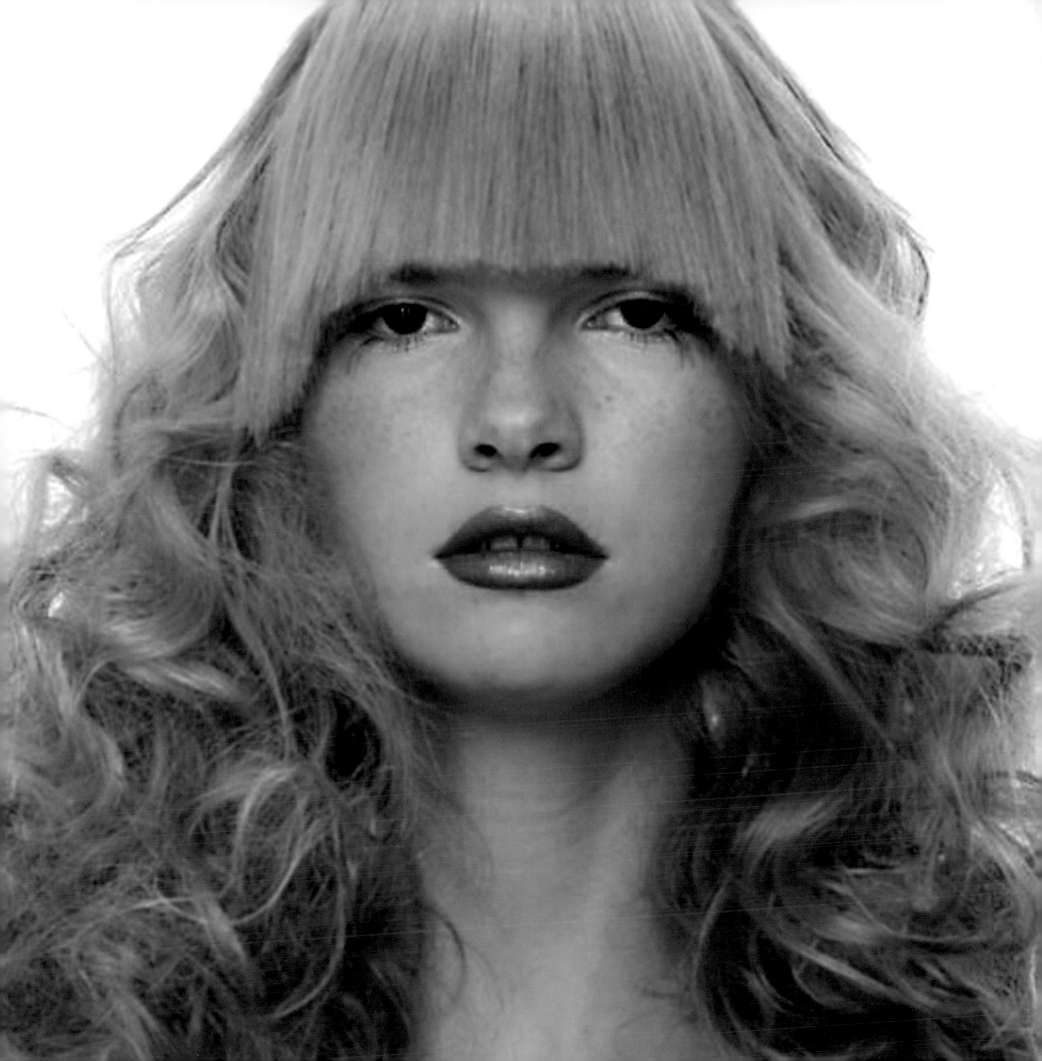

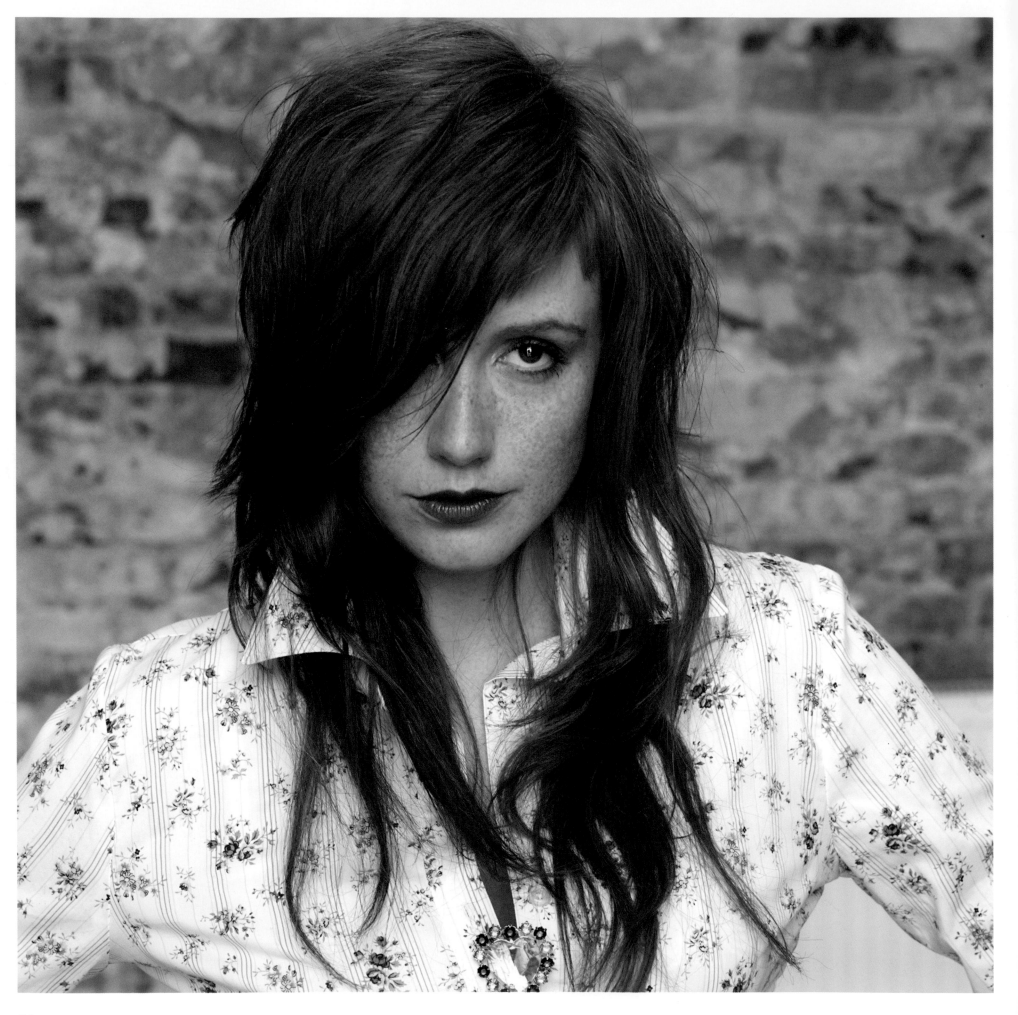

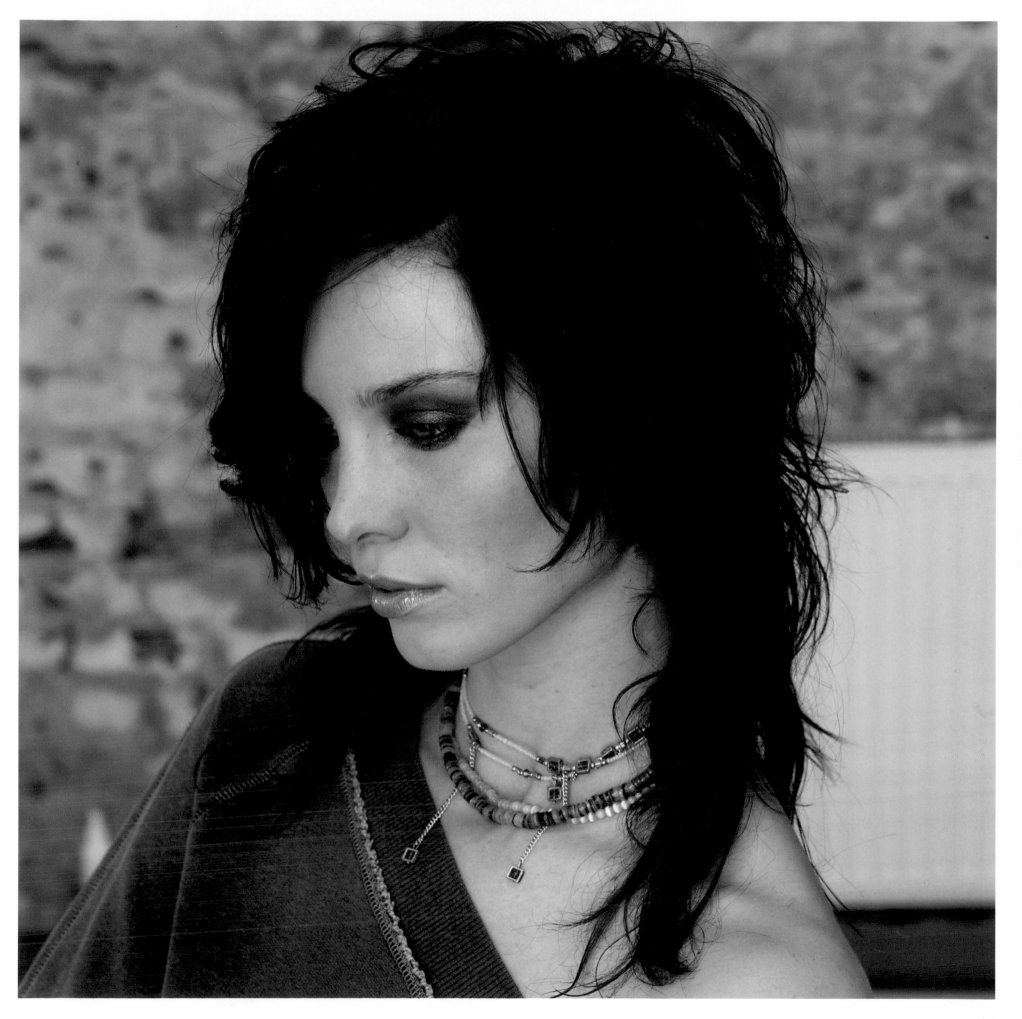

JAMES HAIR FASHION CLUB pages 56–59

Via M. Curie 1/A, 42100 Reggio Emilia, Italy, www.jameshairdiffusion.it

Hair: James Hair Fashion Club
Make-up: Keros
Styling: Fun & Fashion
Photography: Roberto Covi
Model Agency: Why not, Model Management, Woman, Riccardo Gay
Products: High Hair from Wella

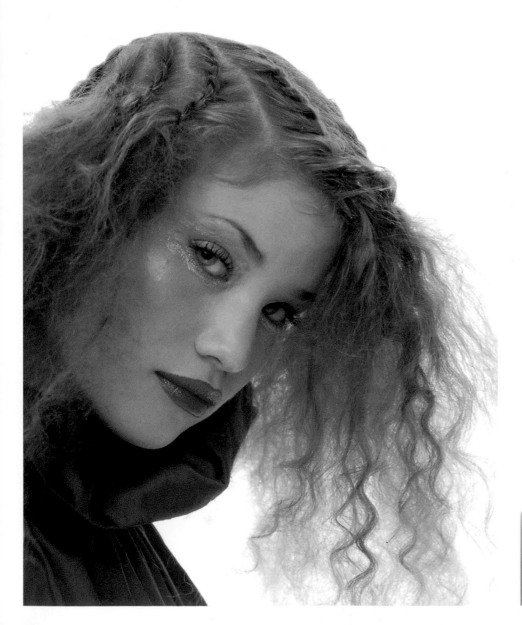

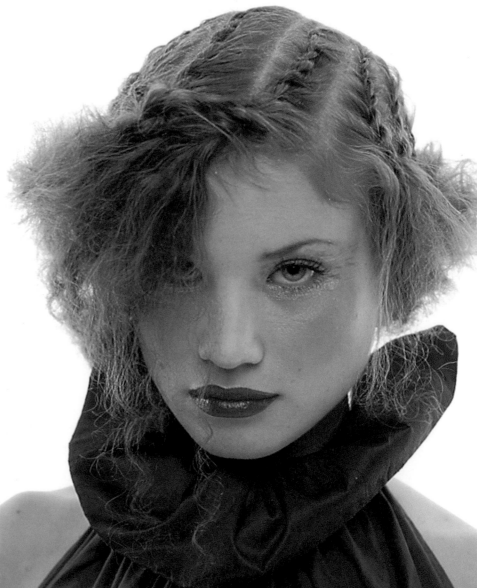

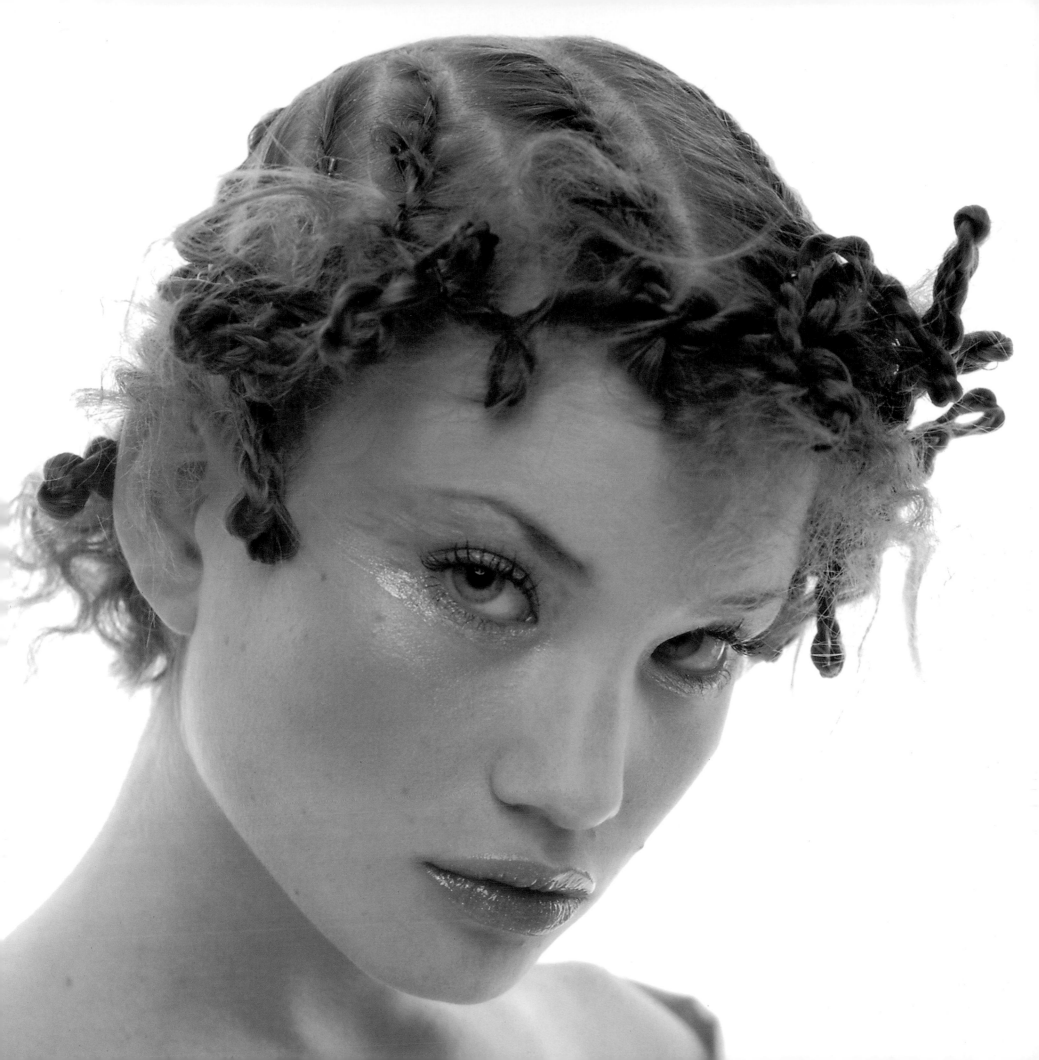

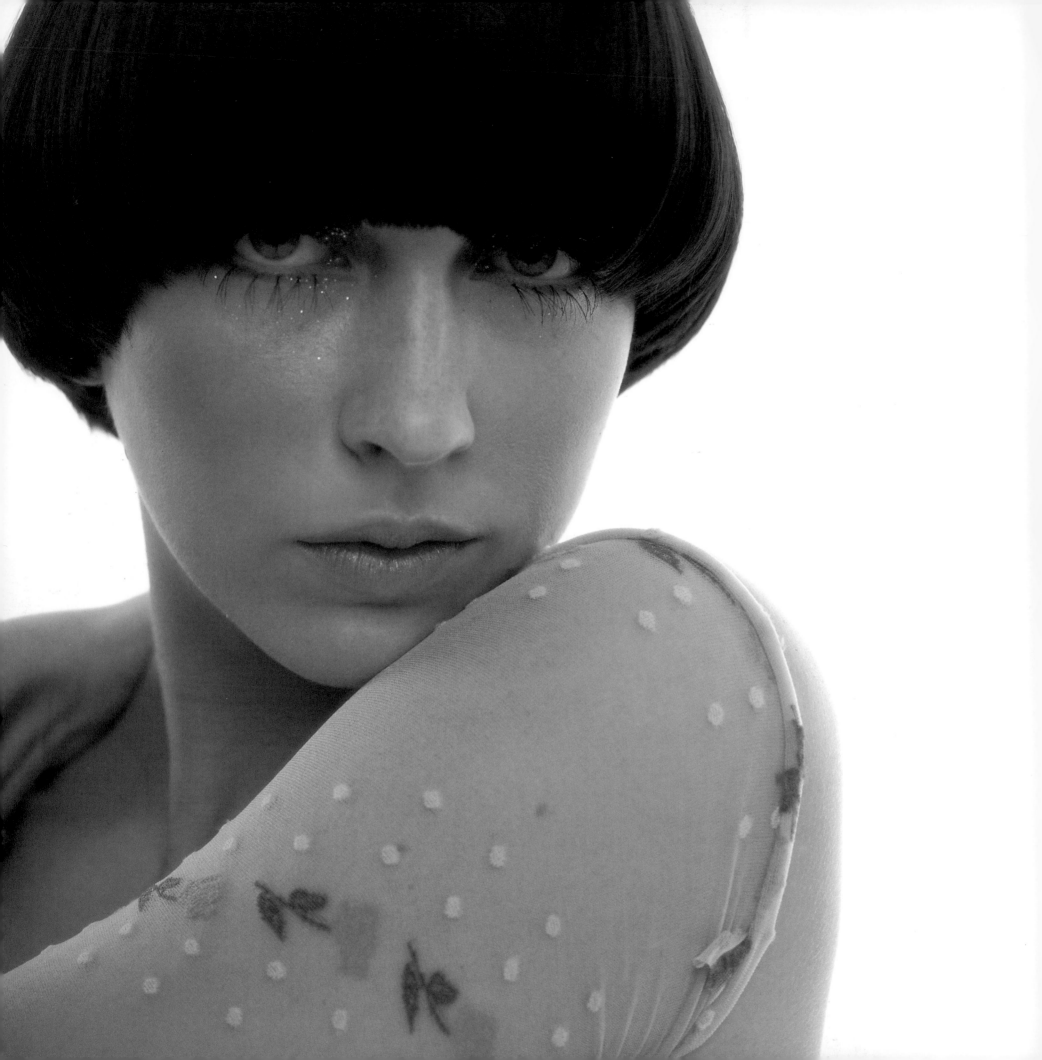

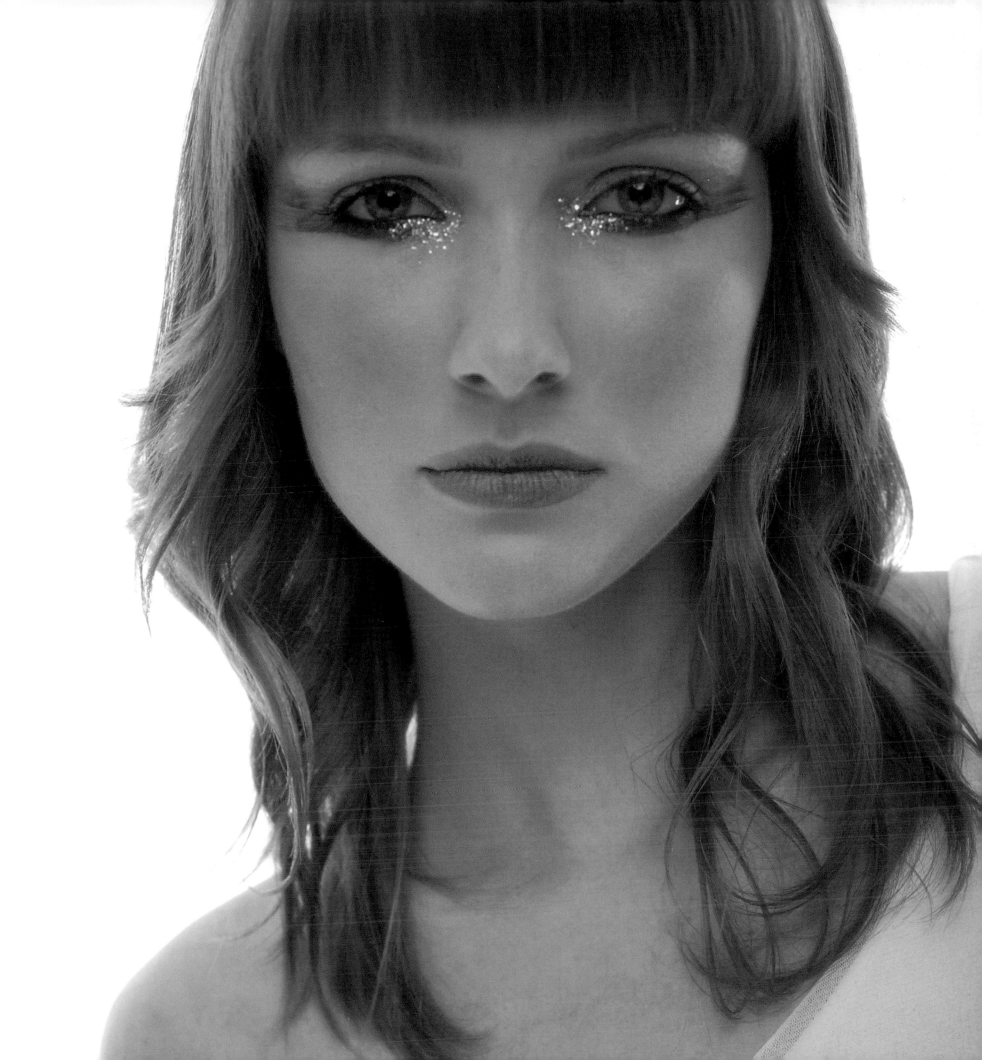

BARIKISU LARSEN pages 60–61

Fælledvej 14C, 4th, DK 2200 København N, Denmark, www.barikisu.com

Hair: Barikisu Larsen
Photography: Jacob Crawfurd, www.crawfurd.dk
Model: Susan

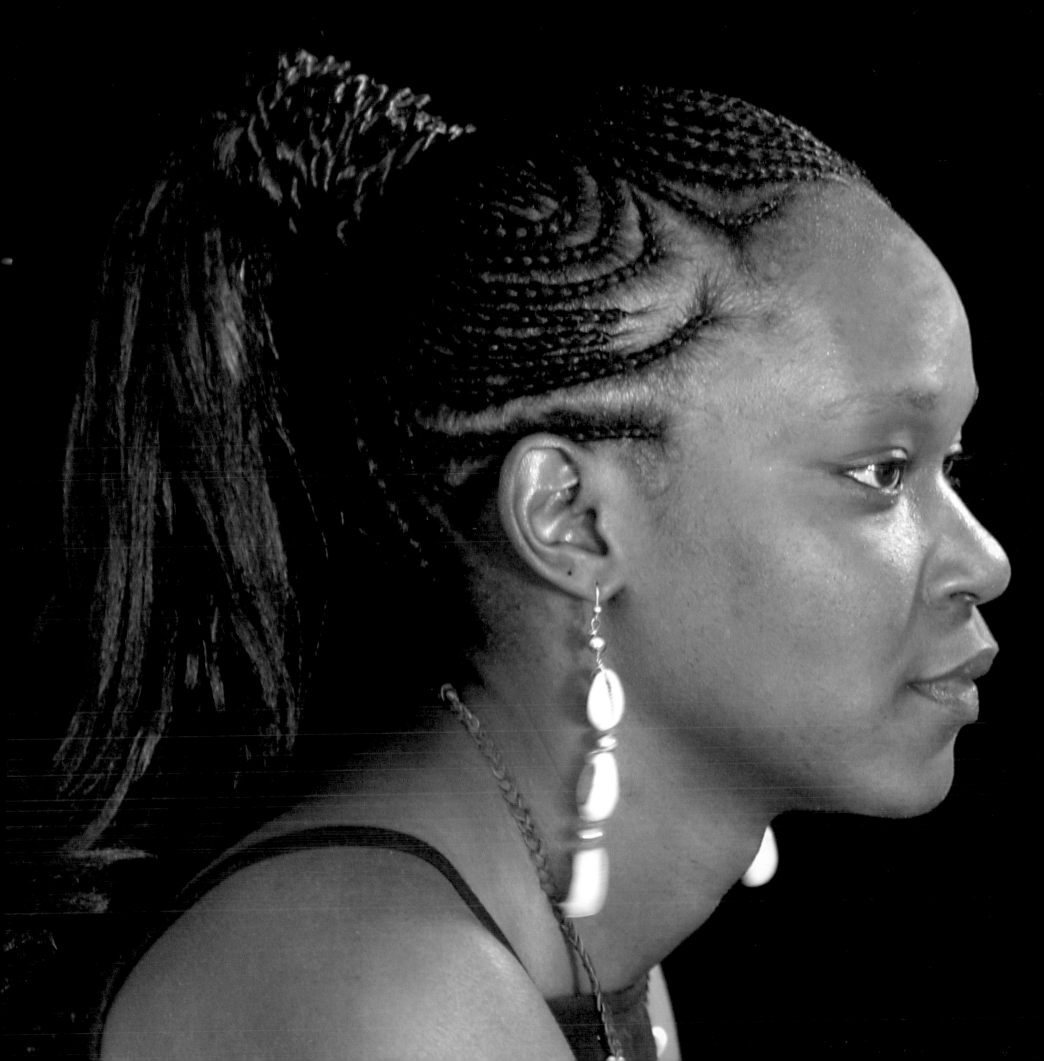

KHAMIT KINKS pages 62–65

4 Leonard Street, New York N.Y. 10013, USA, www.khamitkinks.com

Hair: Solange (p. 62, 63, 65) Khady Mbaye (p. 64) Nicola (p. 65)
Salon: Khamit Kinks
Make-up: Ashunta Sheriff for D.W.M.
Photography: Eric von Lockhart Photography
Models: Kali Hawk (p. 62, 63, 65) Kandiss Edmundson (p. 65) Joanna Goodwin (p. 64) Jahmilla Collier (p. 64)

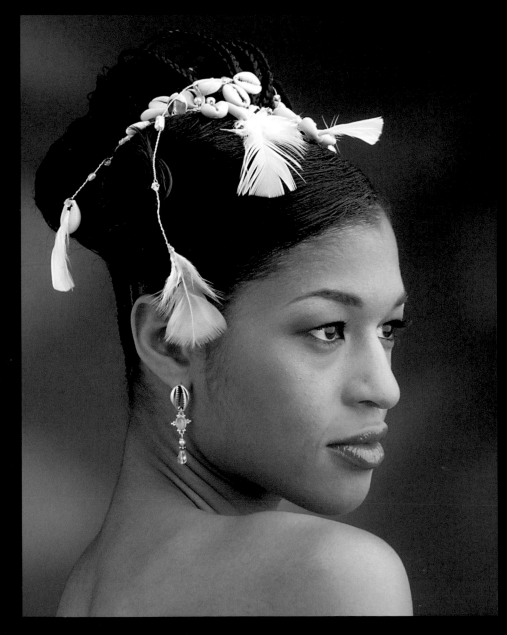

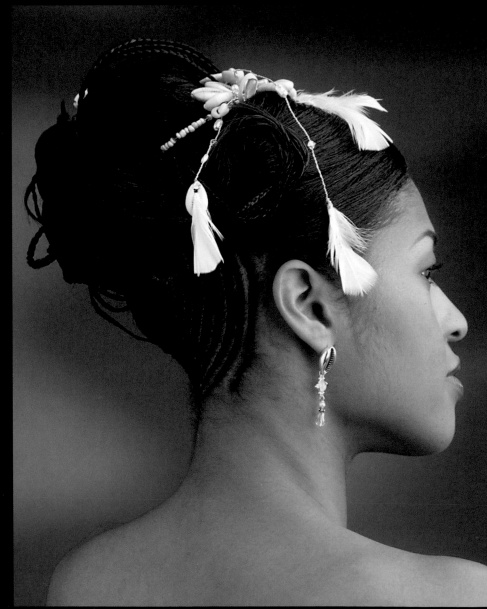

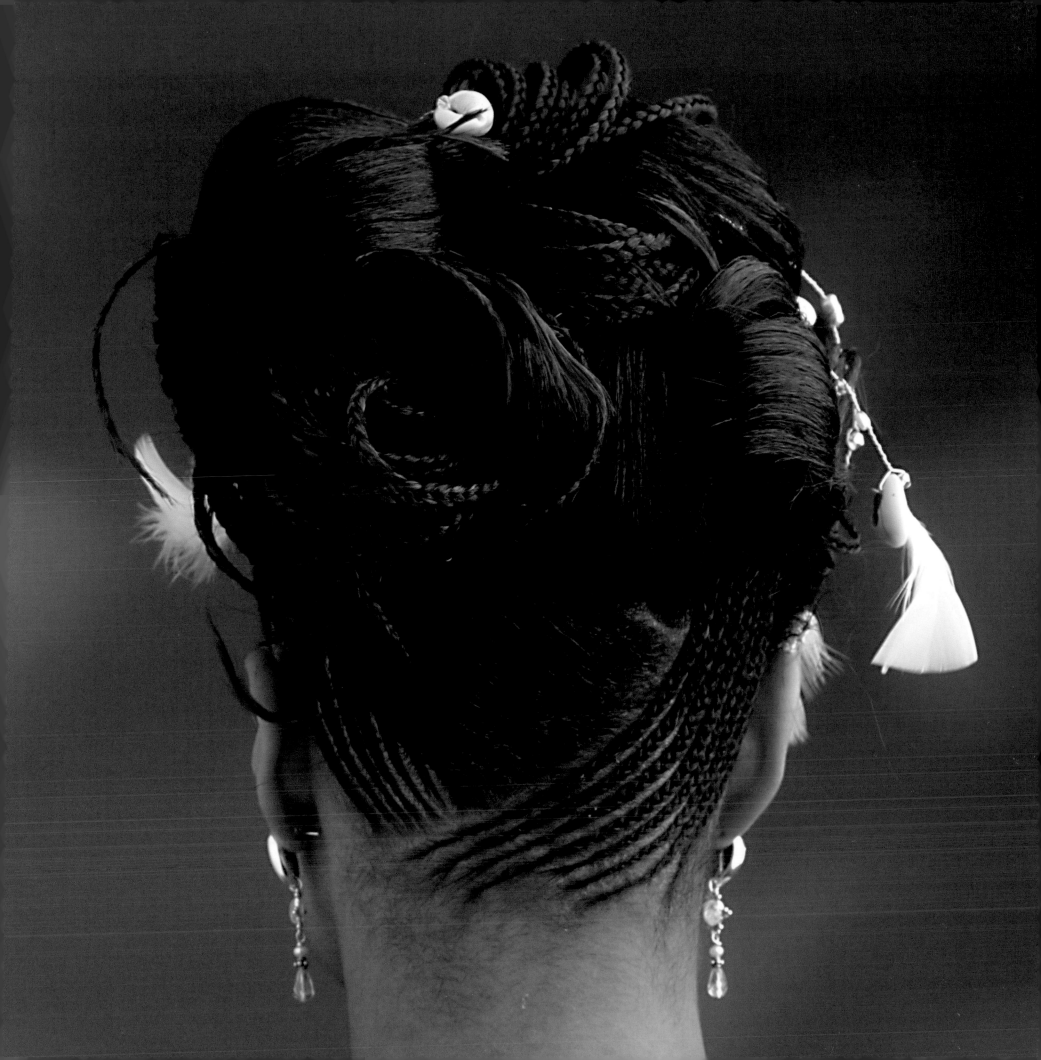

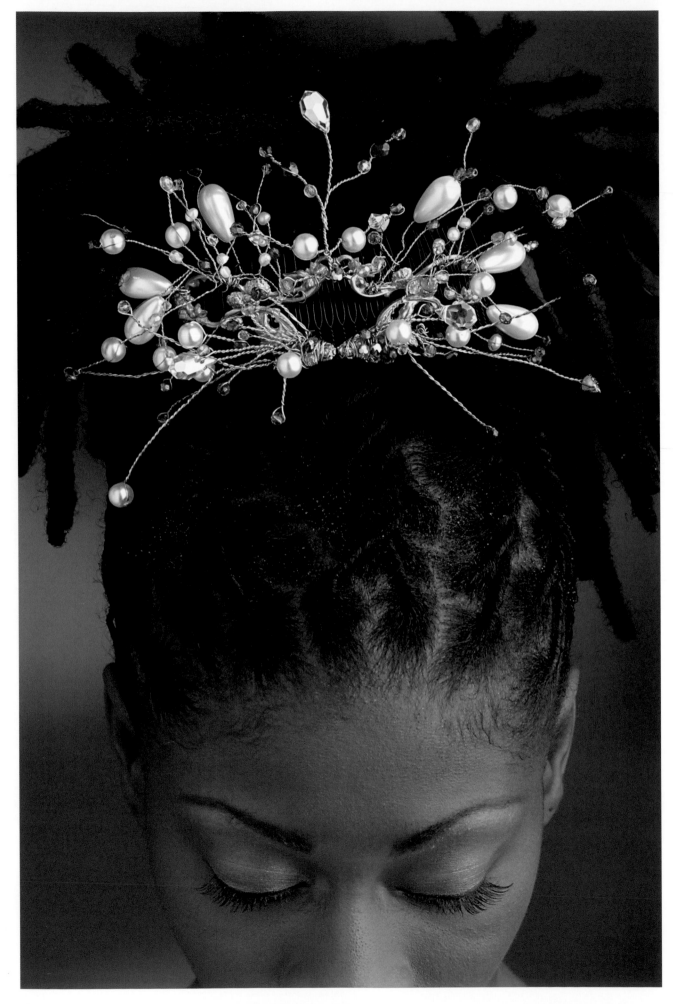

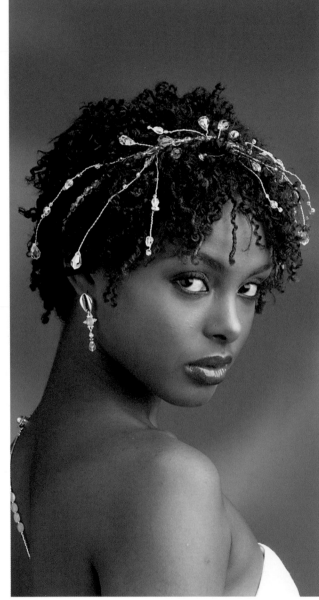

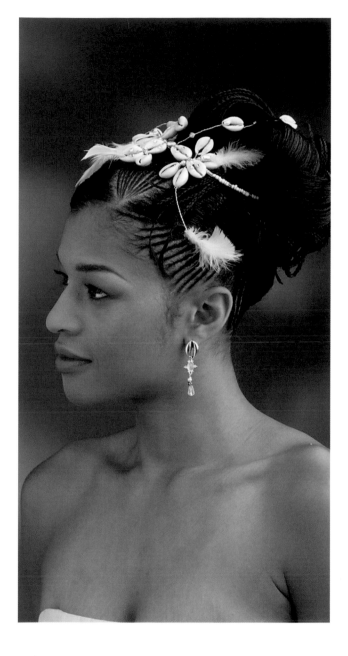

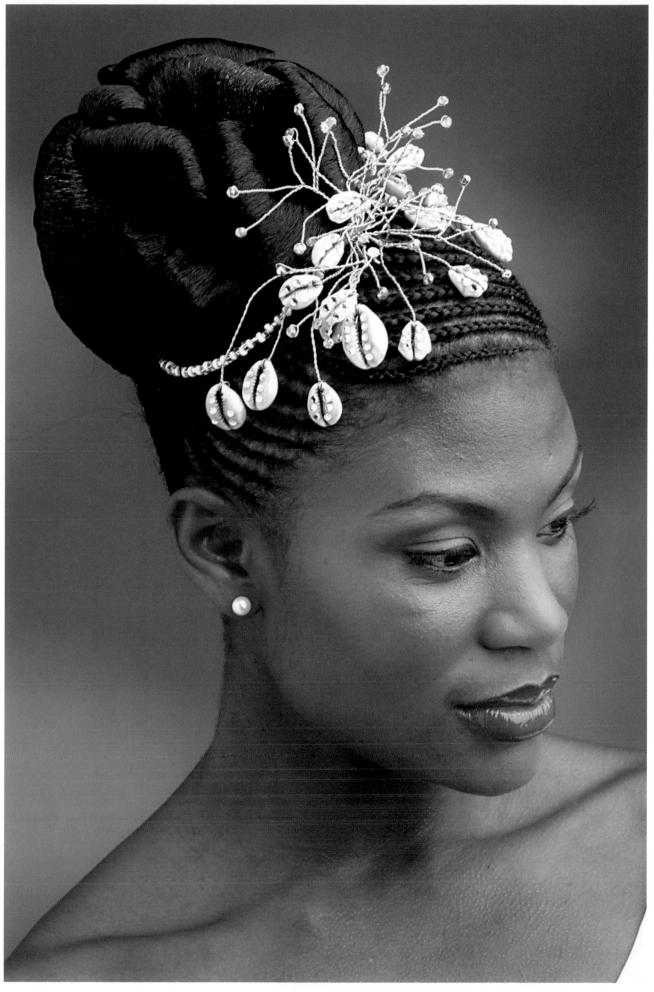

Hair: Svetlana Ryzhkova
Academy: Academy of Hairdressing Art

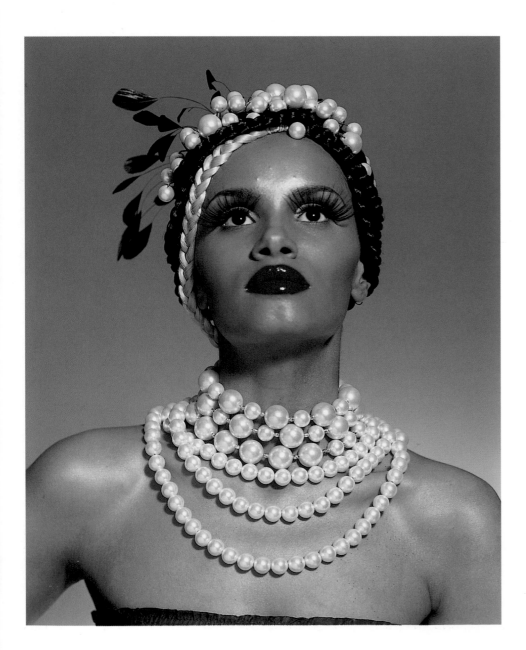

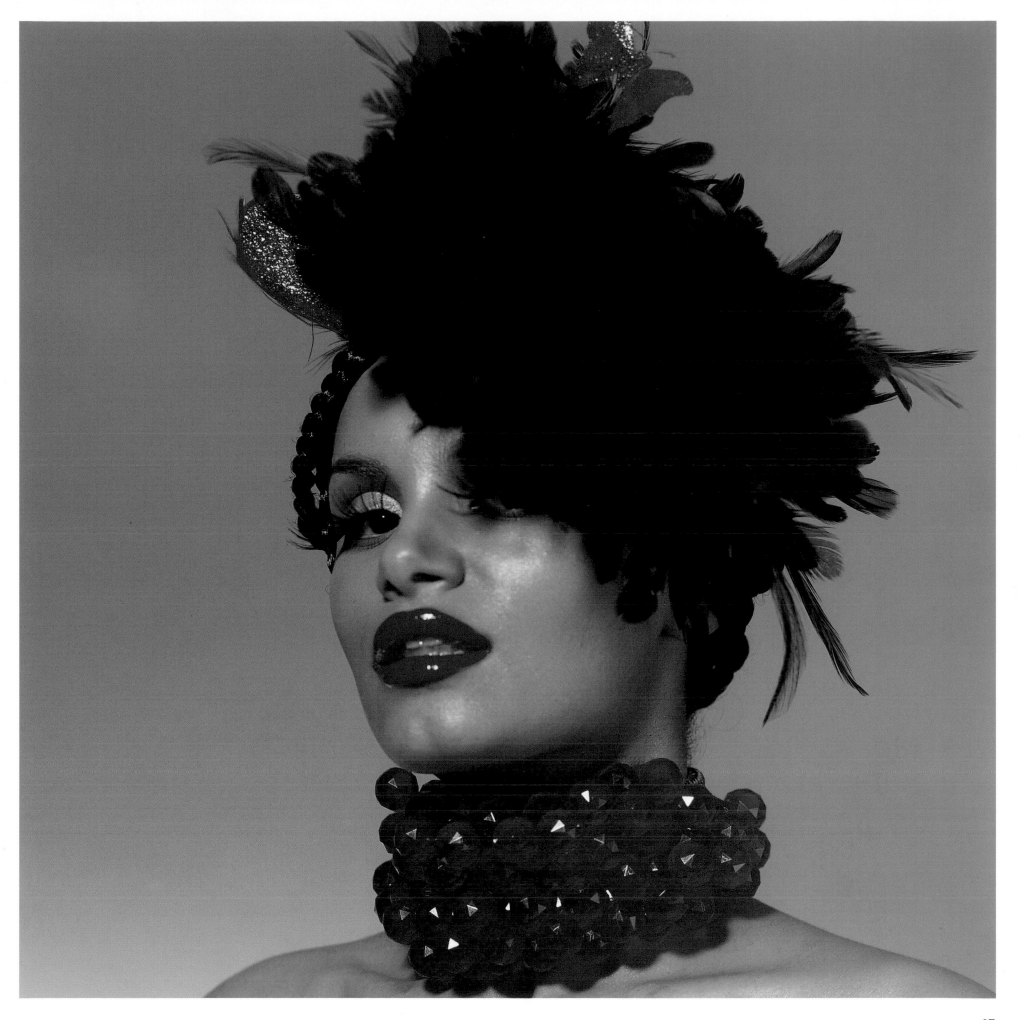

STAN MILTON SALON pages 68–69

721 Miami Circle, Suite 102, Atlanta Georgia 30324, USA, www.stanmiltonsalon.com

Hair: Stan Milton
Color: Kyle Montague (p. 68)
Salon: Stan Milton Salon
Make-up: Karin Robinson
Styling: Laundry by Shelli Segal (p. 68)
Photography: Tom Carson (p. 68) Ben Cornford (p. 69)
Model: Angela Harding, Elite (p. 68) Heather Donaldson (p. 69)
Products: Rene Furterer

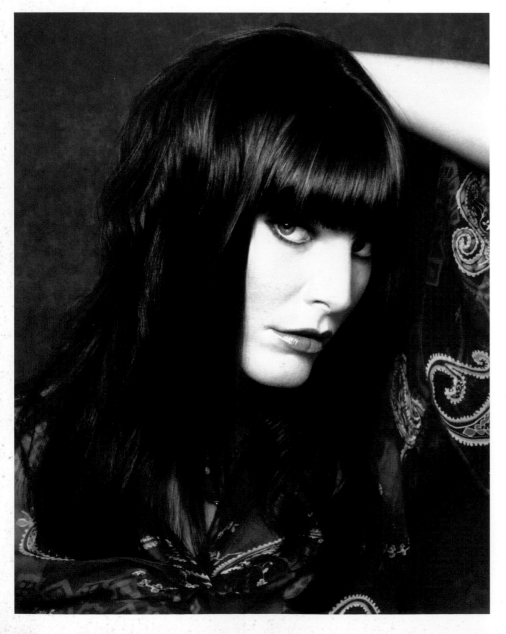

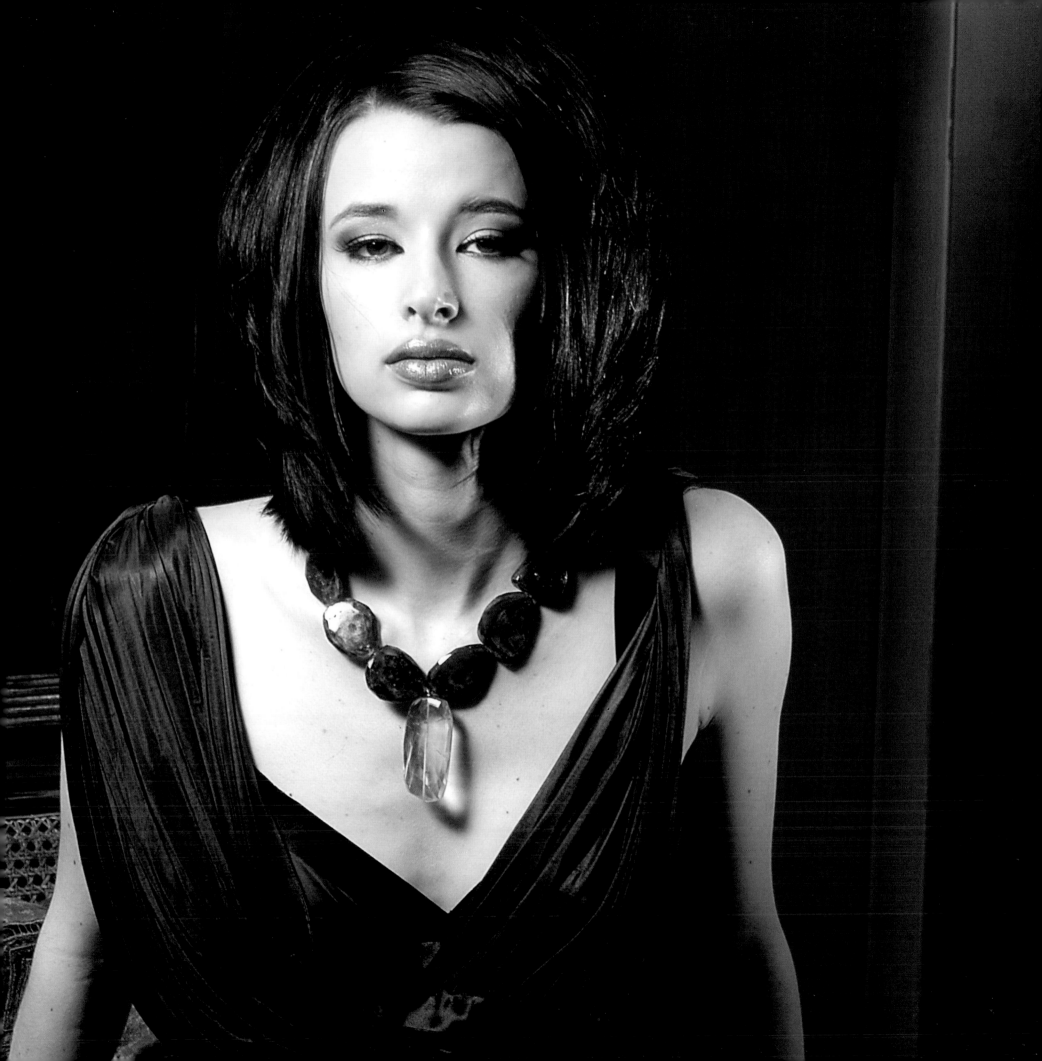

PETRA MECHUROVA pages 70–71

Petra Mechurova Hair Design, Královdorská 12, 11000 Praha 1, Czech Republic, www.petra.mechurova.cz

Hair: Petra Mechurova Hair Design
Salon: Petra Mechurova Hair Design
Make-up: Adriana Bartosová
Styling: Hanka Zárubová
Photography: Anna Kovacicová
Model Agency: Ag. Exit, Slovakia
Production: Milan Dockal

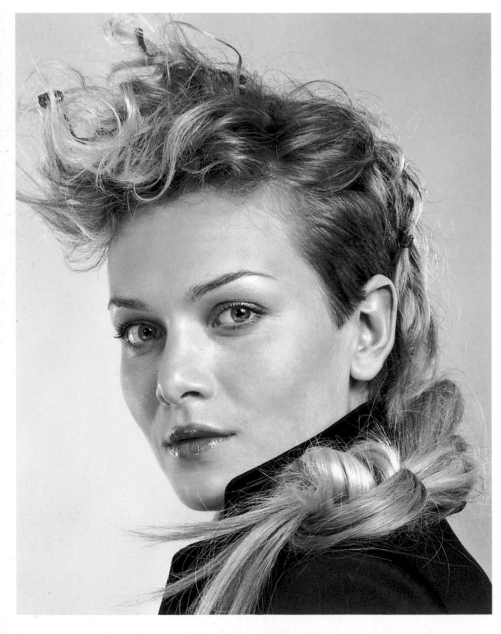

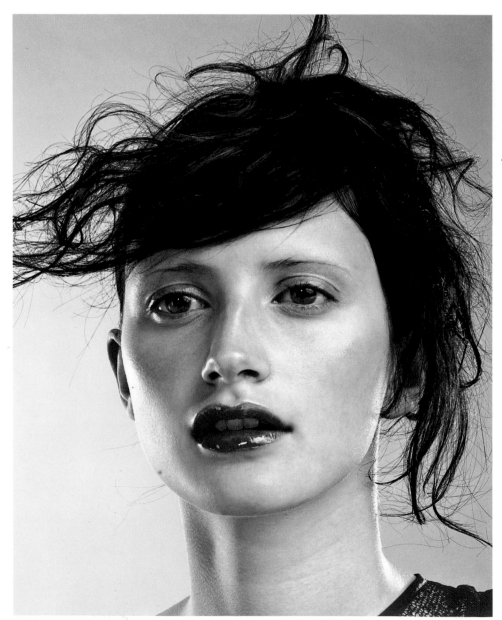

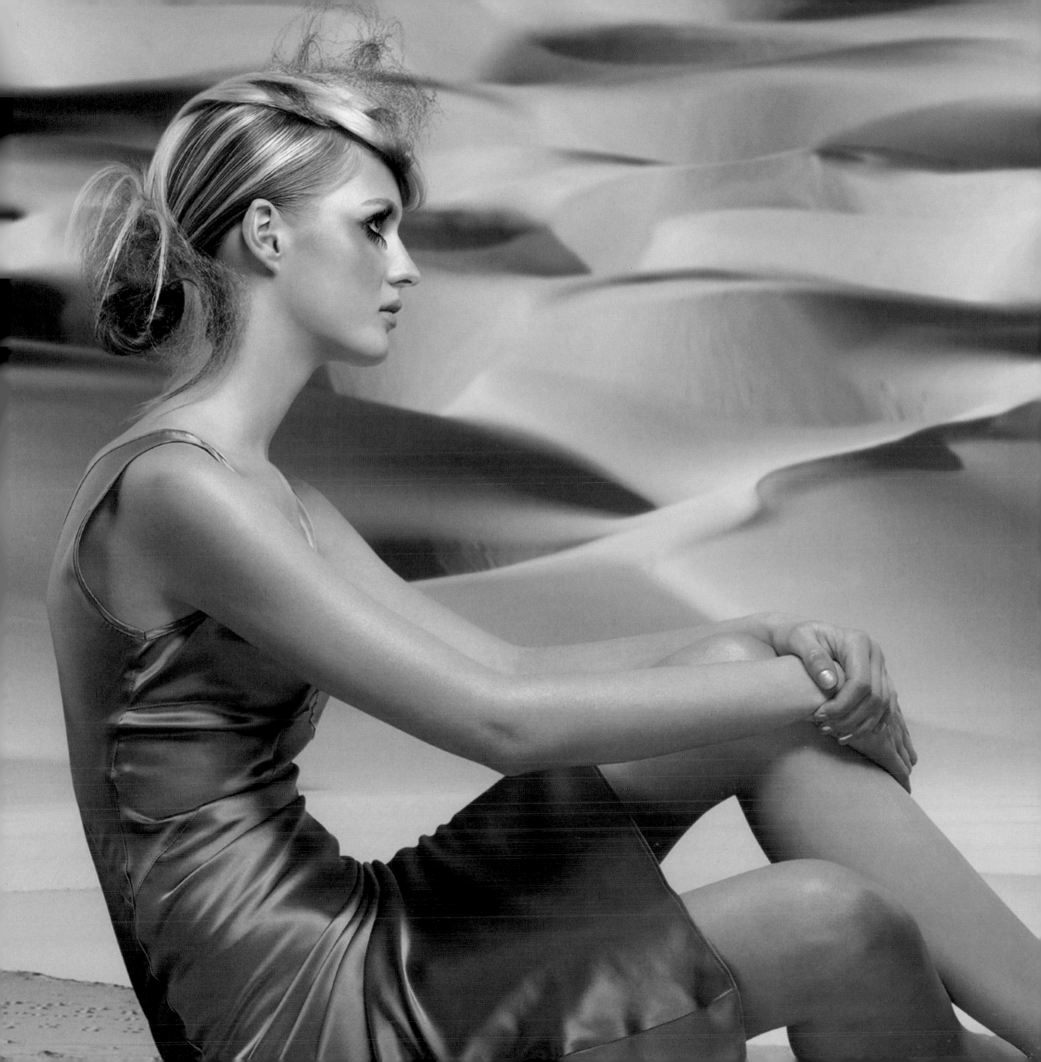

GINGER MEGG'S pages 72–73

Ginger Megg's & Associates, No. 7 St. Albans Street, Merival, Christchurch, New Zealand, wwwgingermeggs.co.nz

Hair: Mike Hamel
Salon: Ginger Megg's
Photography: John Doogan (p. 72) Anthony Mckee (p. 73)

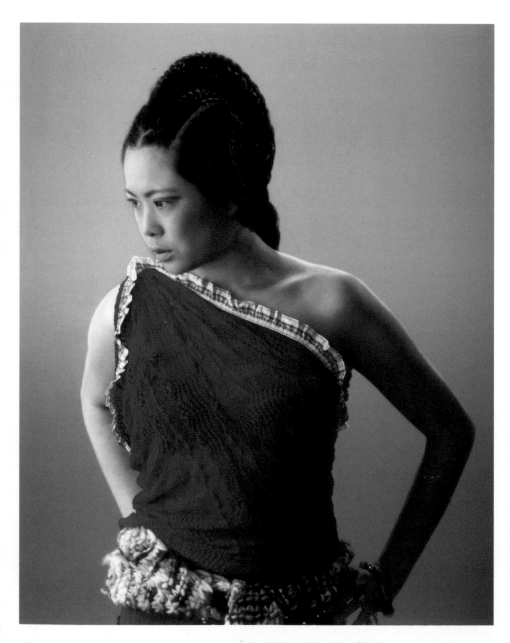
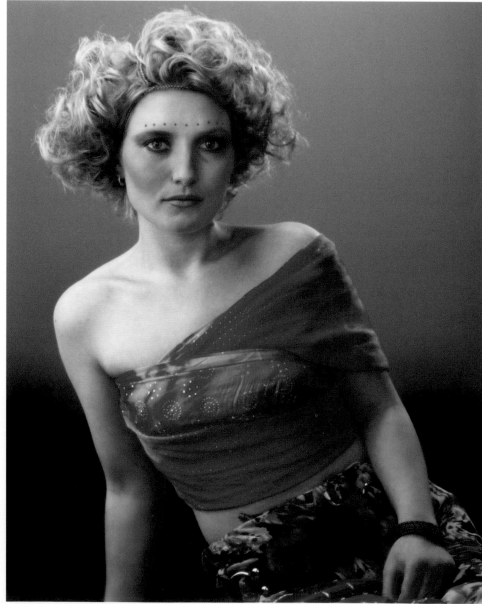

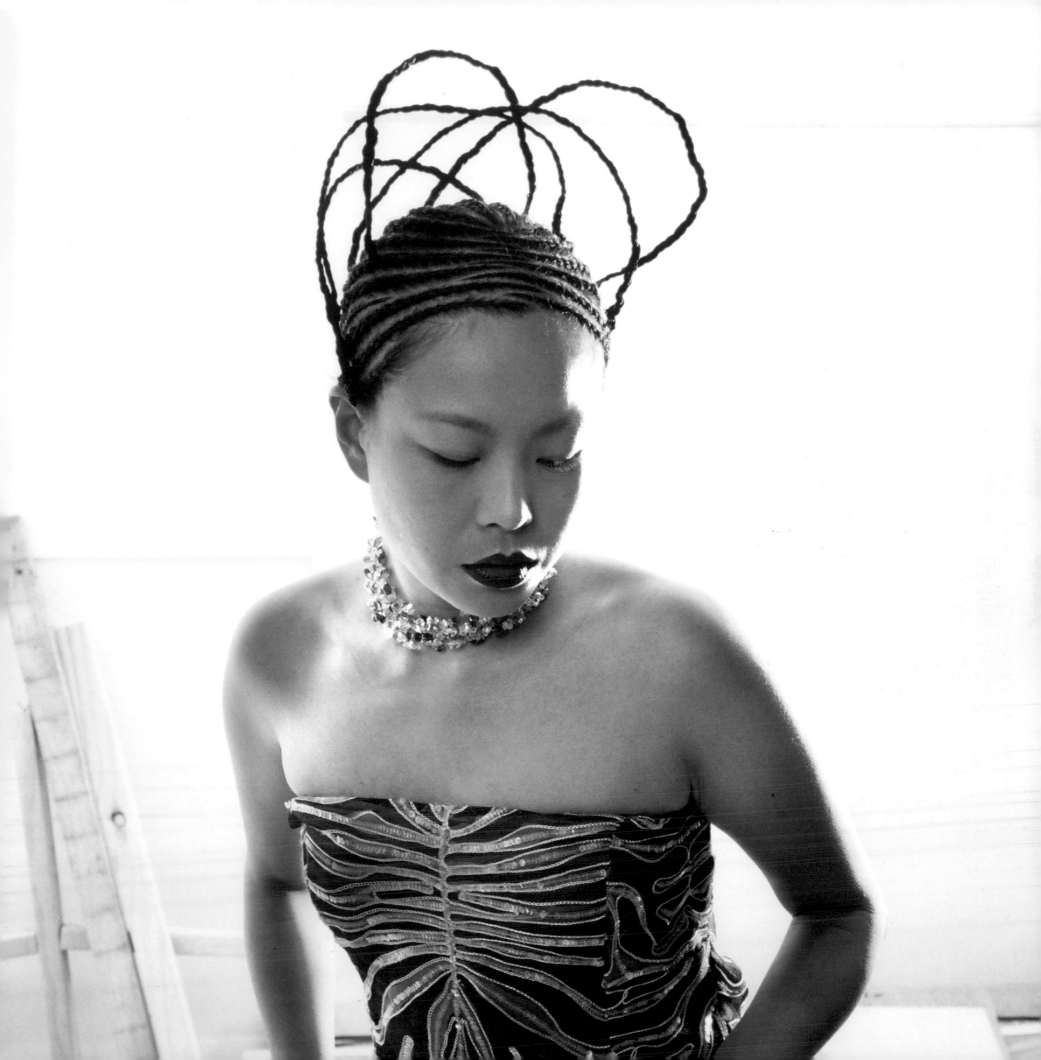

DESMOND MURRAY pages 74–81

Hair & Beauty Partnership, 60 Baker Street, London, United Kingdom

Hair: Desmond Murray for Black Like me (p. 74 - 77) and for Renbow International (p. 78 - 81)
Salon: Hair & Beauty Partnership
Make-up: Denise Rabor (p. 74 - 77) Siobhon Luckie (p. 78 - 81)
Styling: Caroline Summers
Photography: Kevin Mackintosh (p. 78 - 81)

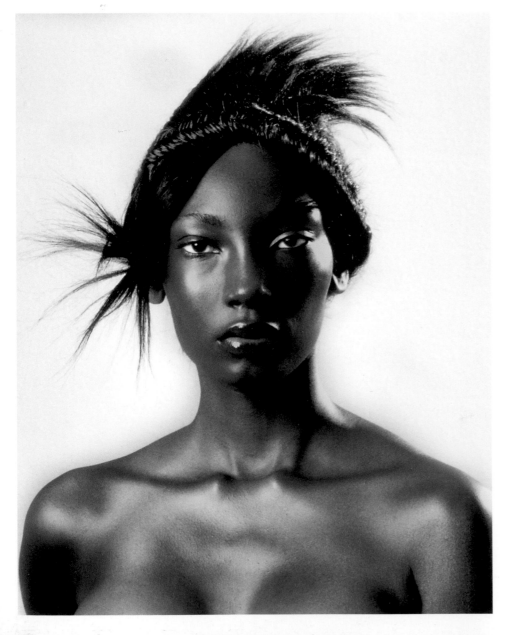

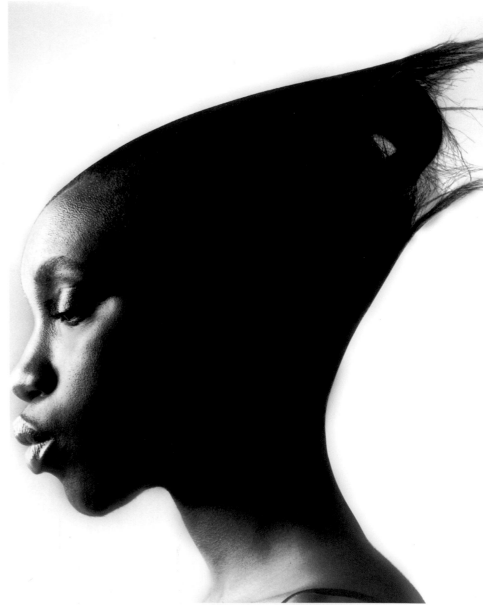

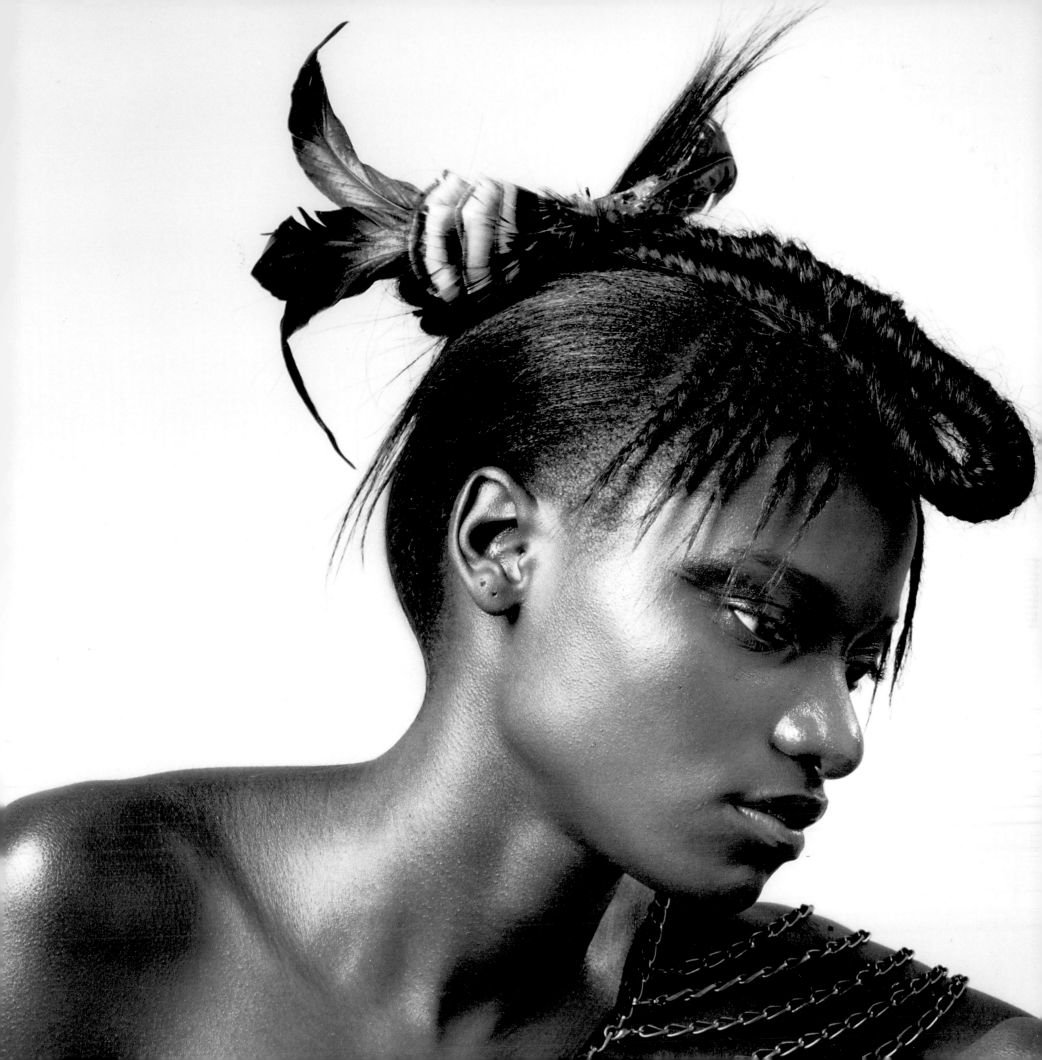

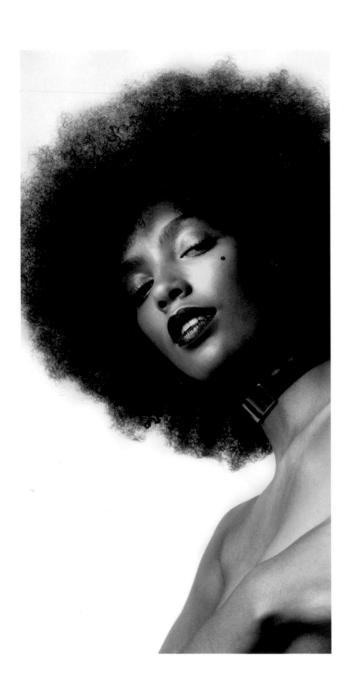

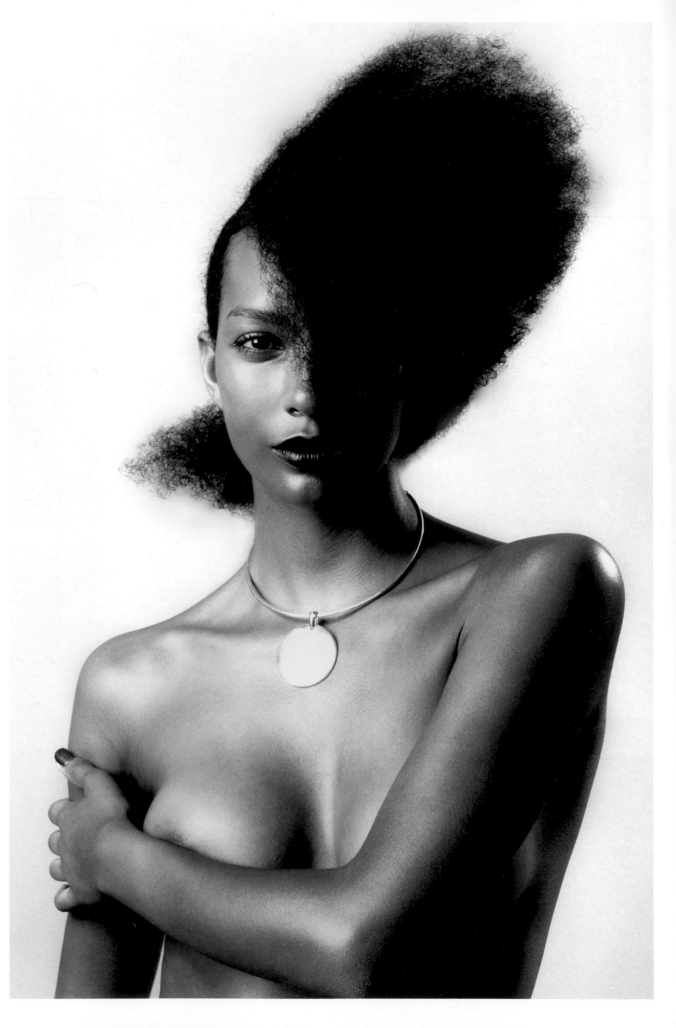

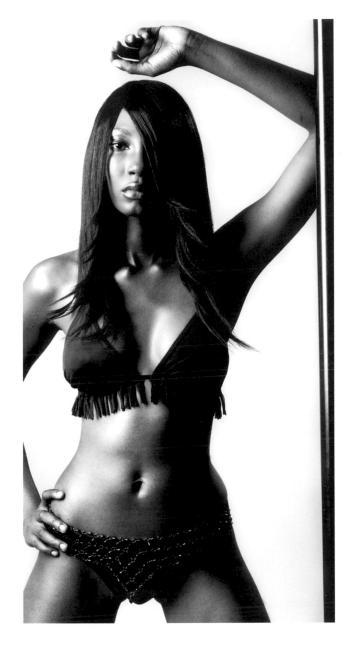
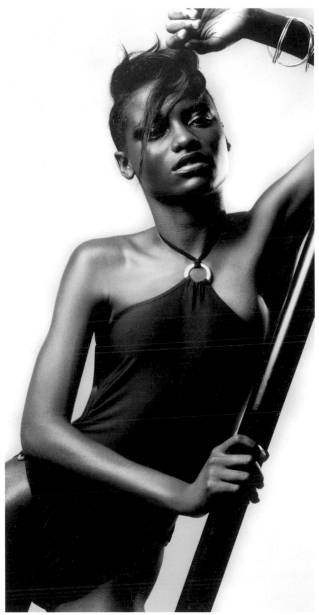
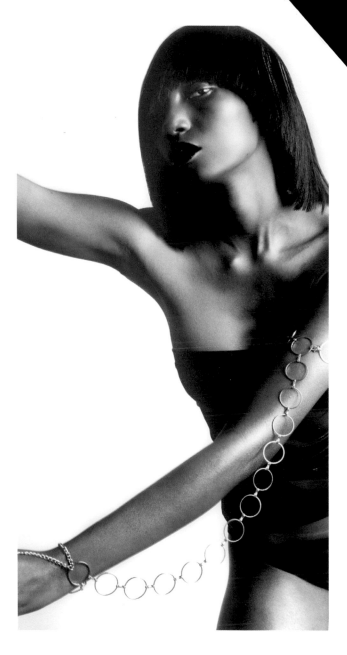

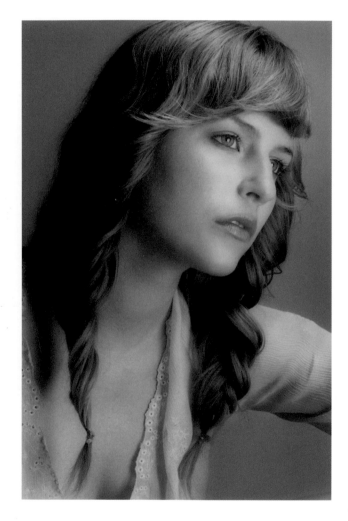
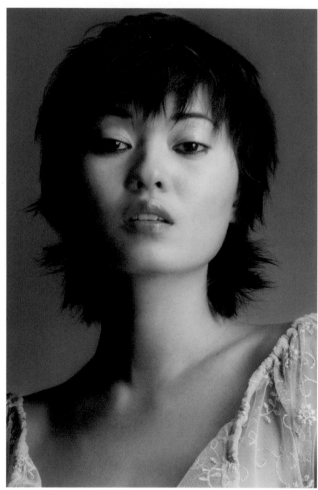
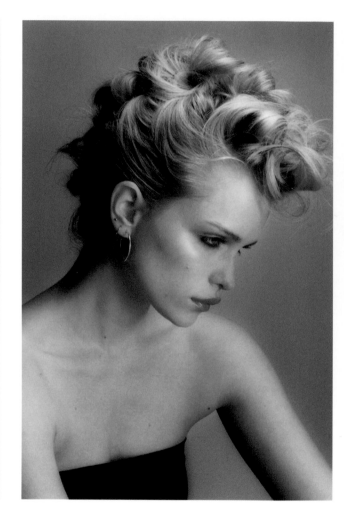

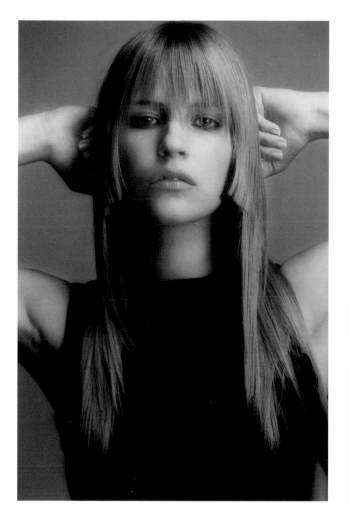
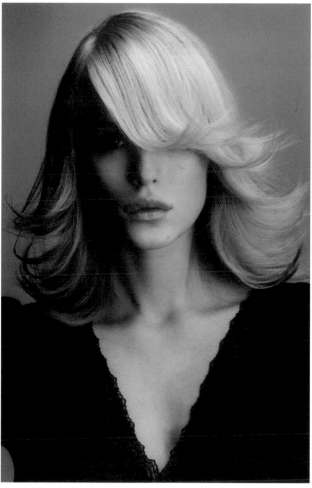
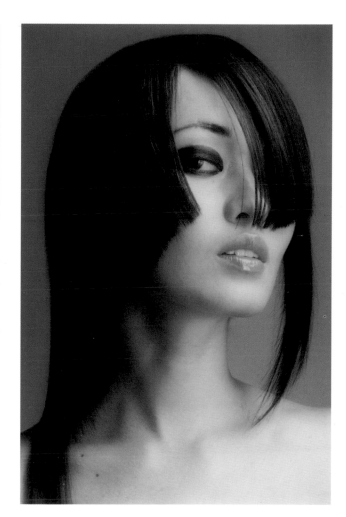

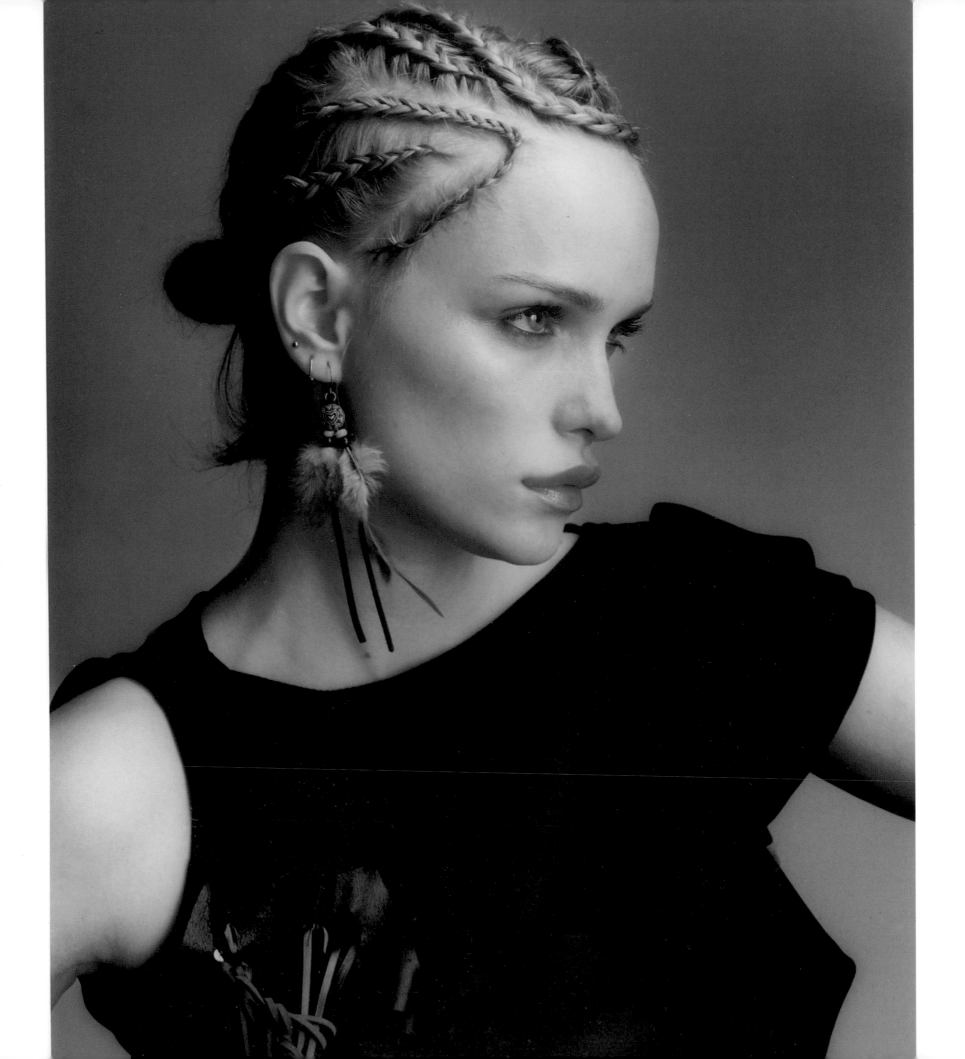

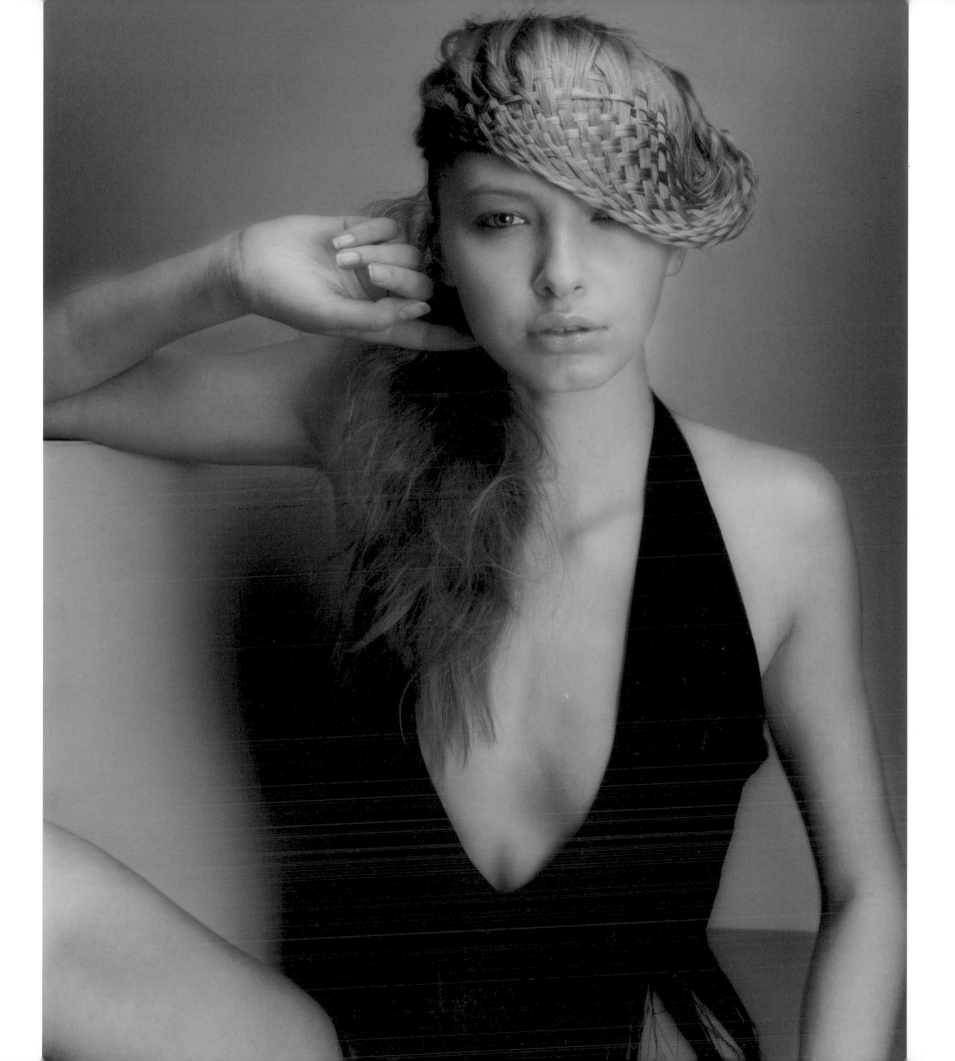

Ad Peters The Haircompany, P.O. Box 603, 7400 AP Deventer, The Netherlands, www.adpeters.nl

Hair: Ad and Jane Peters for L'Oréal Professional
Salon: Ad Peters The Haircompany
Make-up: Lindsey Hop for Lancôme
Styling: Sherida Augustin
Photography: Govert de Roos
Products: L'Oréal

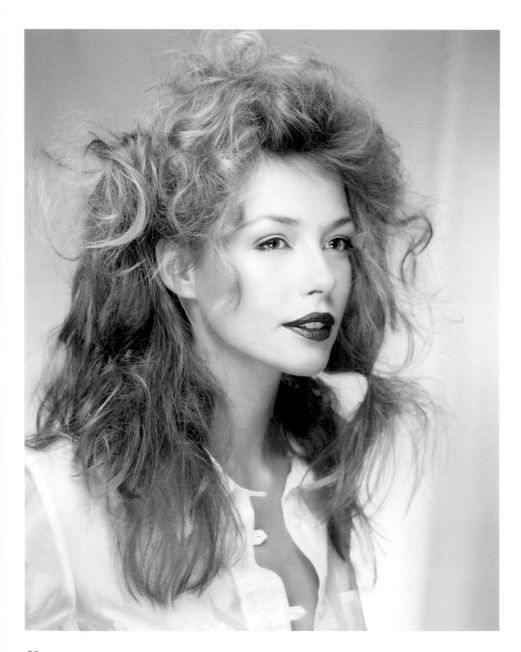

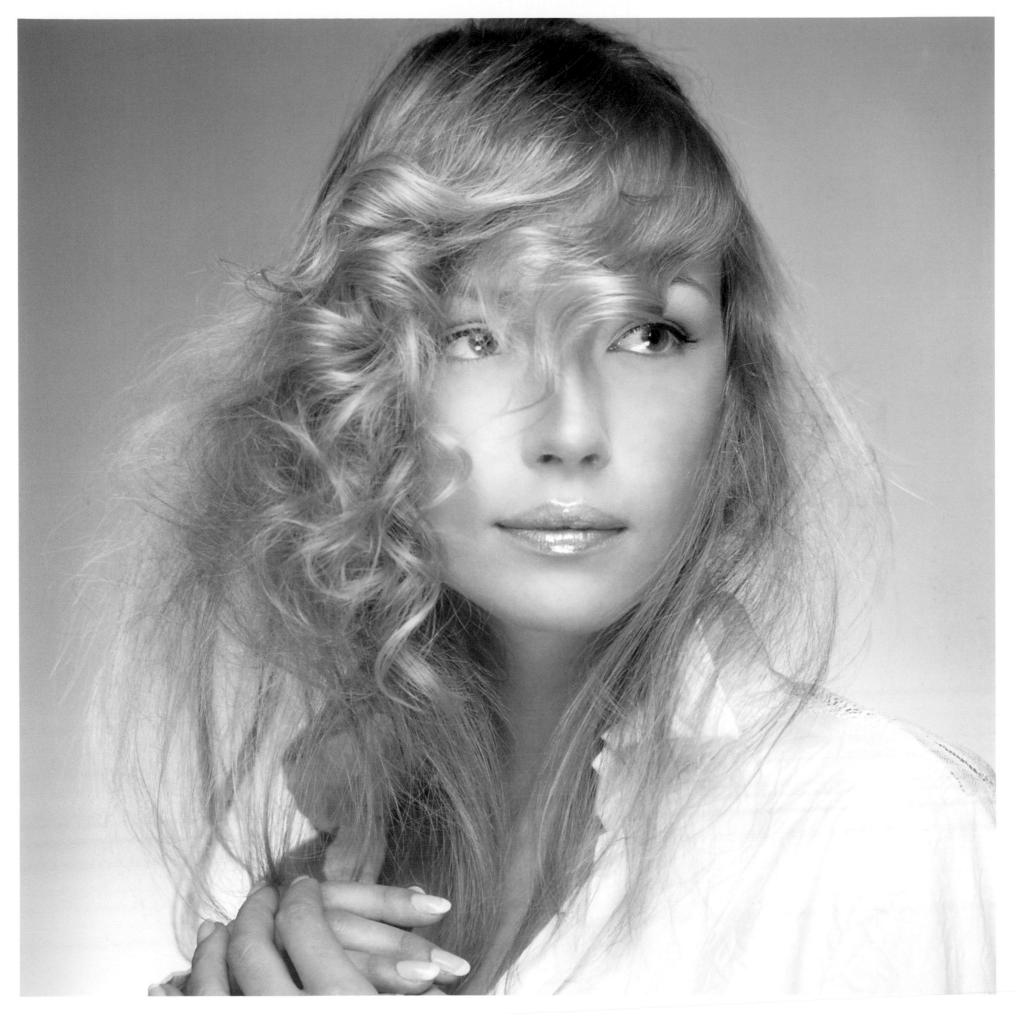

PATRICK CAMERON pages 84–87

Patrick Cameron Ltd, The Paddocks, Woodbank Lane, Chester Ch1 6JD, United Kingdom, www.patrick-cameron.com

Hair: Patrick Cameron
Make-up: Daniel K.
Styling: Marco Erbi
Photography: Alistair Huges
Products: Wella

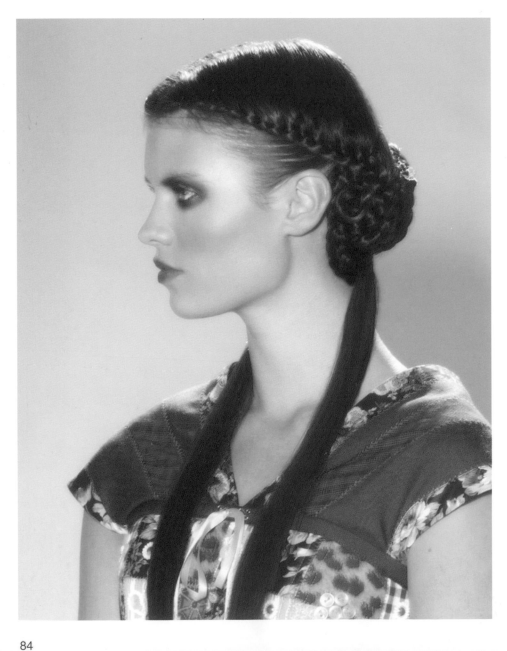

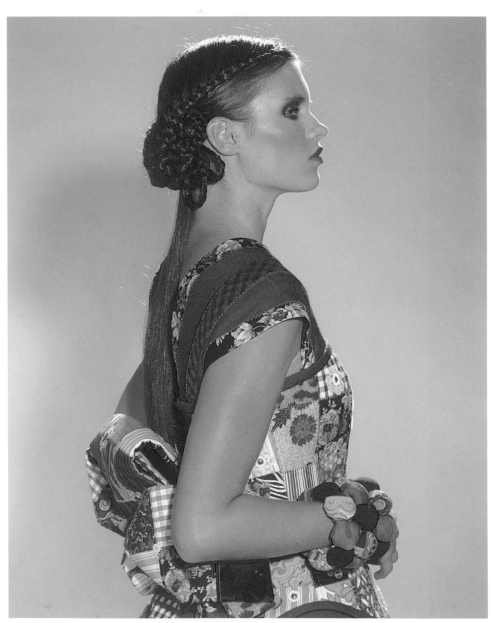

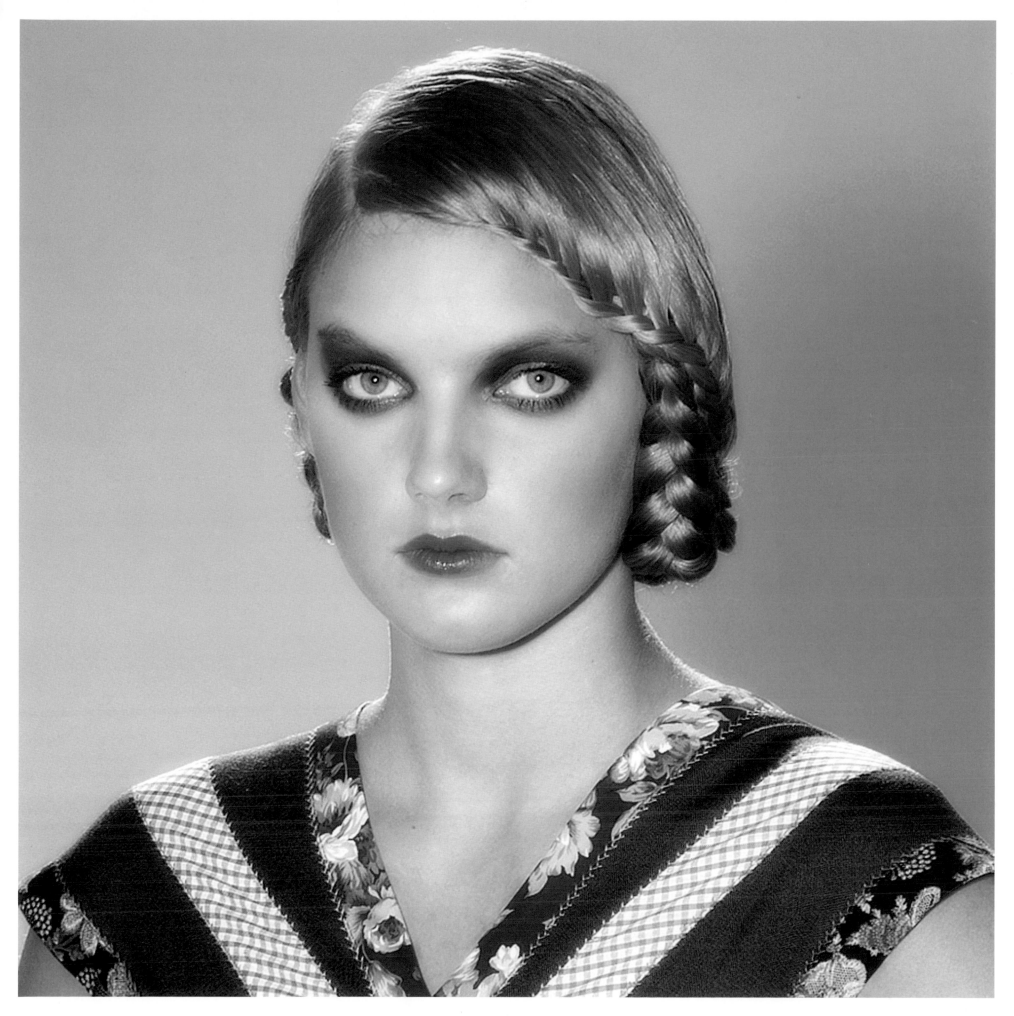

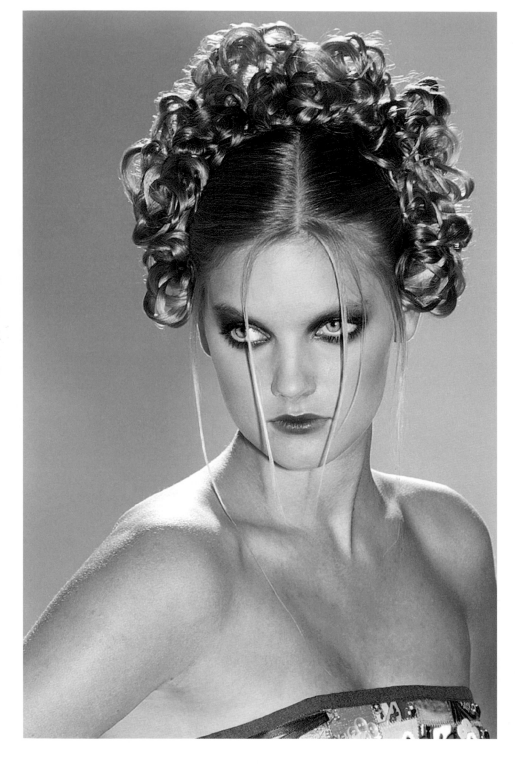
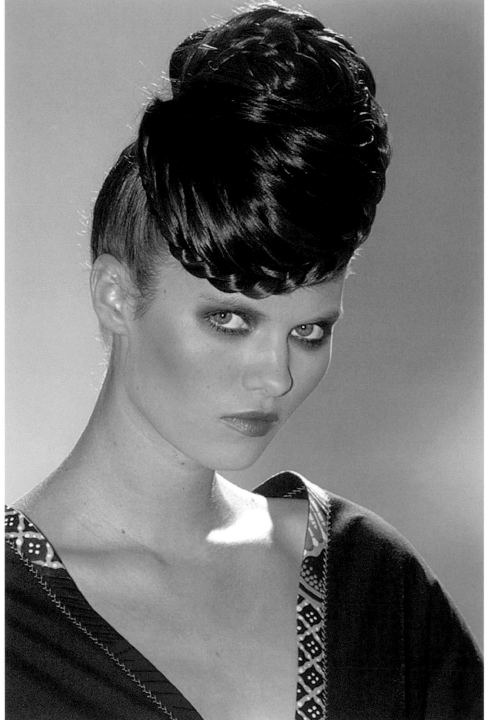

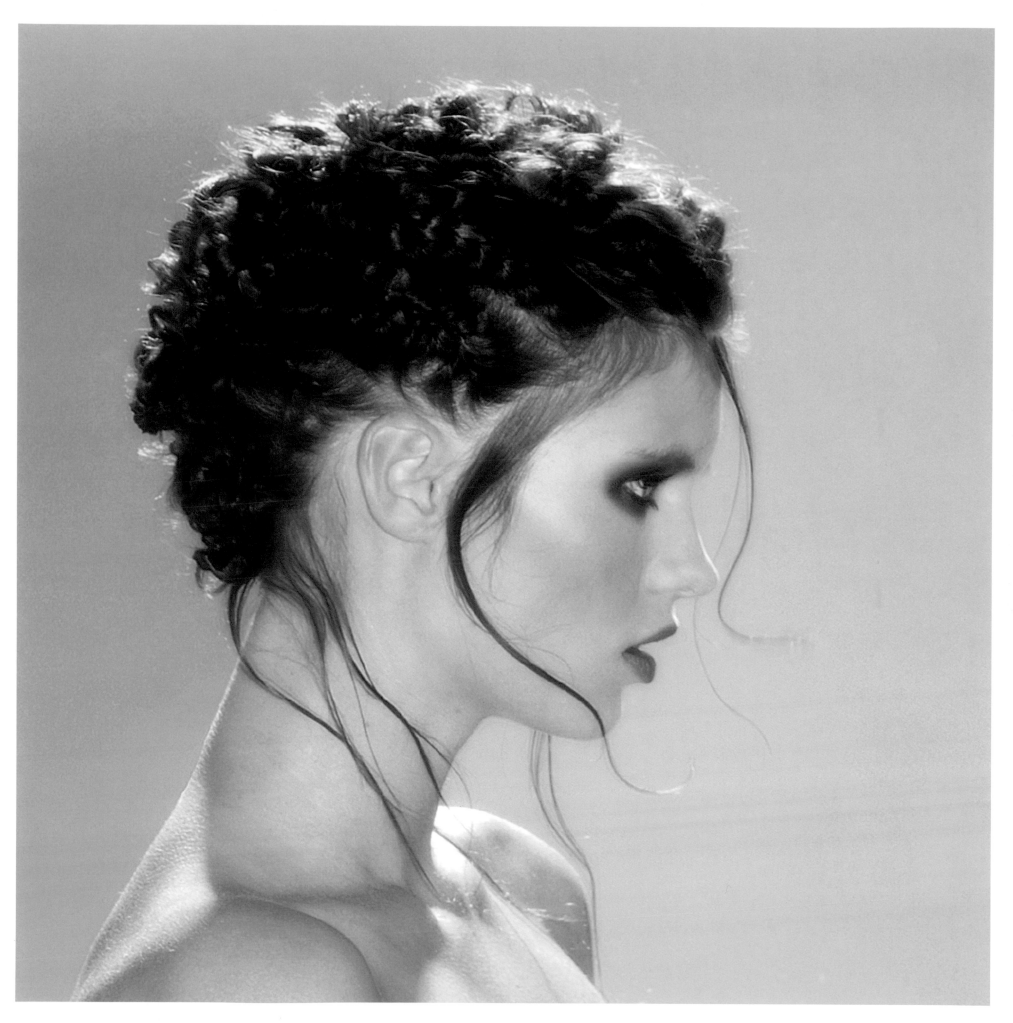

Gandini Club, Località Foroni 12, 37067 Valeggio S/M (VR) Italy, www.gandiniteam.com

Hair: Stefano
Salon: Gandini Club
Photography: Marco Masotti

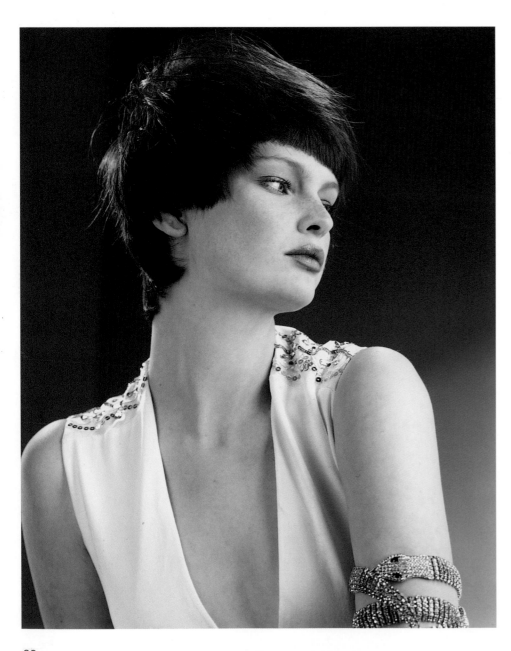

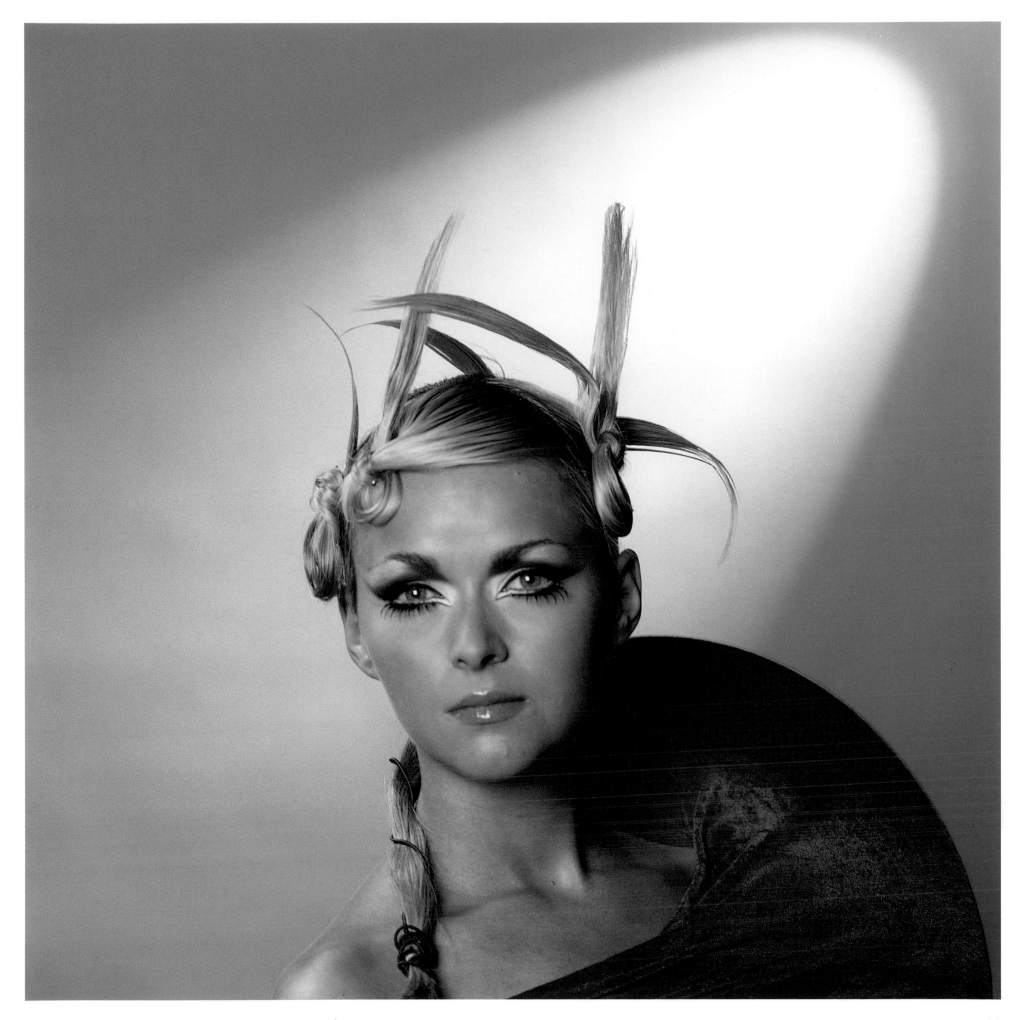

HAIR LOUNGE pages 90–91

437 Portobello Road, Nottinghill Gate, London W10 5SA, United Kingdom

Hair: Charlotte Mensah
Salon: Hair Lounge
Make-up: Maria Sanchez
Photography: Michele Jorsling
Models: Mayen and Lorna
Products: Goldwell Trendline

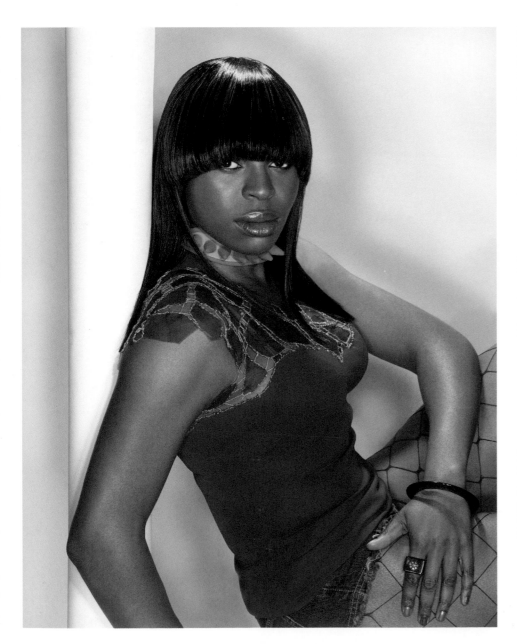
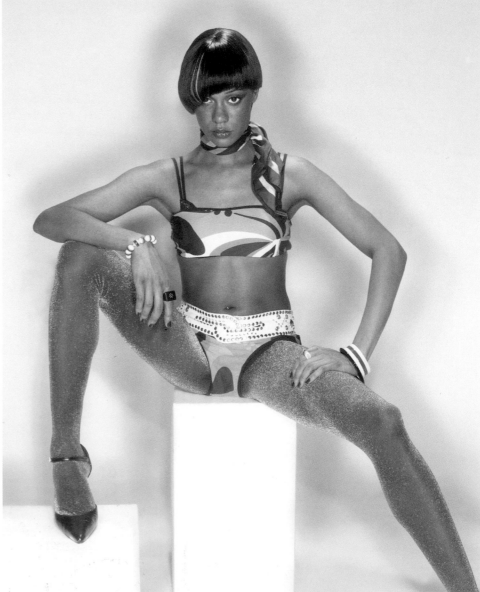

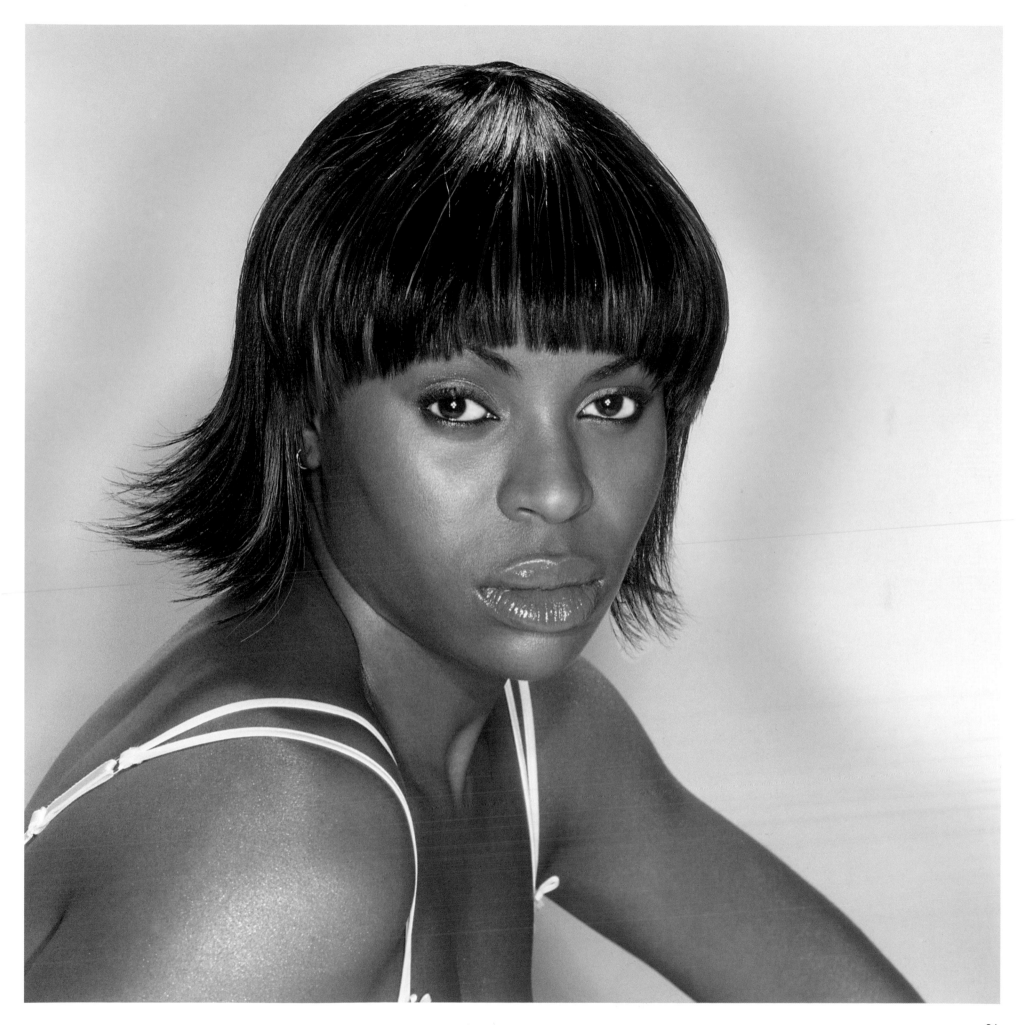

HYPE COIFFURE

17 Tulse Hill, London SW2 2TH, United Kingdom

Hair: Hype Coiffure
Salon: Hype Coiffure

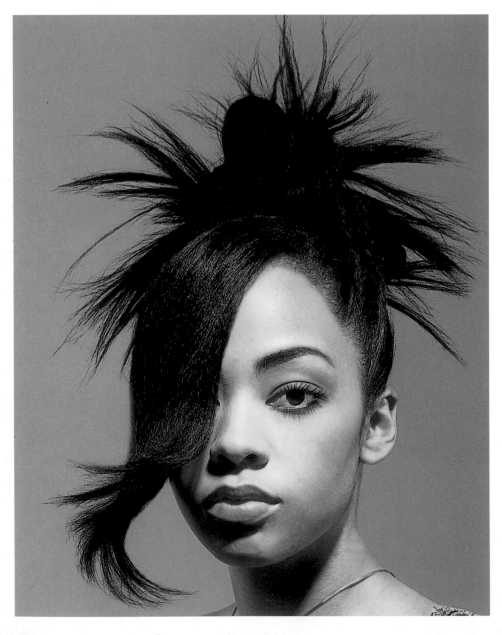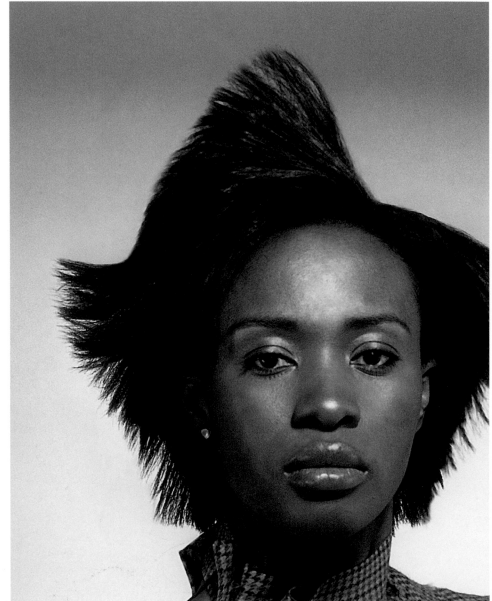

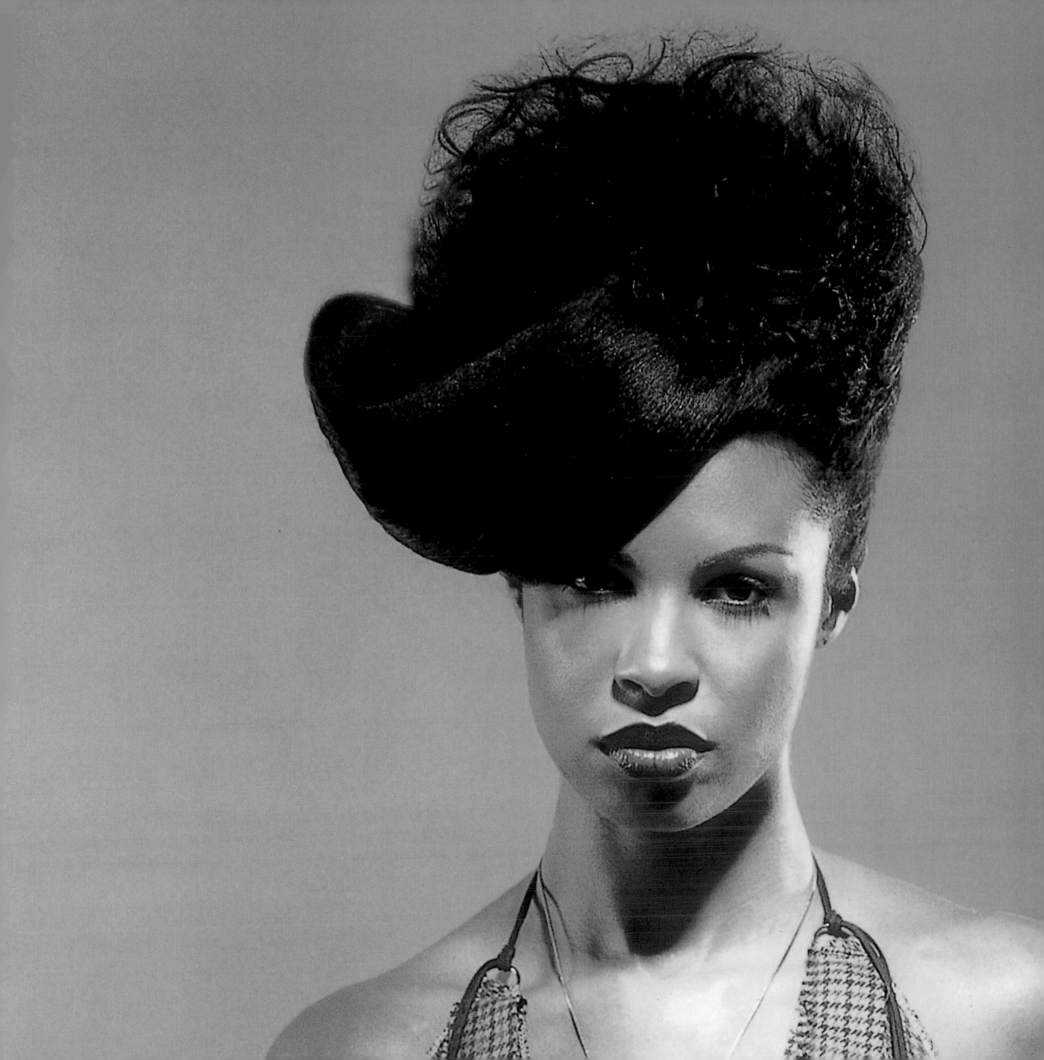

NODDY'S ON KING pages 94–97

88 King Street, Newton NWS, 2042 Sydney, Australia

Hair: David McCulloch (p. 94, 95) Shane Henning (p. 96, 97)
Color: Jodi Fisher (p. 94, 95)
Salon: Noddy's on King
Make-up: Caroline Travaglia (p. 94, 95) Laura Nolan (p. 96, 97)
Photography: Michelle Holden (p. 94, 95) David Gubert (p. 96, 97)

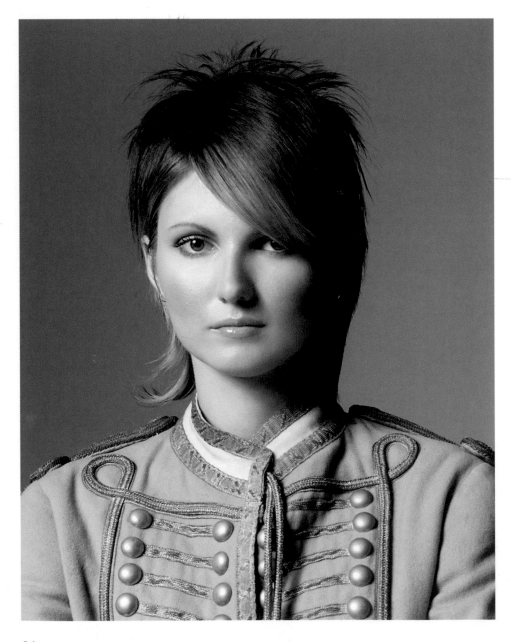

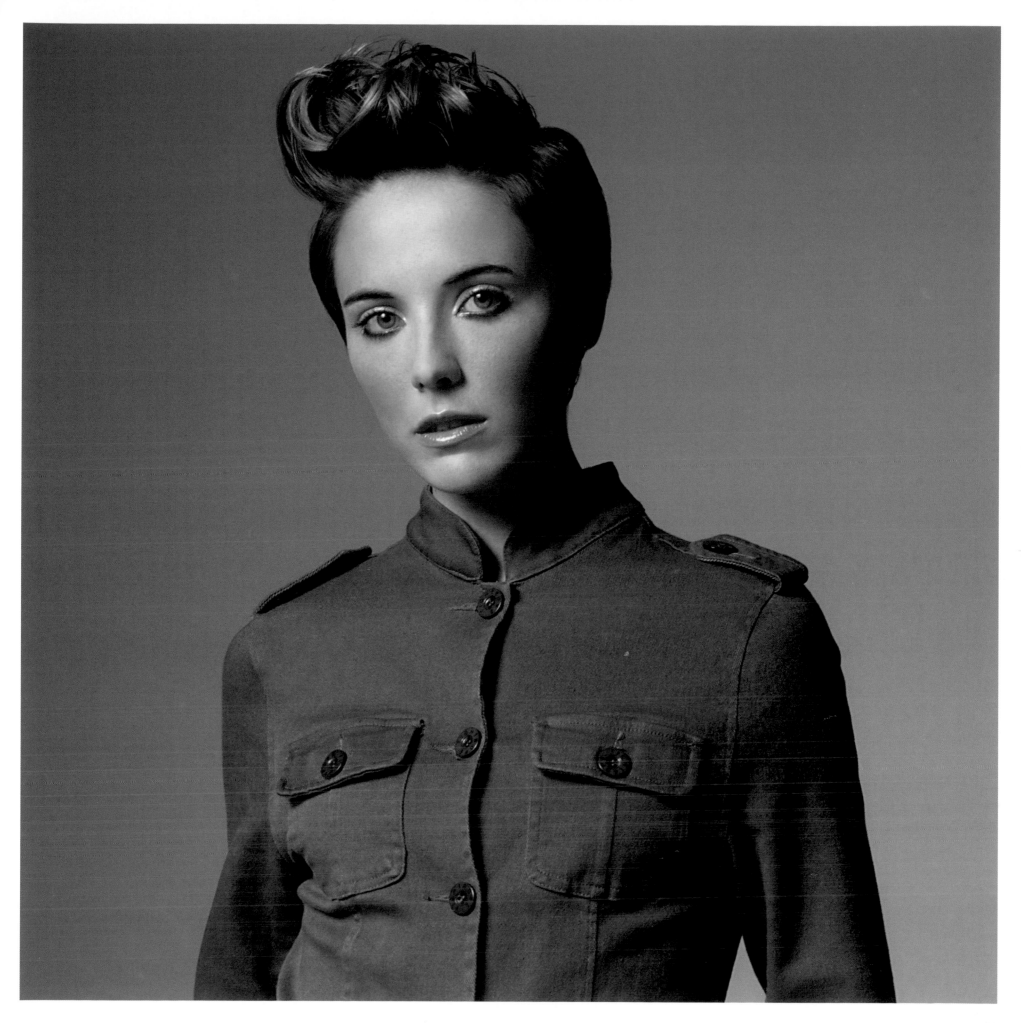

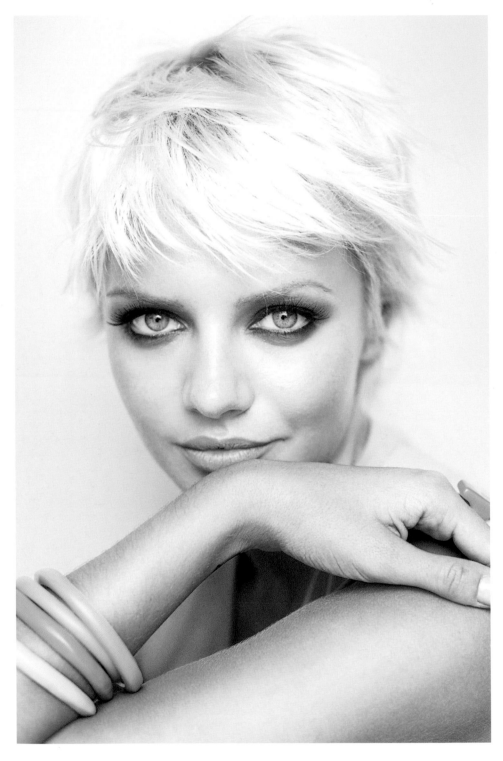
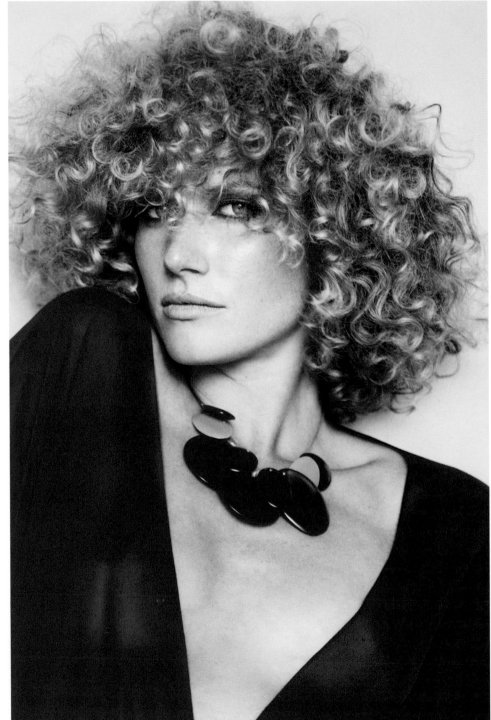

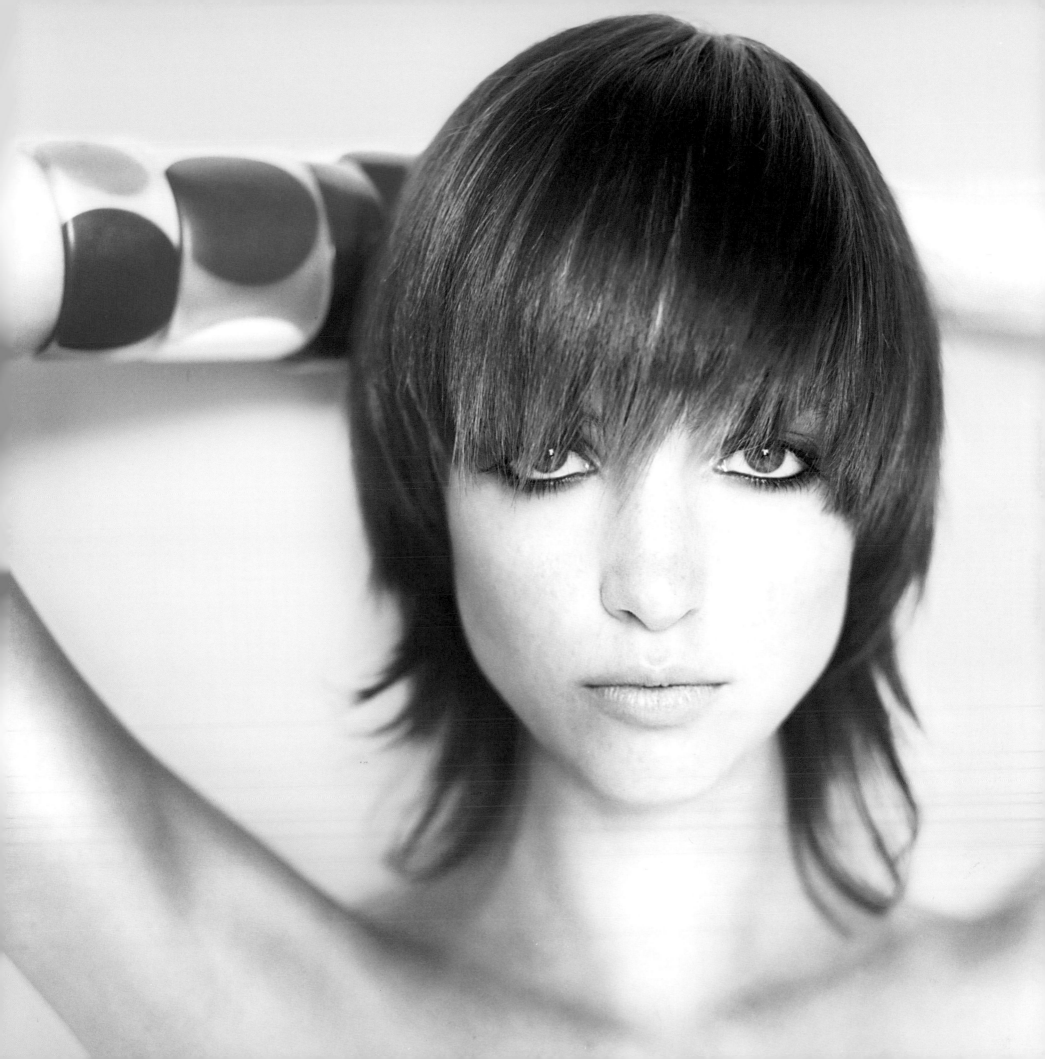

MAY LTD.

Zanevskiy pr. 37, 195112 St. Petersburg, Russia, www.may.spb.ru

Hair: Olga Piljushenko (p. 99) Anton Harebov and Denis Kartashov (p. 100, 101)
Colour: Elena Sukhopara and Zoya Ljubtseva (p. 100, 101)
Academy: May International Hair Stylist Training Centre
Photography: Sergey Narchuck (p. 99) Sergey Narchuck and Konstantin Sterkhov (p. 100, 101)

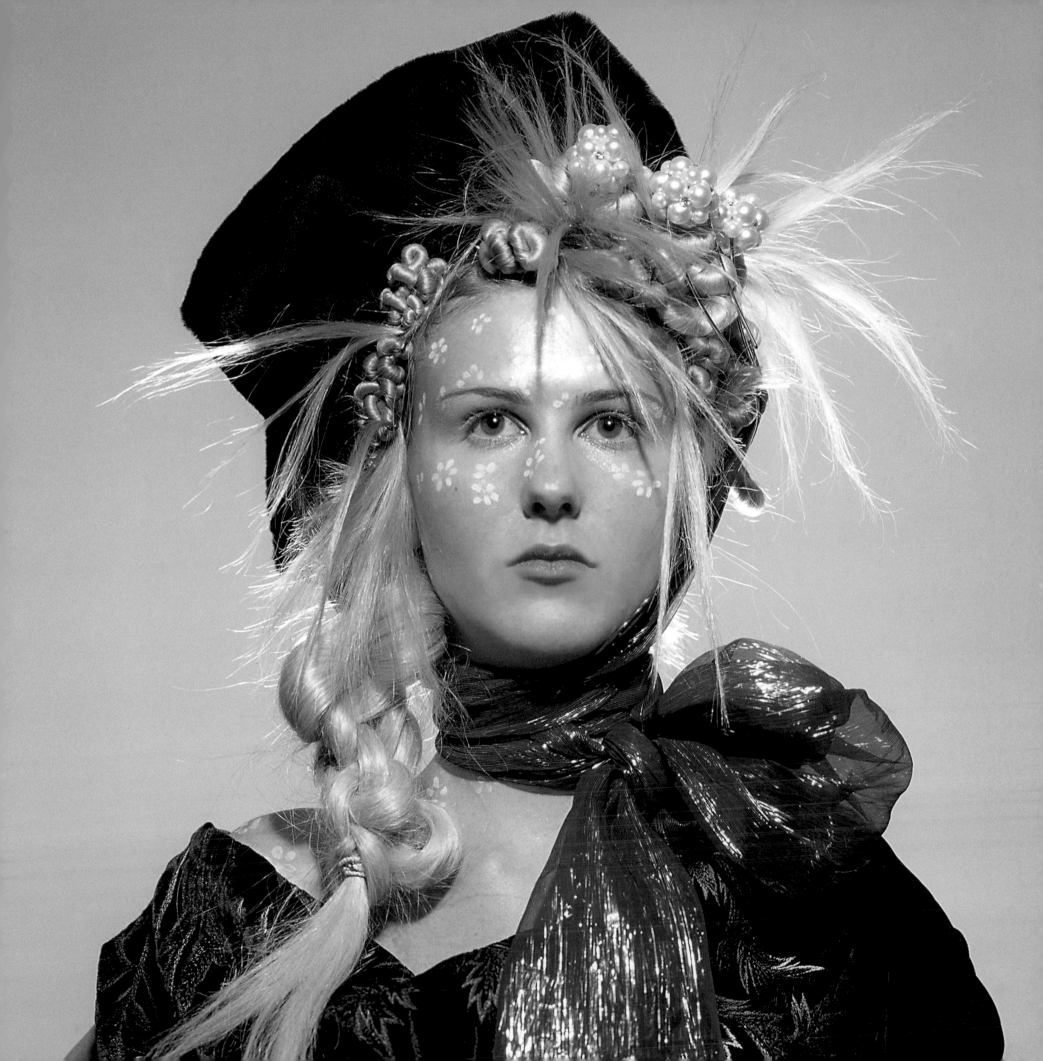

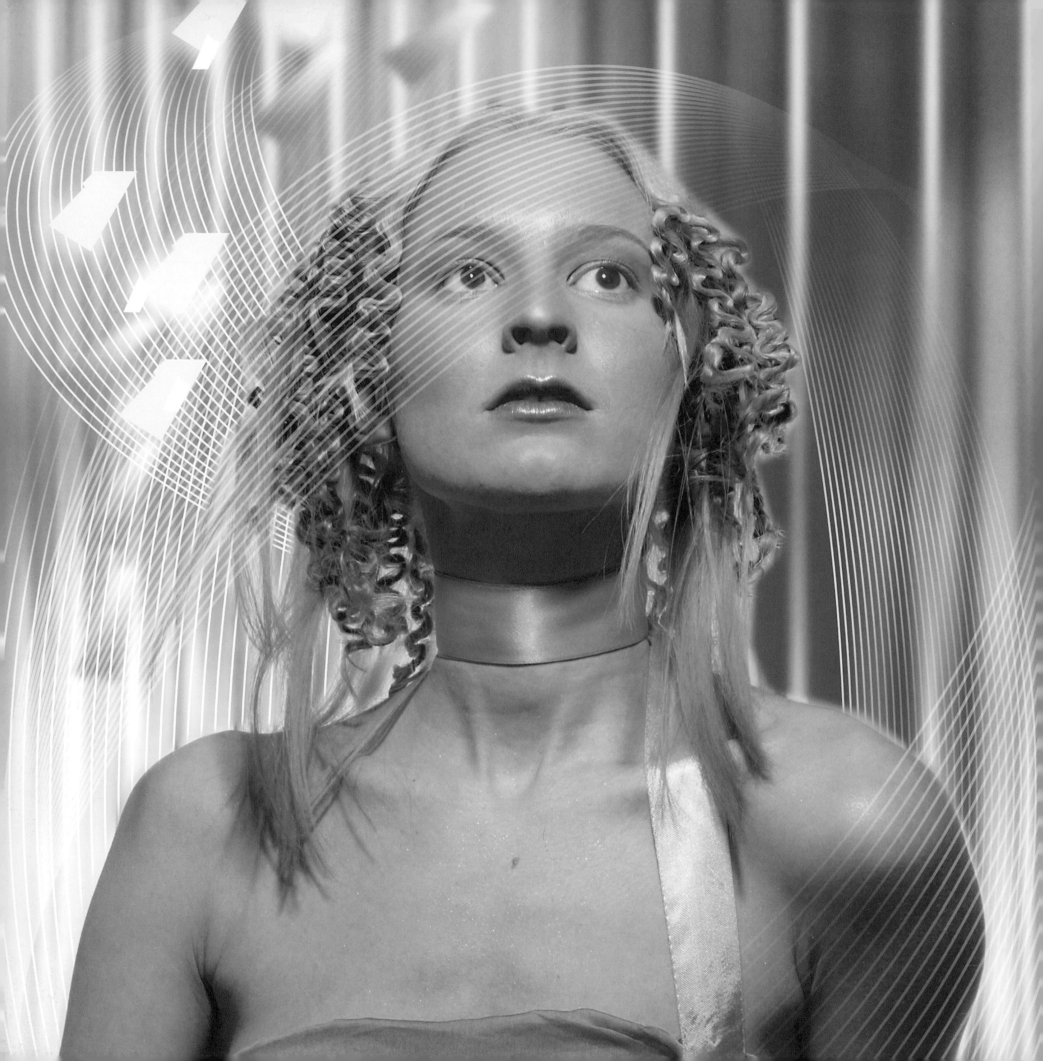

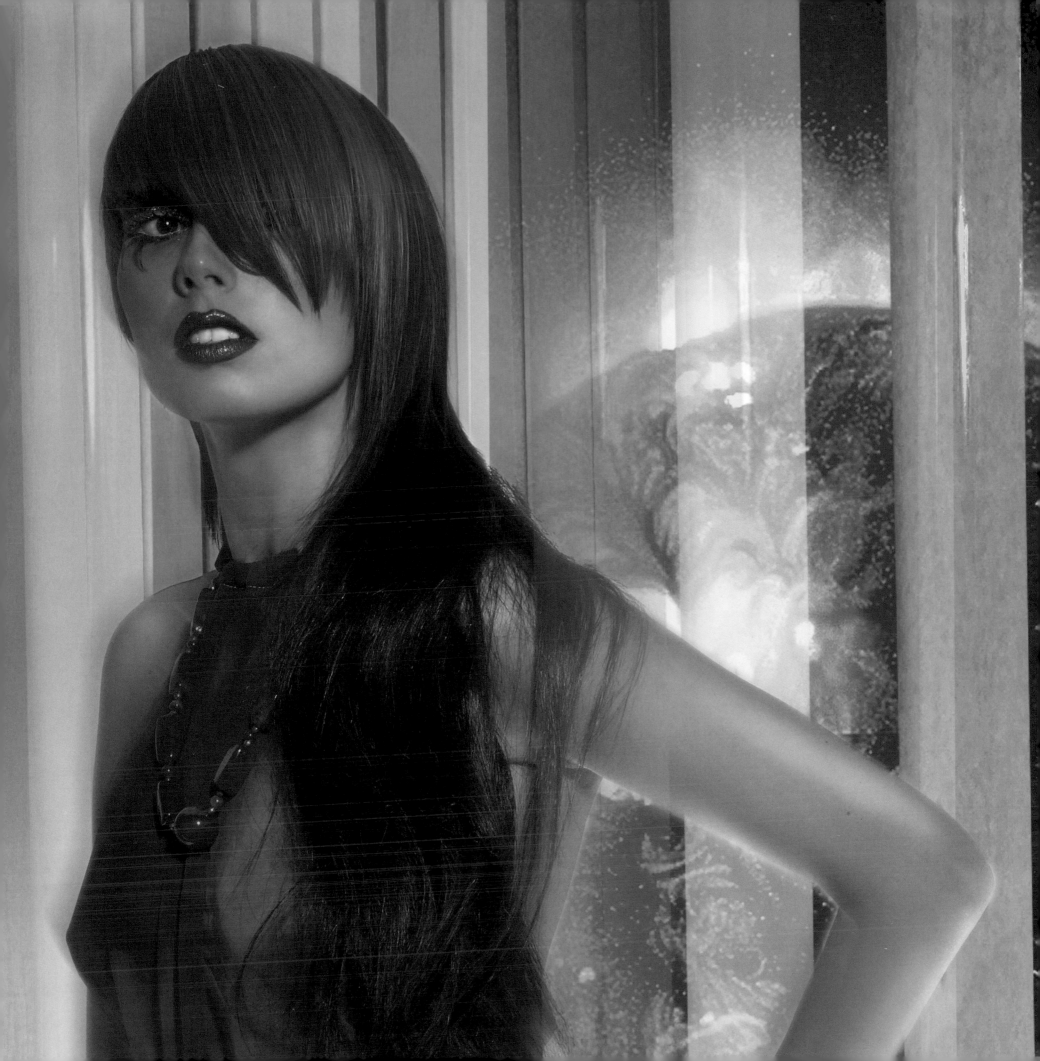

ANTONIO BELLVER pages 102–111

Av. Coyoacán No. 425, Col del valle, Entre Division del Norte y Torres Adalid, C.P. 03100, Mexico D.F, Benito Juárez, Mexico, www.antoniobellver.com

Hair: Antonio Bellver
Salon: Jossclaude & Bellver, Barcelona, Mexico
Make-up: Marian Vera
Styling: Ester Fernandez
Photography: Luis Vidal byglobal

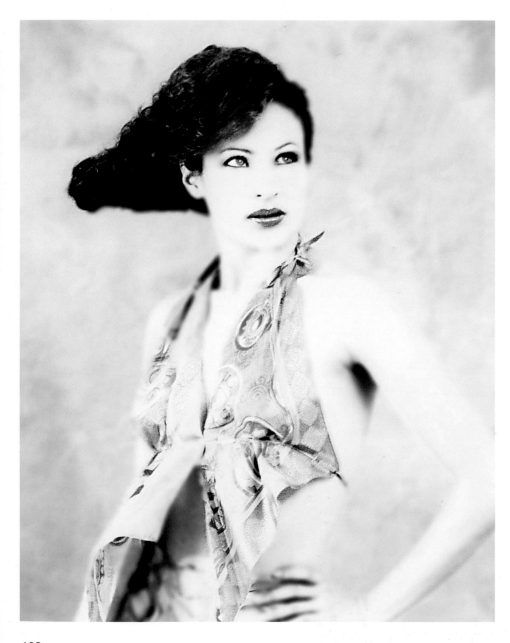

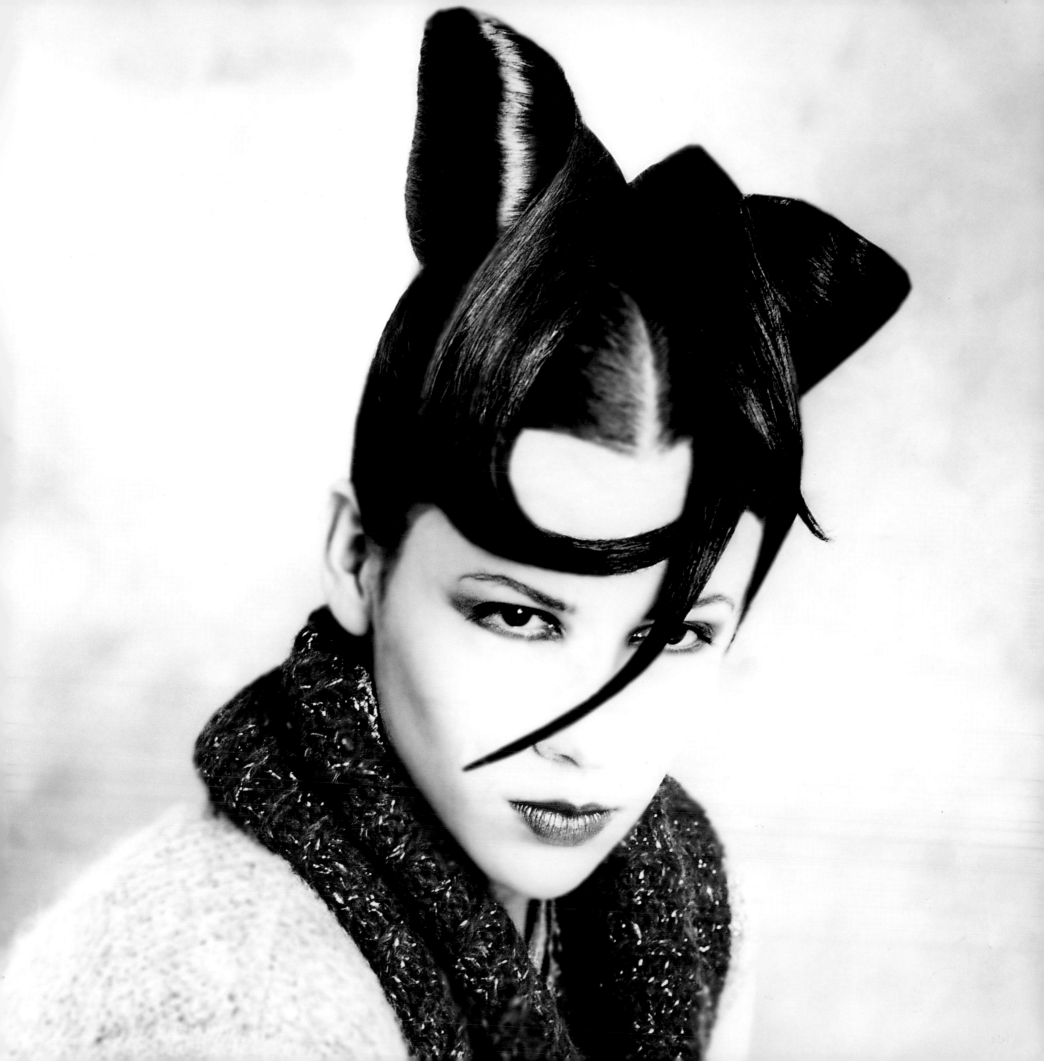

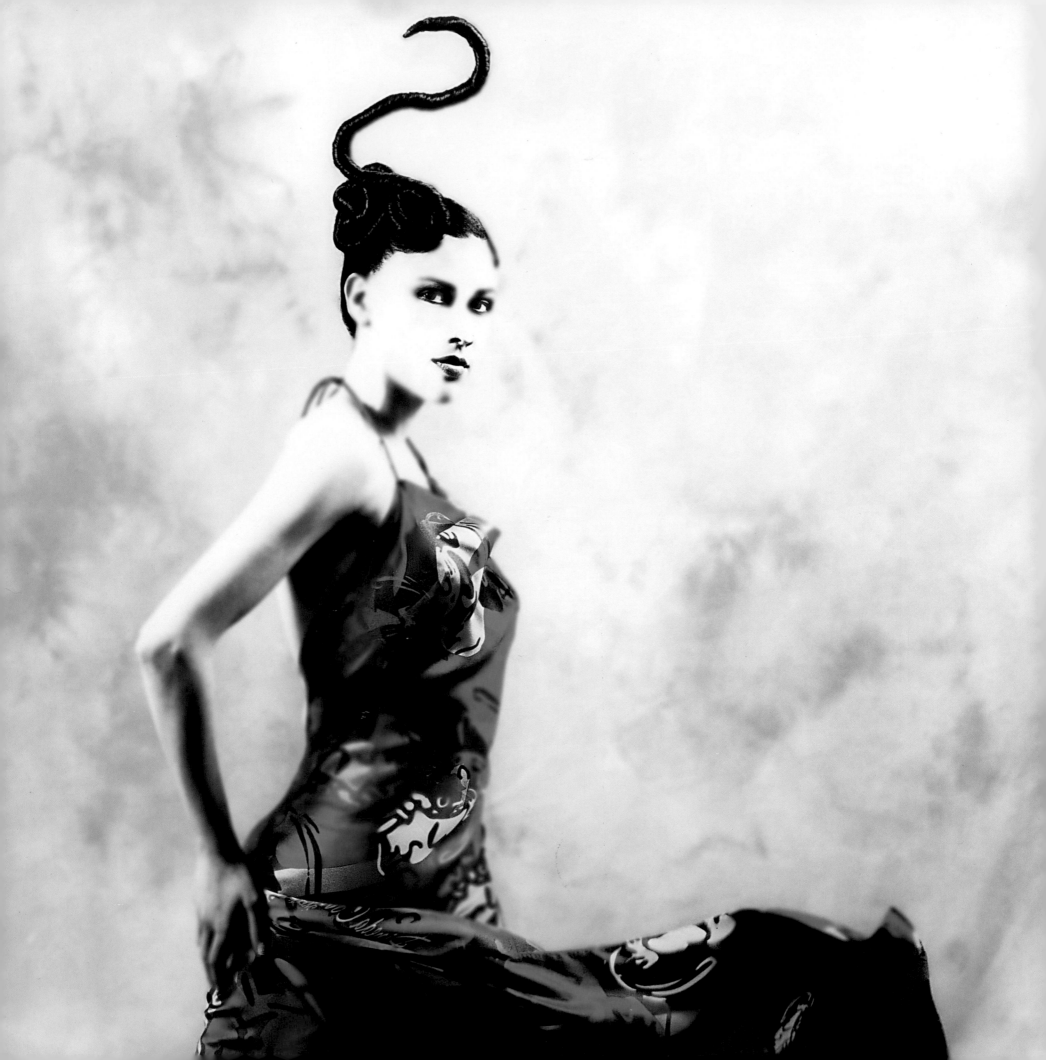

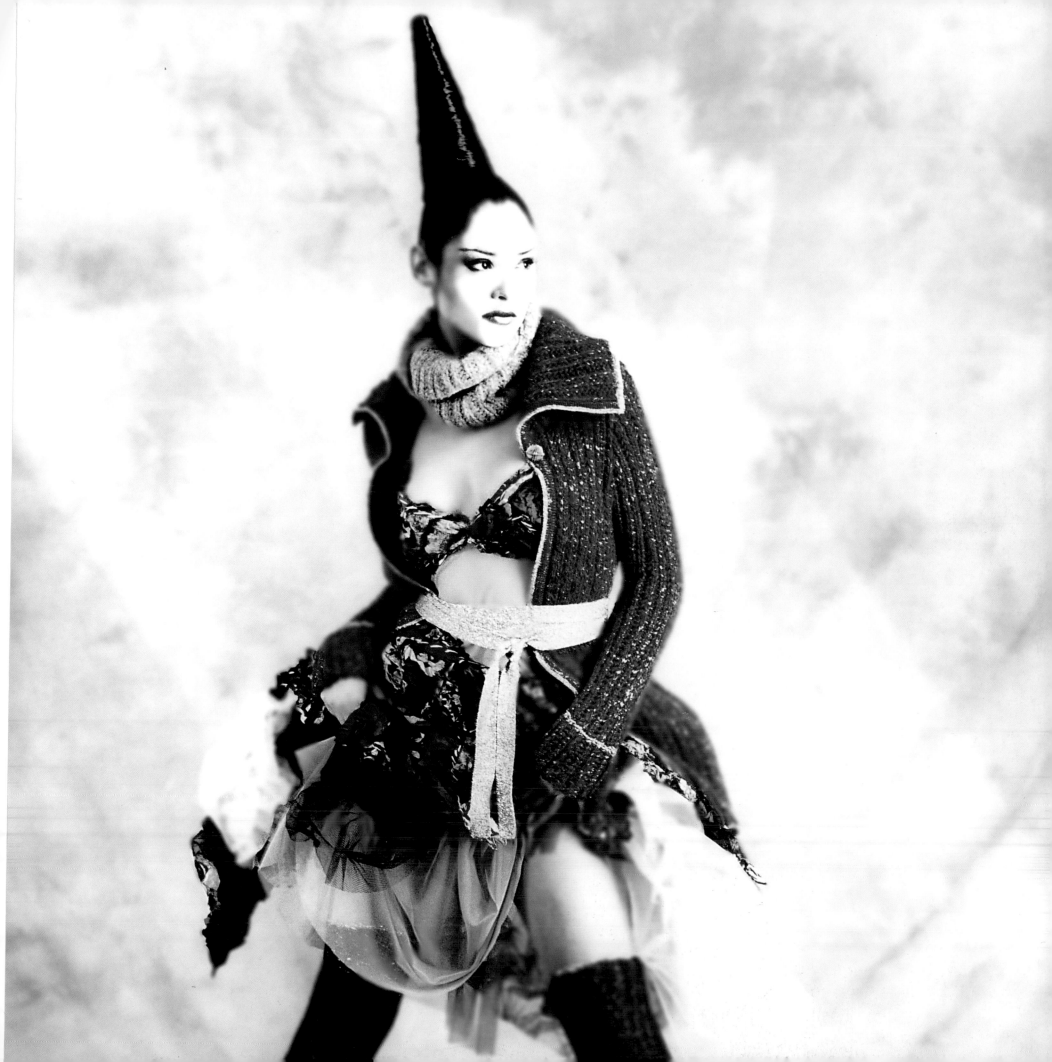

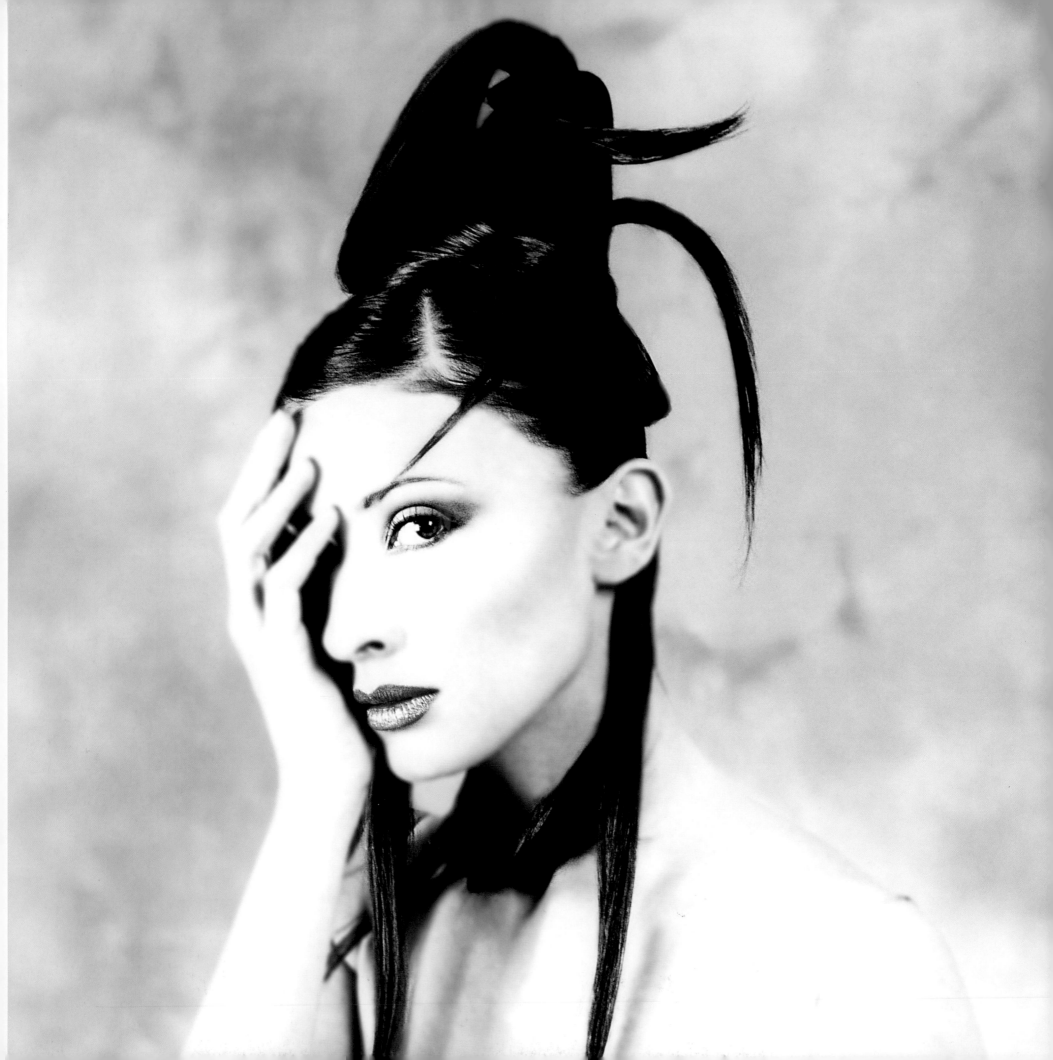

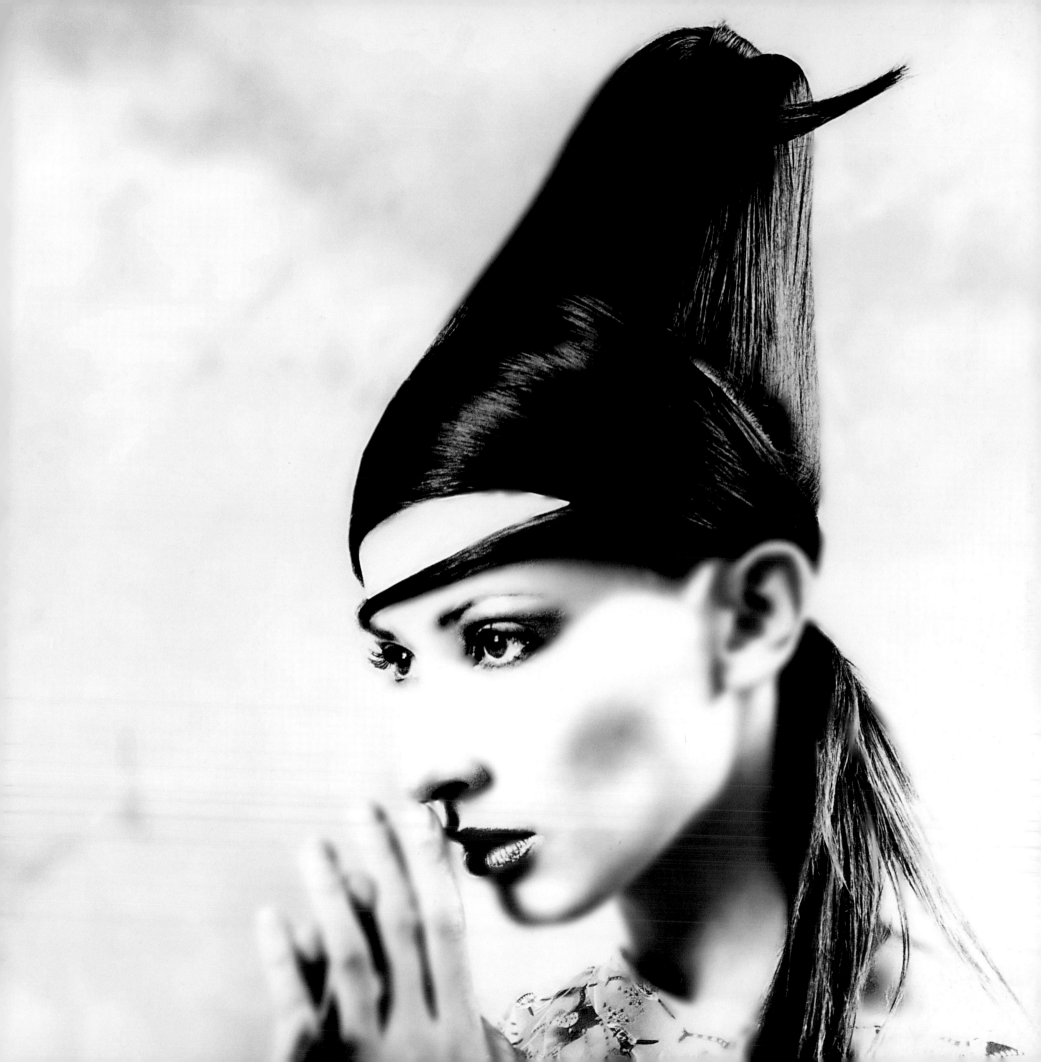

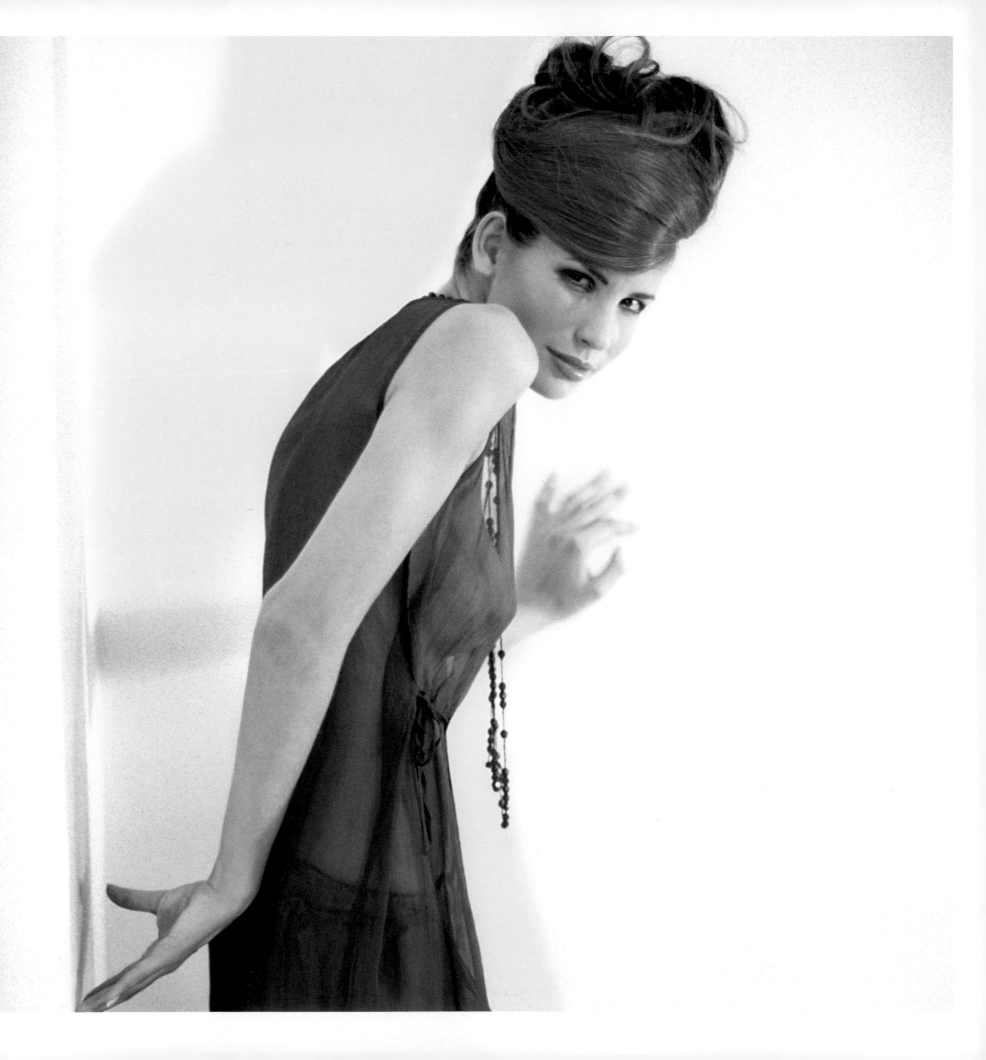

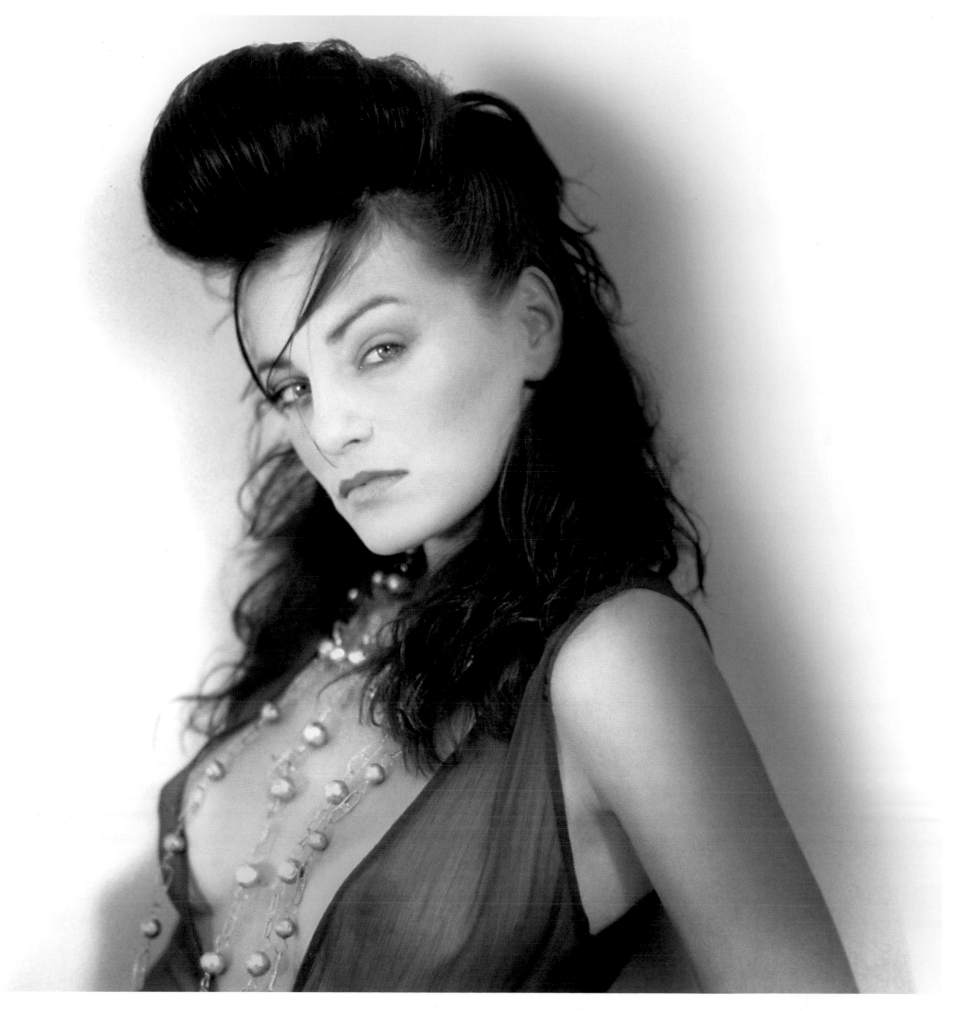

CARL WATKINS pages 112–113

Carl Watkins and Associates, 74 Victoria Street, Christchurch, New Zealand, www.carlwatkins.co.nz

Hair: Carl Watkins
Salon: Carl Watkins and Associates

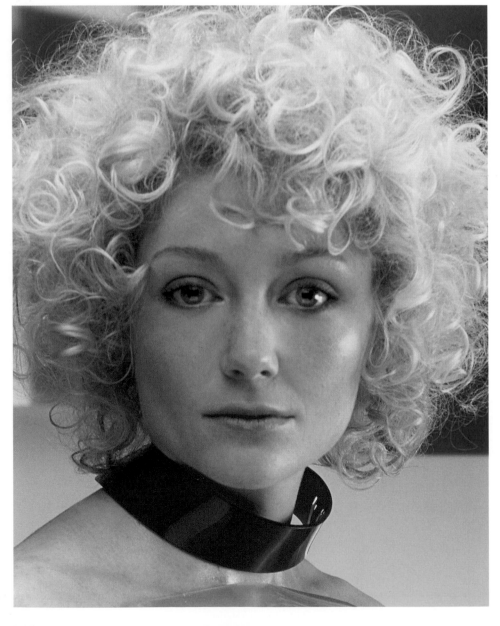

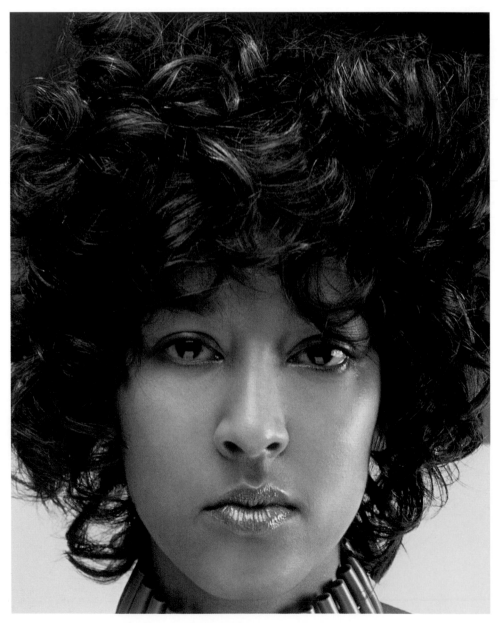

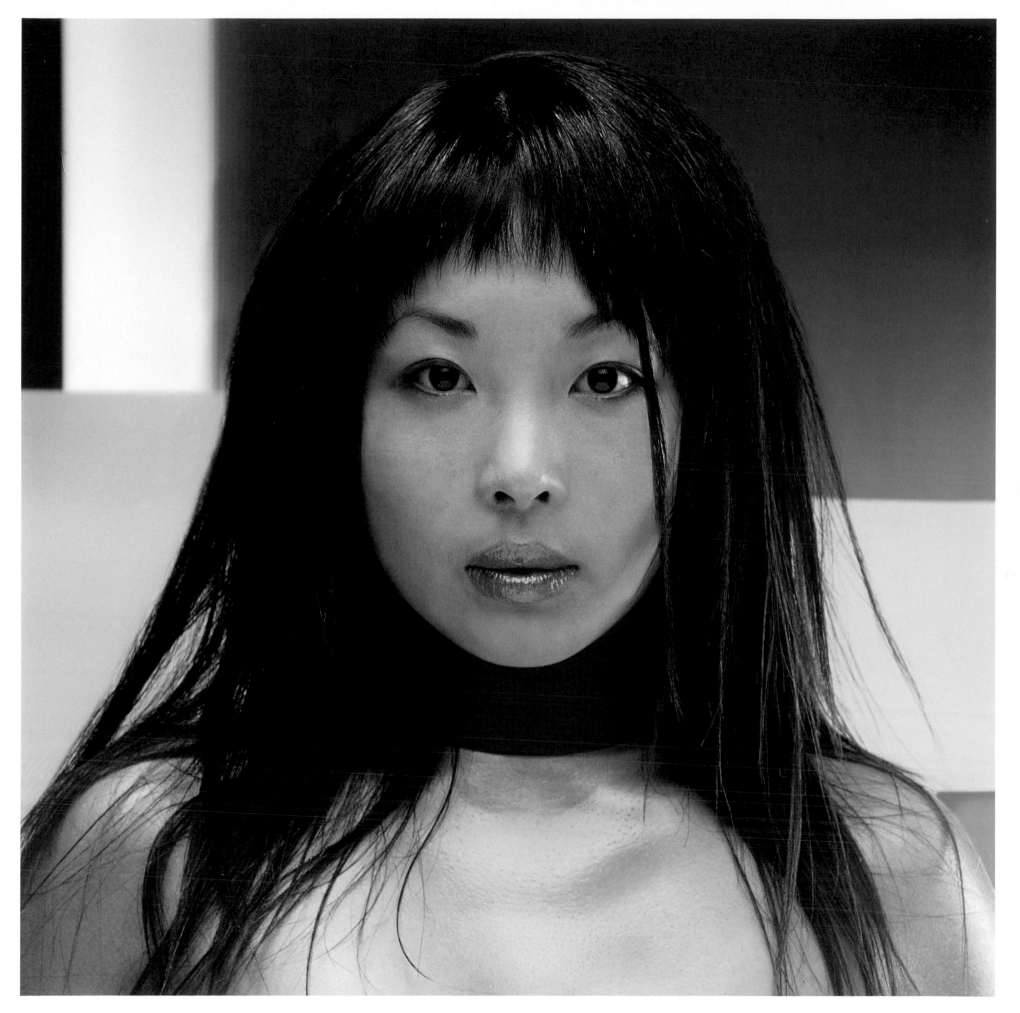

GRITTI PALACE pages 114–115

66 Gawler Place, Adelaide SA 5000, Australia, www.grittypalace.com.au

Hair: Grant Nelson (p. 114) Tania Scar Sella (p. 114) Ross Leondiou (p. 115)
Salon: Gritty Palace
Make-up: Liz McFarland (p. 114, 115) Jason (p. 114)
Photography: Grant Nelson
Model: Joanne O'Connor (p. 115)

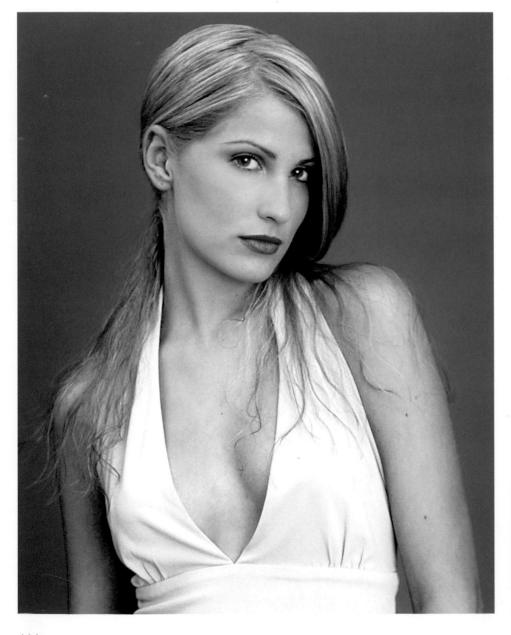

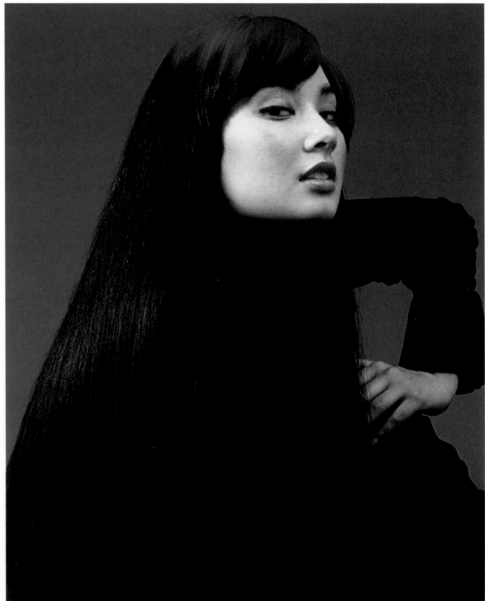

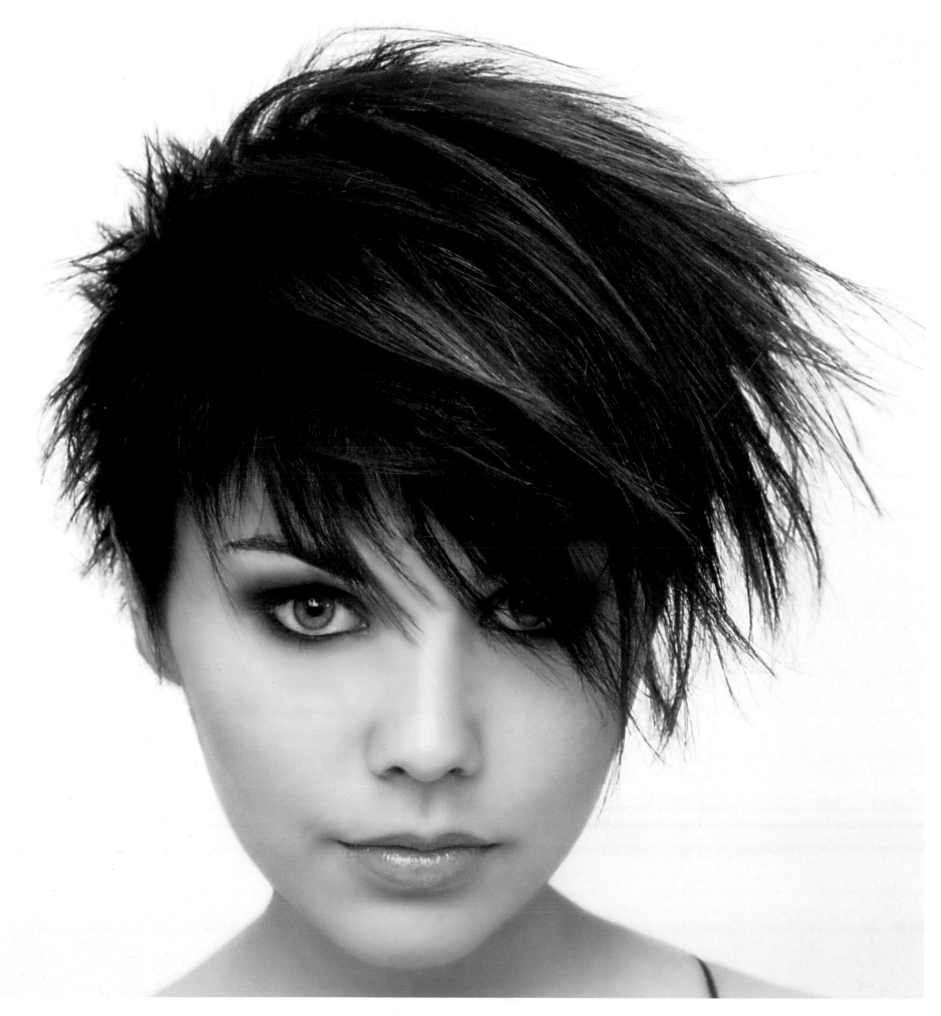

JASON LEA pages 116–117

Jason Lea Hairdressing Group, 11 Lower Bridge Street, Chester, United Kingdom

Hair: Steven Blyth
Make-up: Karen Lockyer
Styling: Vivianna Rullo
Photography: Jim Crone
Products: Tigi and Wella

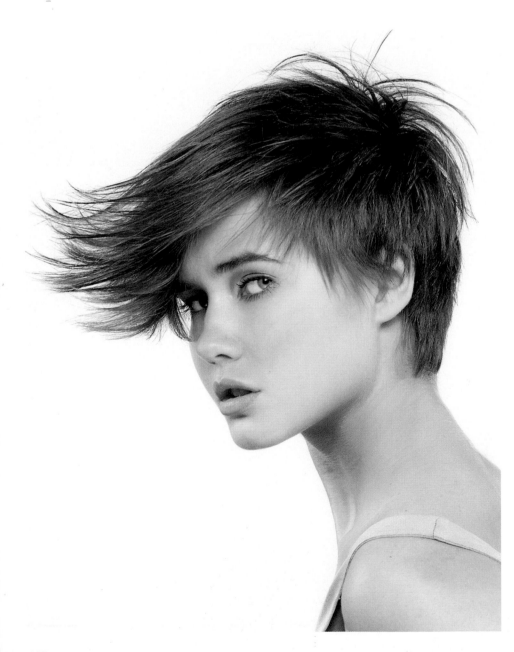
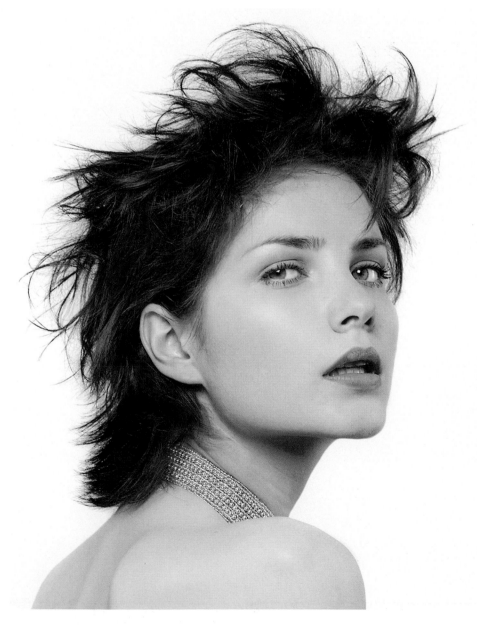

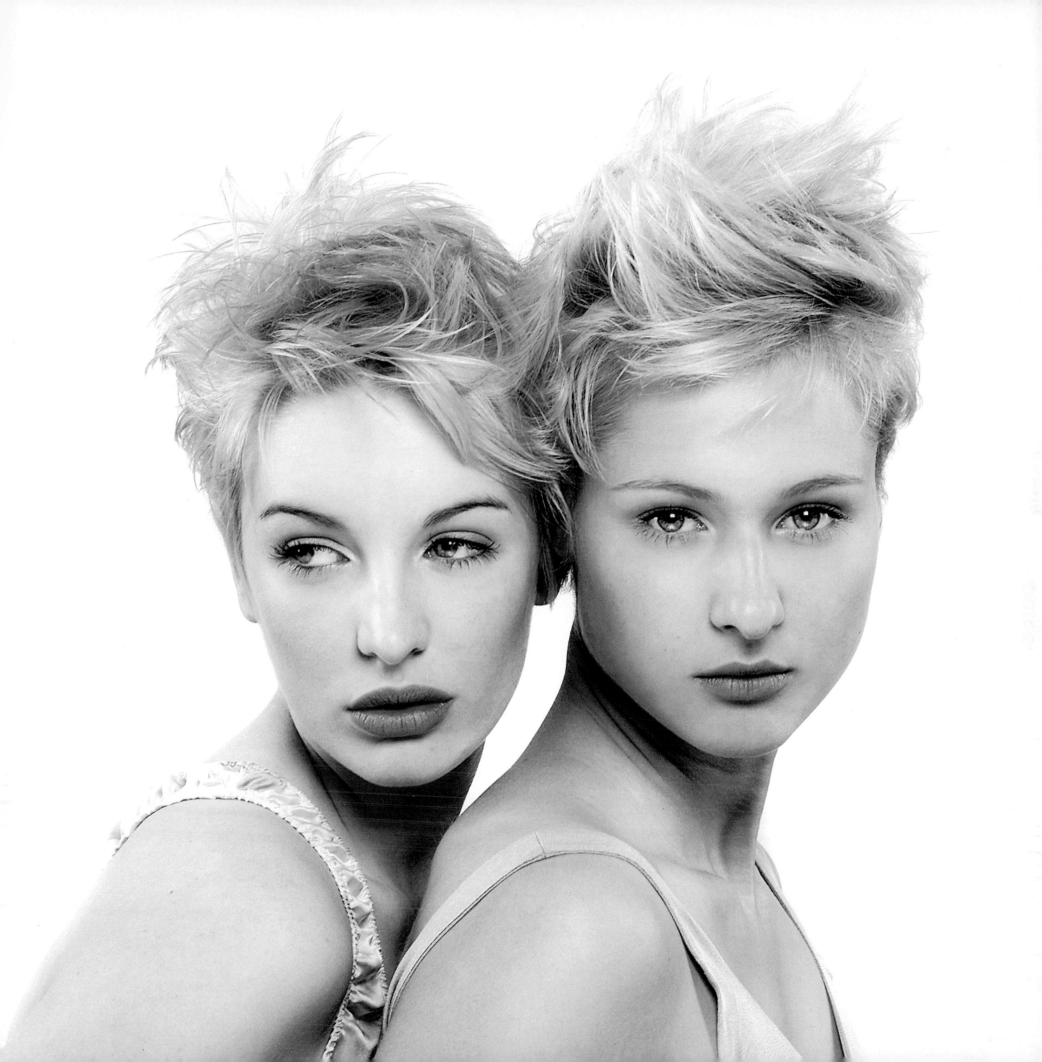

RICHARD KOFFIJBERG pages 118–119

Richard Koffijberg Hairdressers, Scheldestraat 8, 1078 GK Amsterdam, The Netherlands, www.koffijberg.nl

Hair: Richard Koffijberg, Kimm Koffijberg, Frank Koolman, Esther Nieremeijer
Salon: Richard Koffijberg Hairdressers
Make-up: Aron Brouwer
Styling: Nickel Didde and Tiny Houdijk
Photography: Richard Koffijberg
Model Agency: Models@Broadcasting
Products: L'Oréal Professional

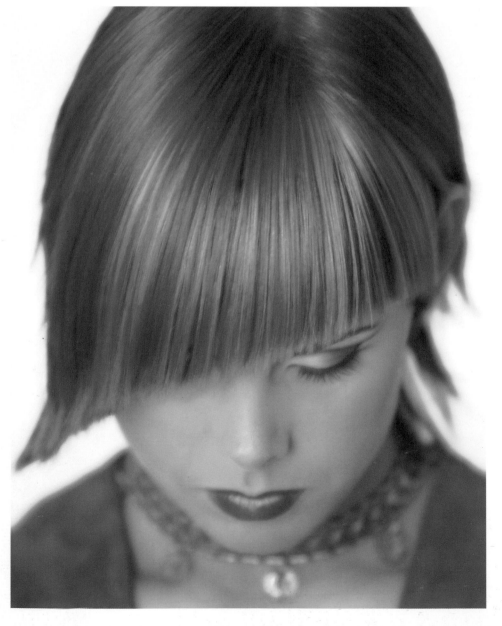 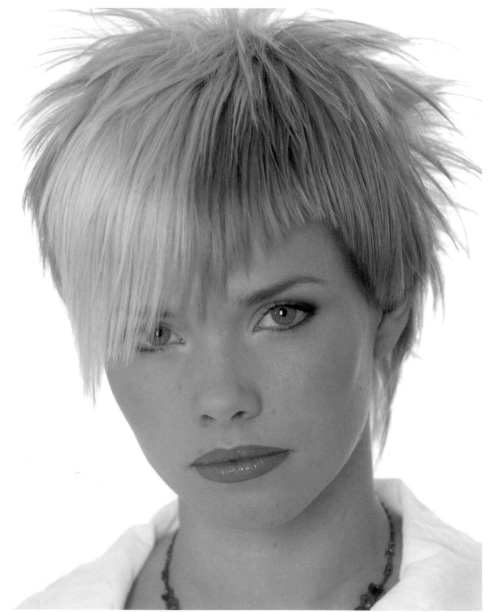

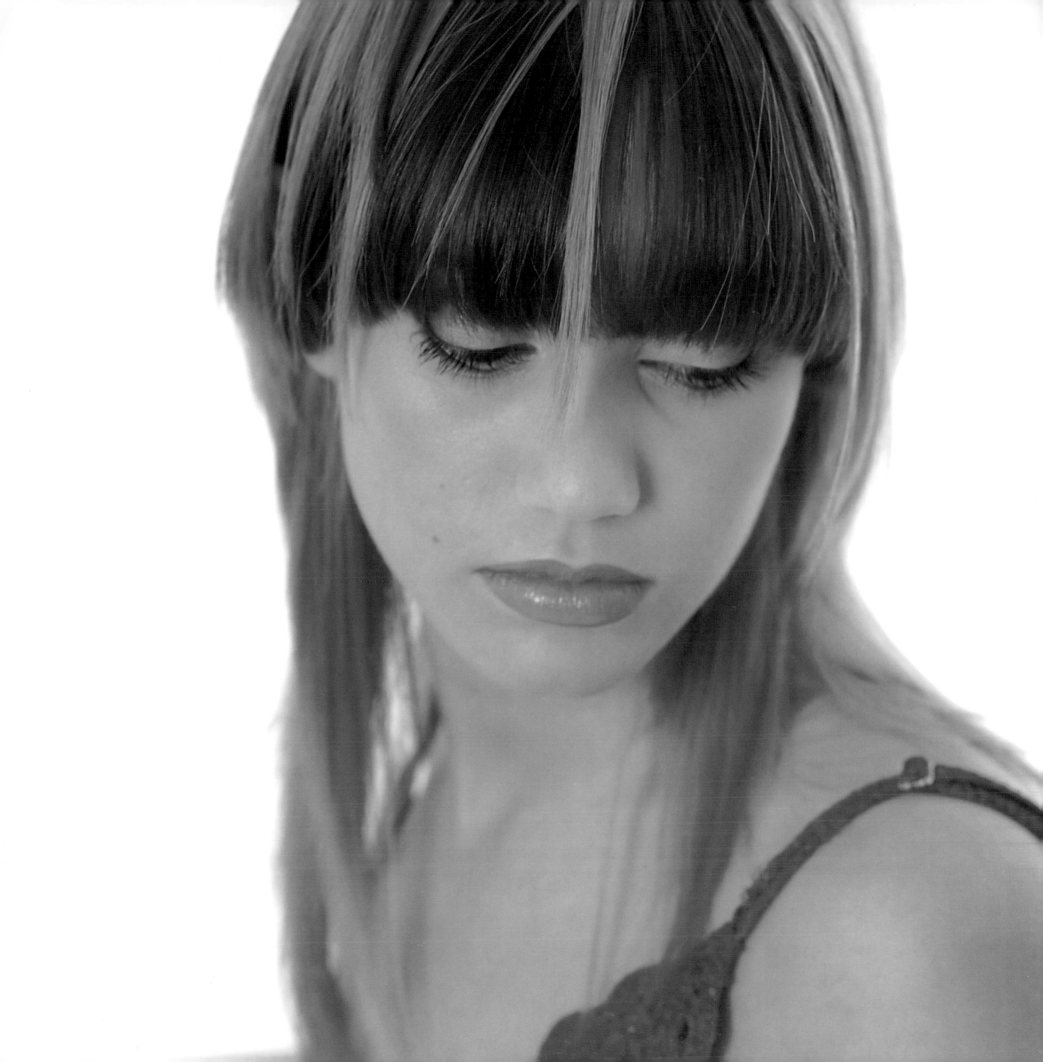

Hair: Medusa Artistic Team
Make-up: Carol Wilson
Styling: Beverley Williams
Photography: Jim Crone
Products: Wella

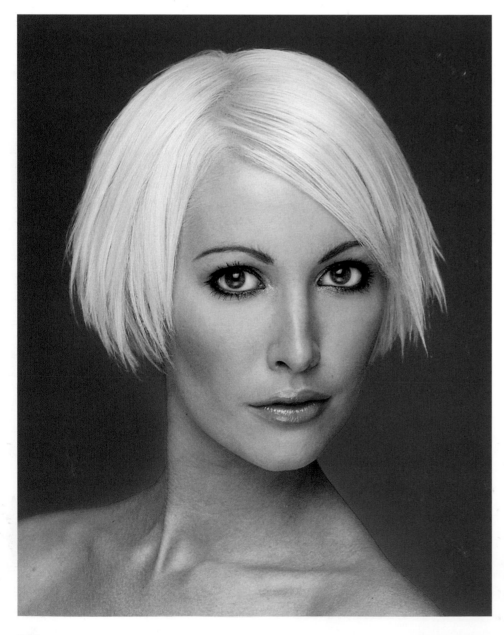
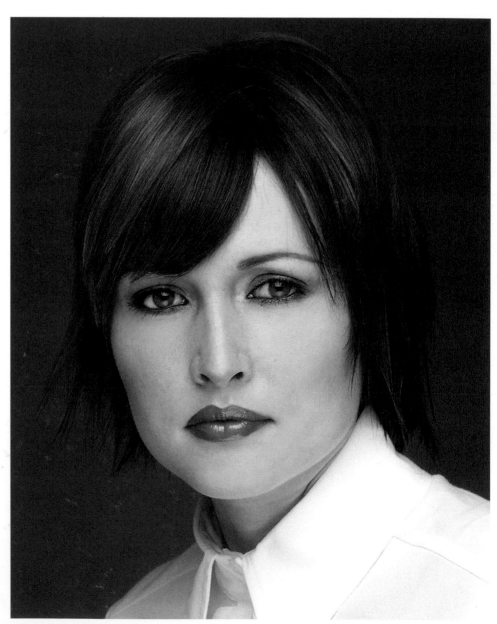

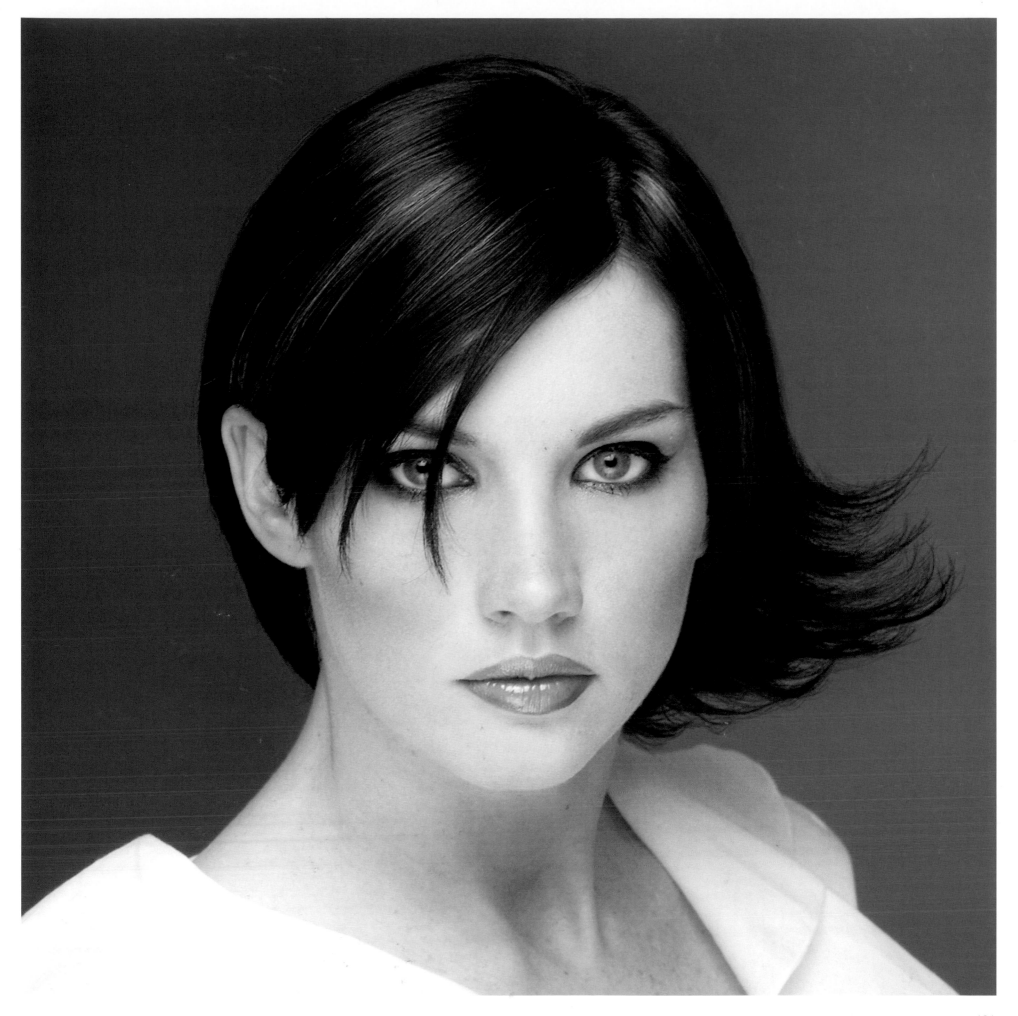

KUHN pages 122–123

Kuhn Intercoiffure, Tramstrasse 15, 8050 Zürich, Switzerland, www.team-kuhn.ch

Hair: Kuhn Artistic Team
Make-up: Jasmin Bossert
Styling: Yvo Aeschlimann
Photography: Adrian Portmann
Products: Sebastian

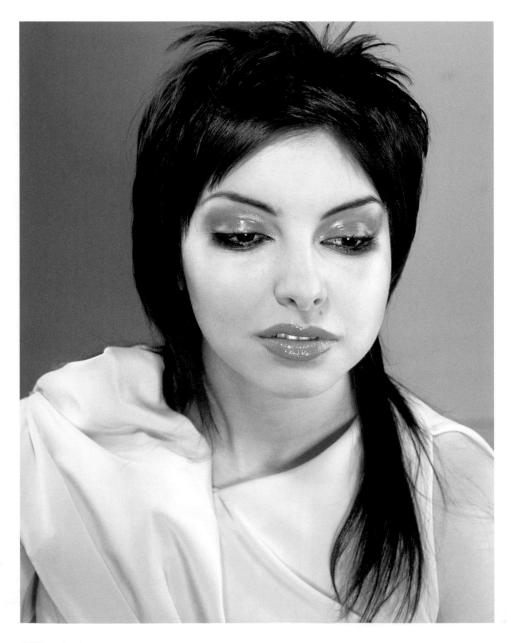
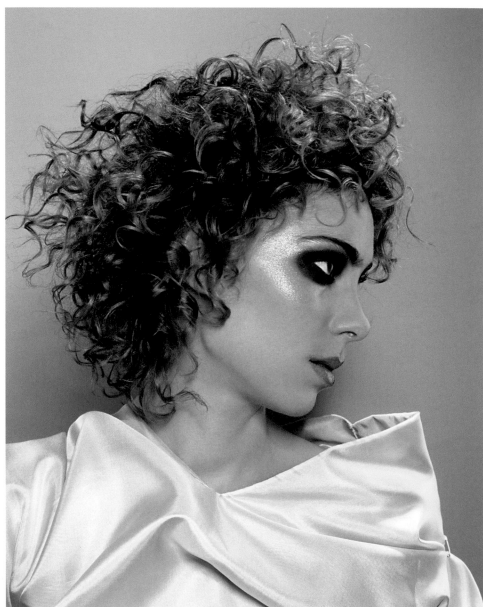

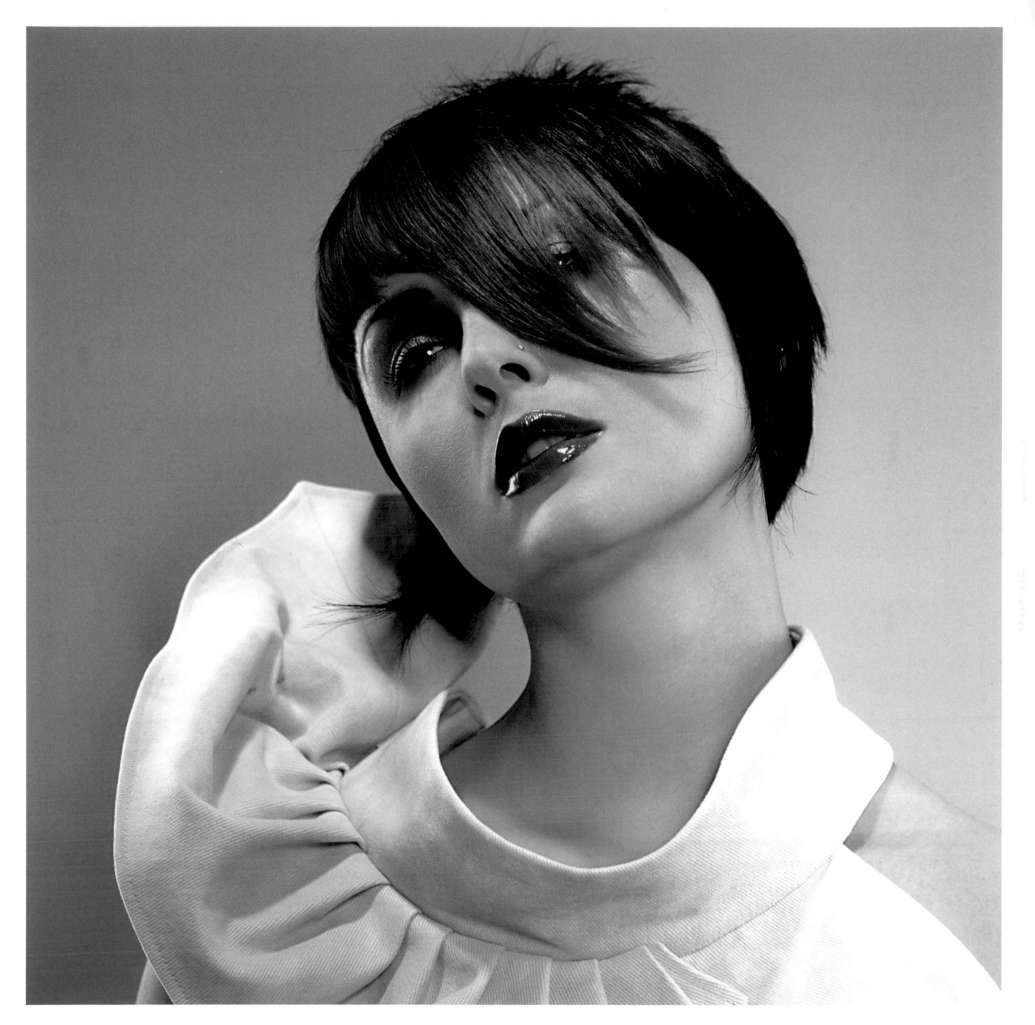

MIEKA HAIRDRESSING pages 124–125

308 Smith Street, Collingwood, Melbourne VIC 3066, Australia

Hair: Tracey Hughes
Make-up: Trudy Joyce
Styling: Michael Angel
Photography: Brett Brogan

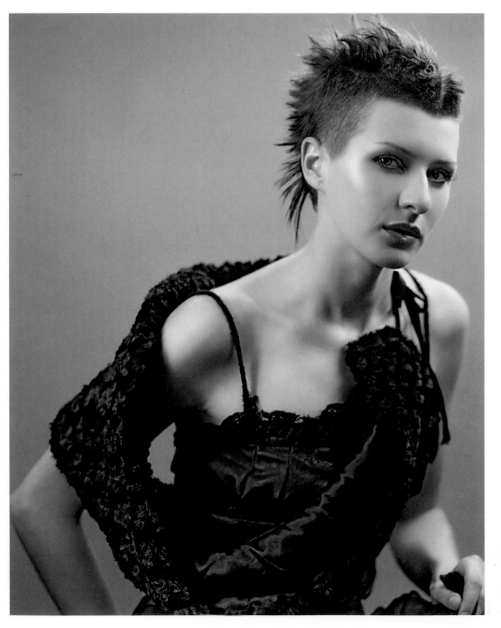
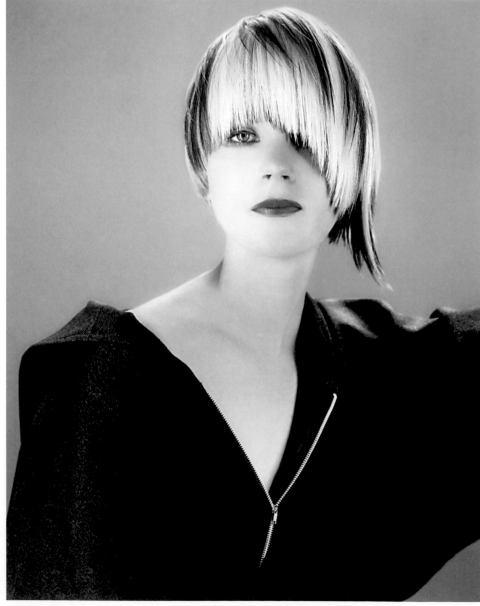

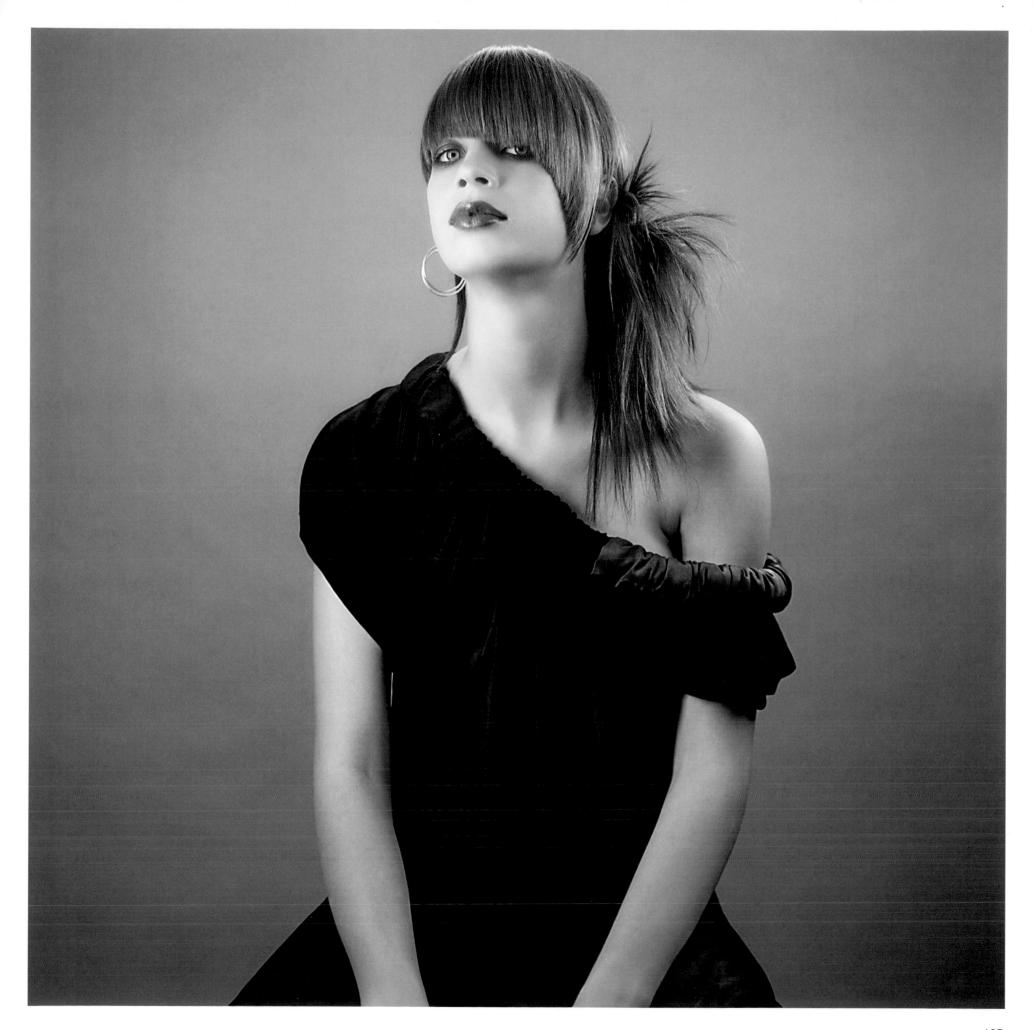

SILVIA ARANZA pages 126–127

Irigoyen 475, 7300 Azul-Buenos Aires, Argentina

Hair: Silvia Aranza
Make-up: Caro Severi
Photography: Guillermo Losio
Model: Augustina
Products: L'Oréal

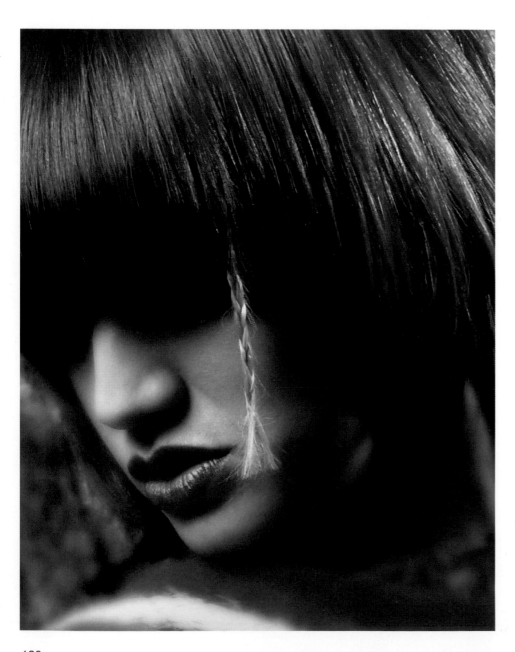

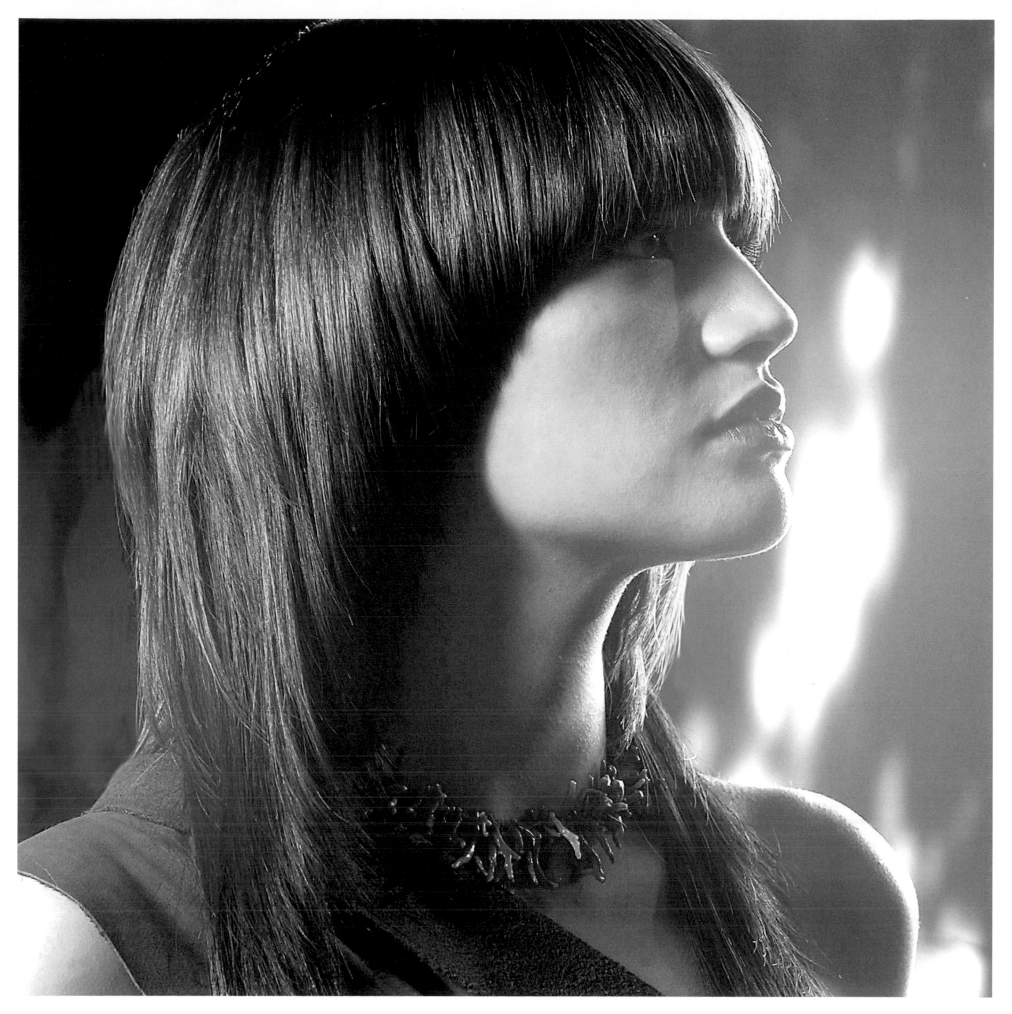

ERIC STIPA pages 128-129

72 rue Nationale, 37000 Tours, France, www.ericstipa.com

Hair: Eric Stipa
Make-up: Vesna
Styling: Christine Birkle for Hut Up Berlin (p. 128)
Photography: Stéfan Kraus

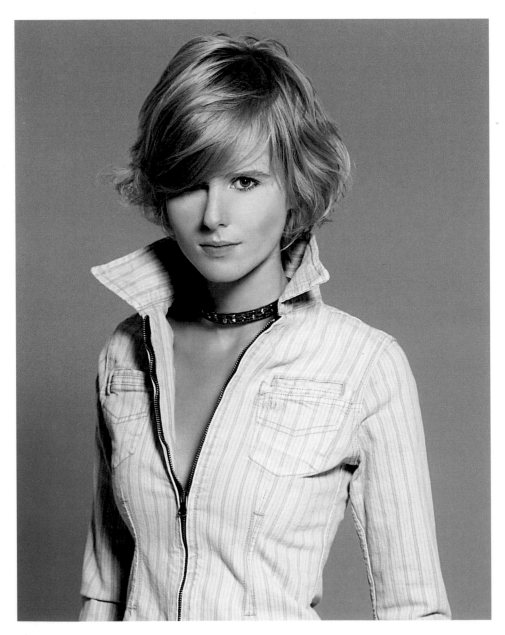

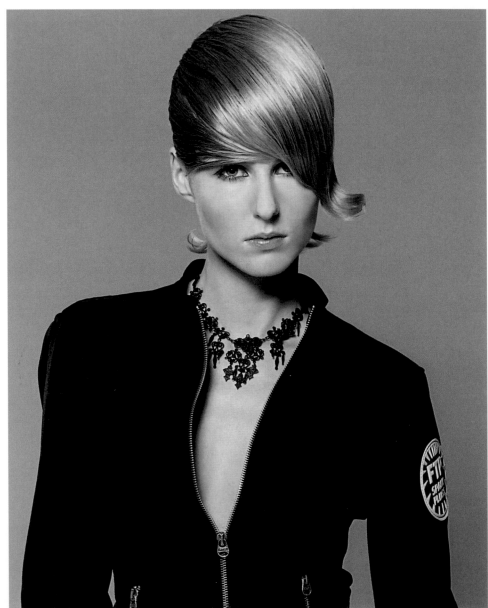

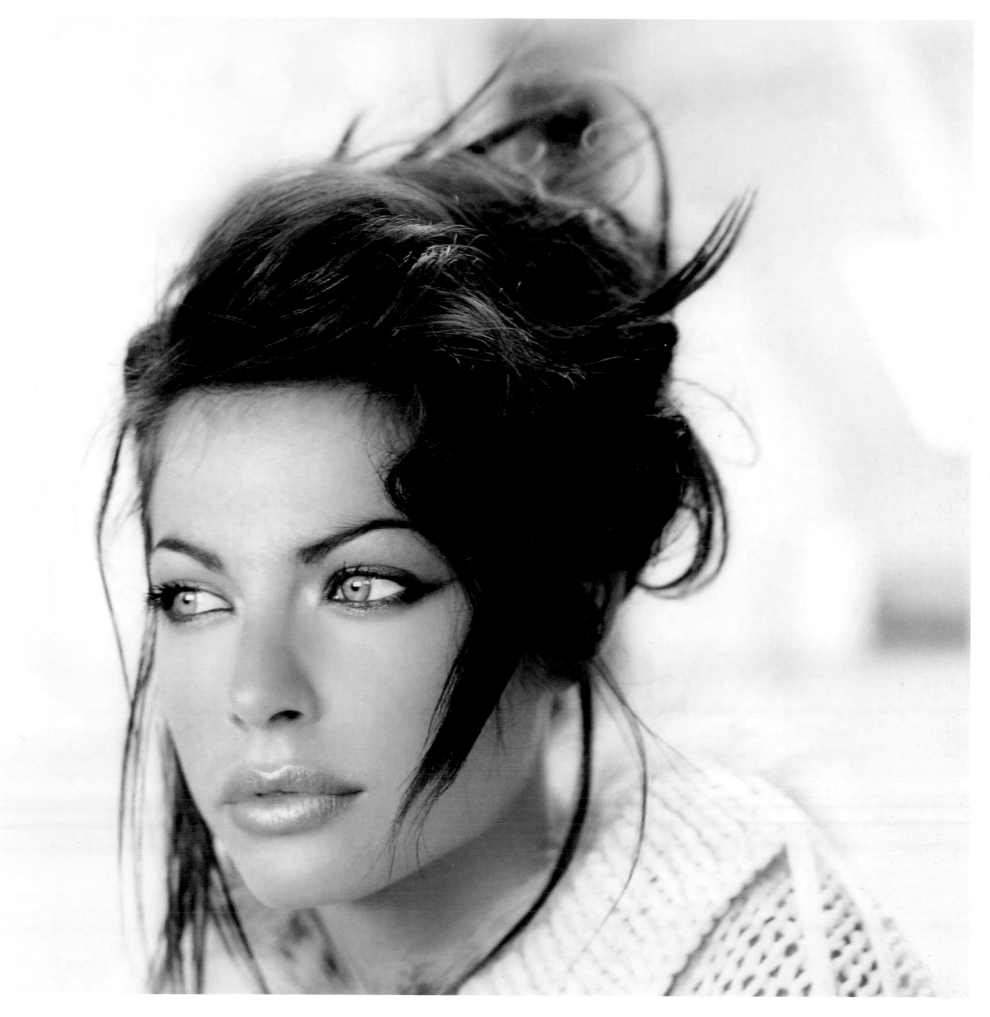

CONTEMPORARY HAIR pages 130–131

2 The Wynd, Marske-by-the-Sea, Saltburn TS11 7LA, United Kingdom

Hair: Alan Simpson and Karen Storr
Make-up: Carol at Carol Hayes
Styling: Rachel Franconi
Photography: Simon Bottomley
Products: L'Oréal Professionnel

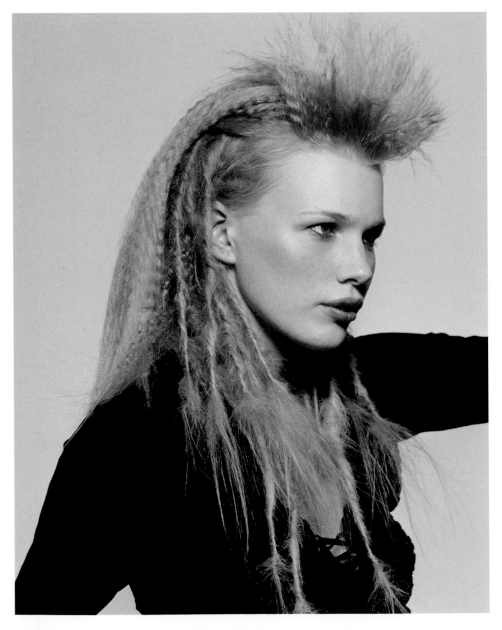

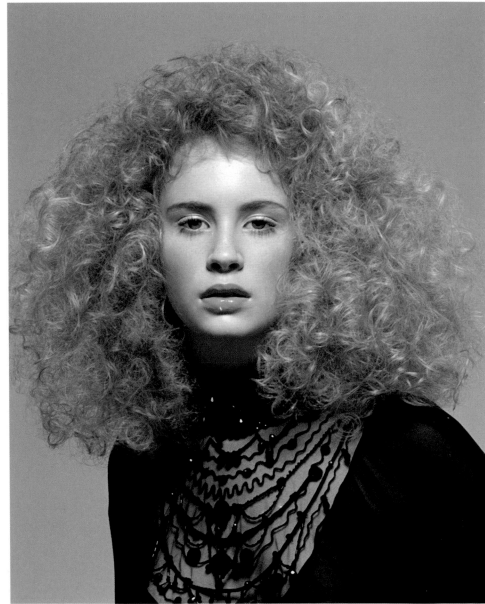

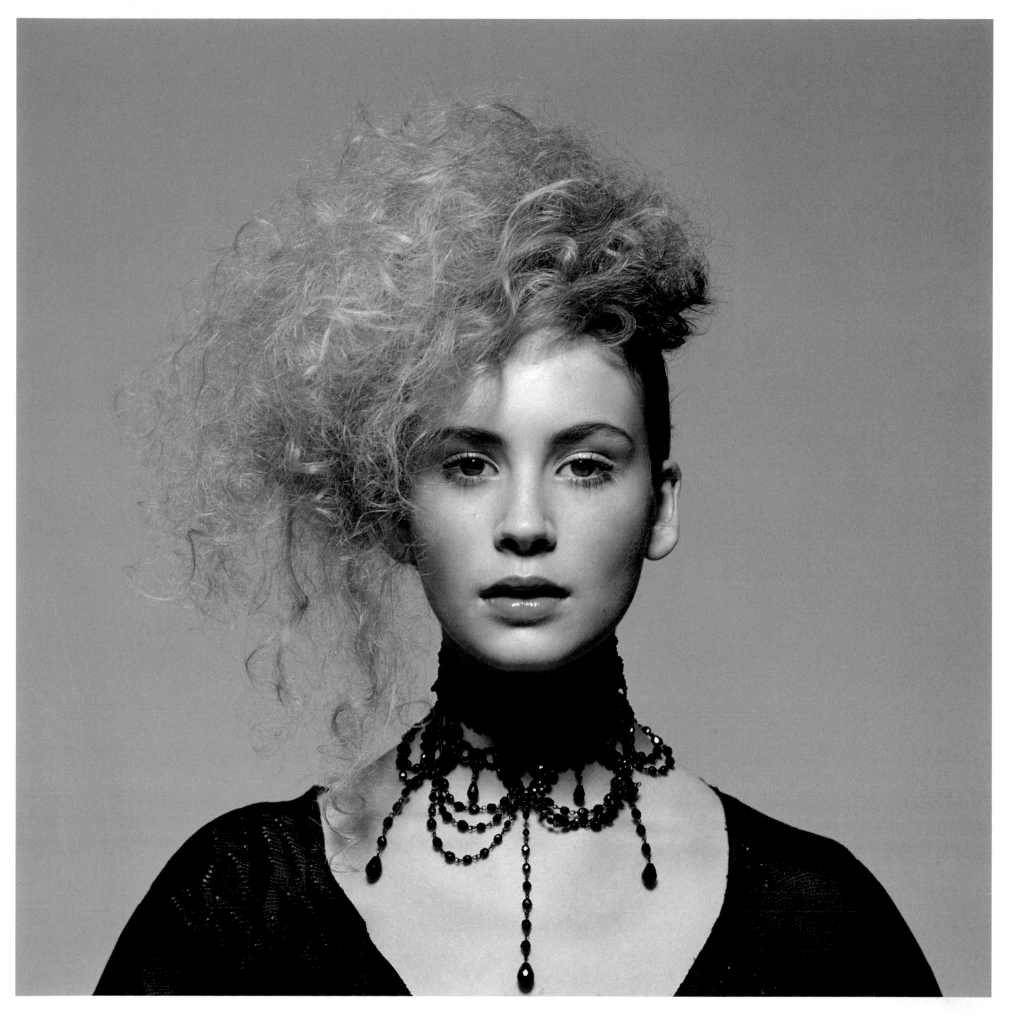

ISHOKA HAIRDRESSING & BEAUTY pages 132–135

11 Albyn Terrace, Aberdeen AB10 1YP, United Kingdom

Hair: Rachel Smith
Make-up: Rhona Stewart
Styling: Ishoka
Photography: Jim Crone
Products: Wella

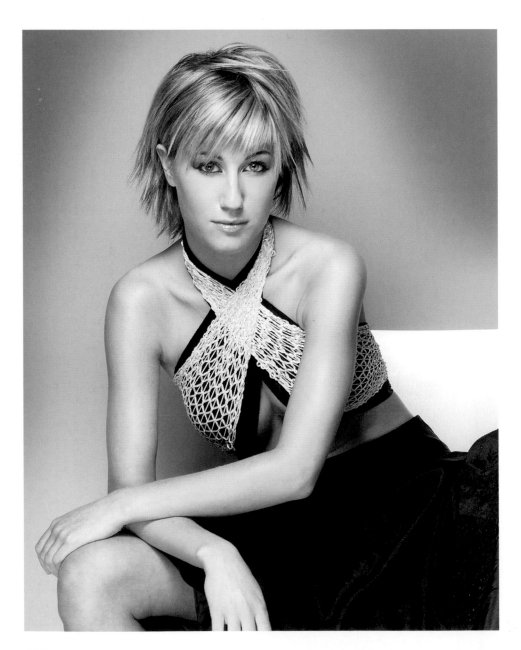

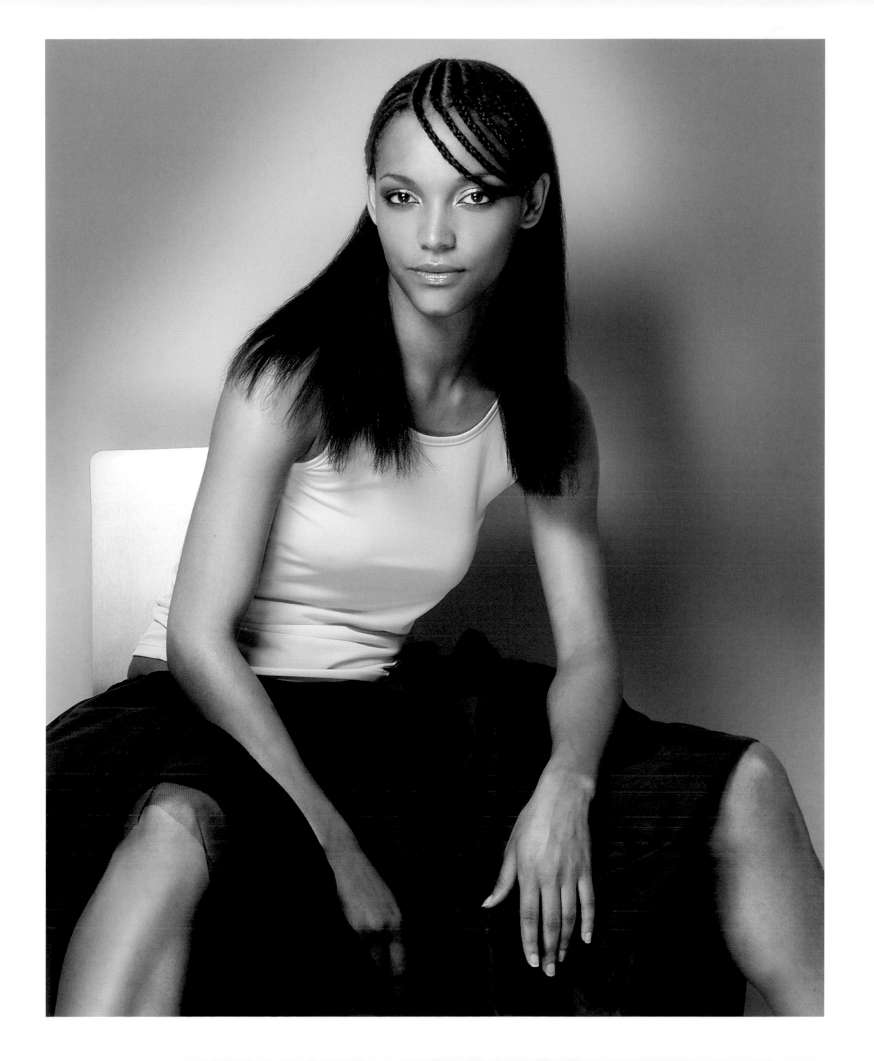

MIC STYLING pages 136–139

Sojer d.o.o. Trzaska 116, 1000 Ljubljana, Slovenia, www.micstyling.com

Hair: Mic Styling Academy
Academy: Mic Styling Academy
Make-up: Mic Styling Beauty
Photography: Franci Virant
Products: L'Oréal Professional

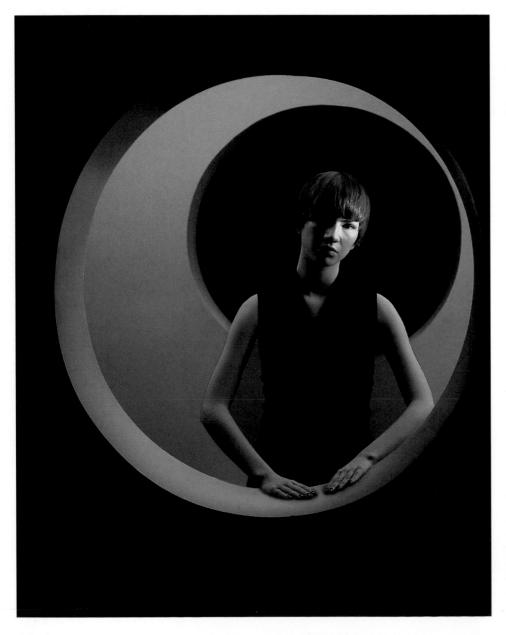

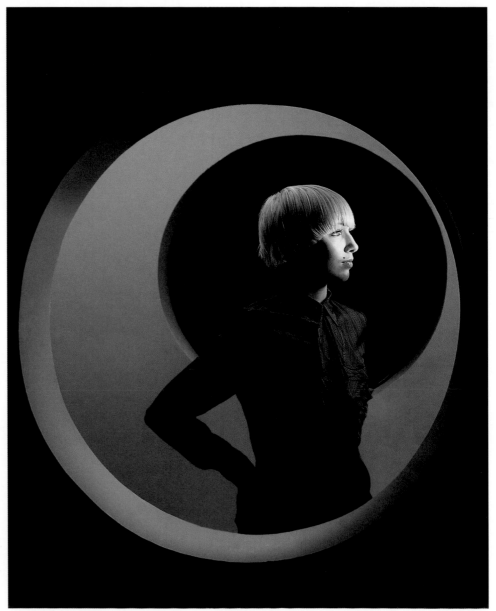

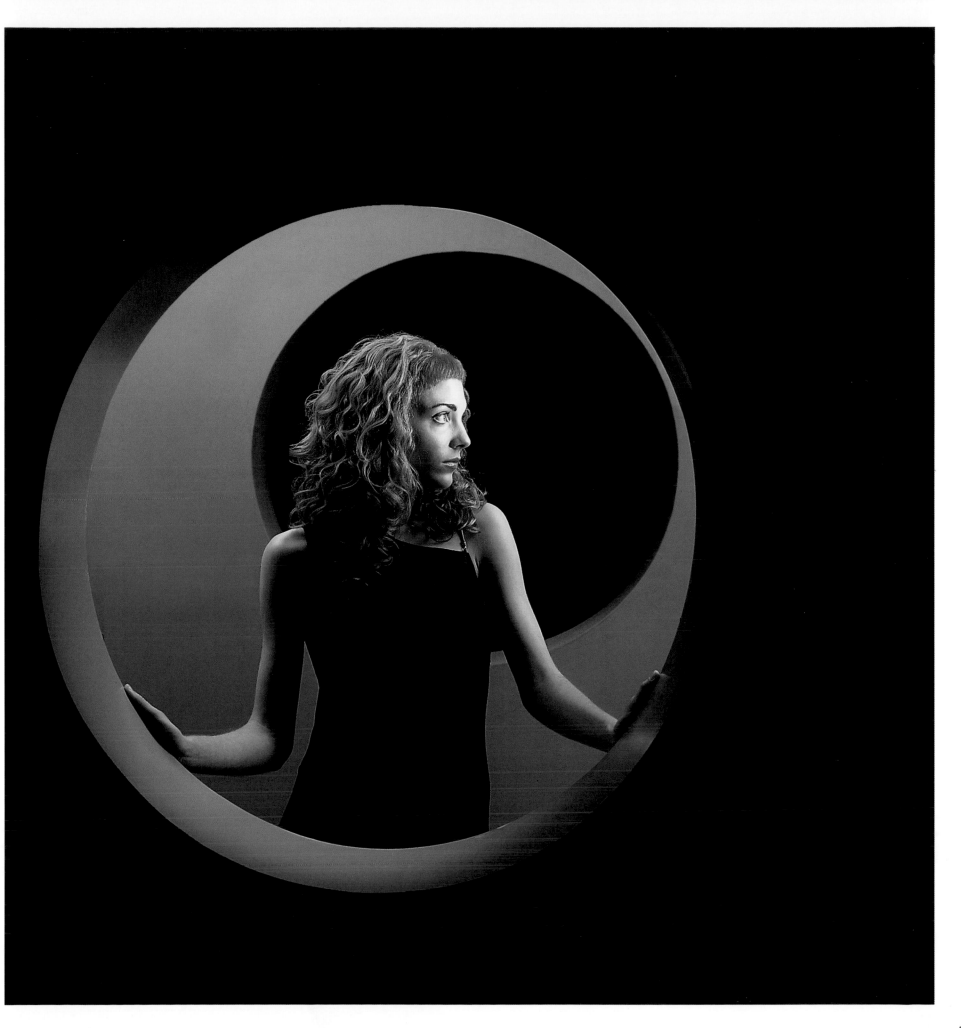

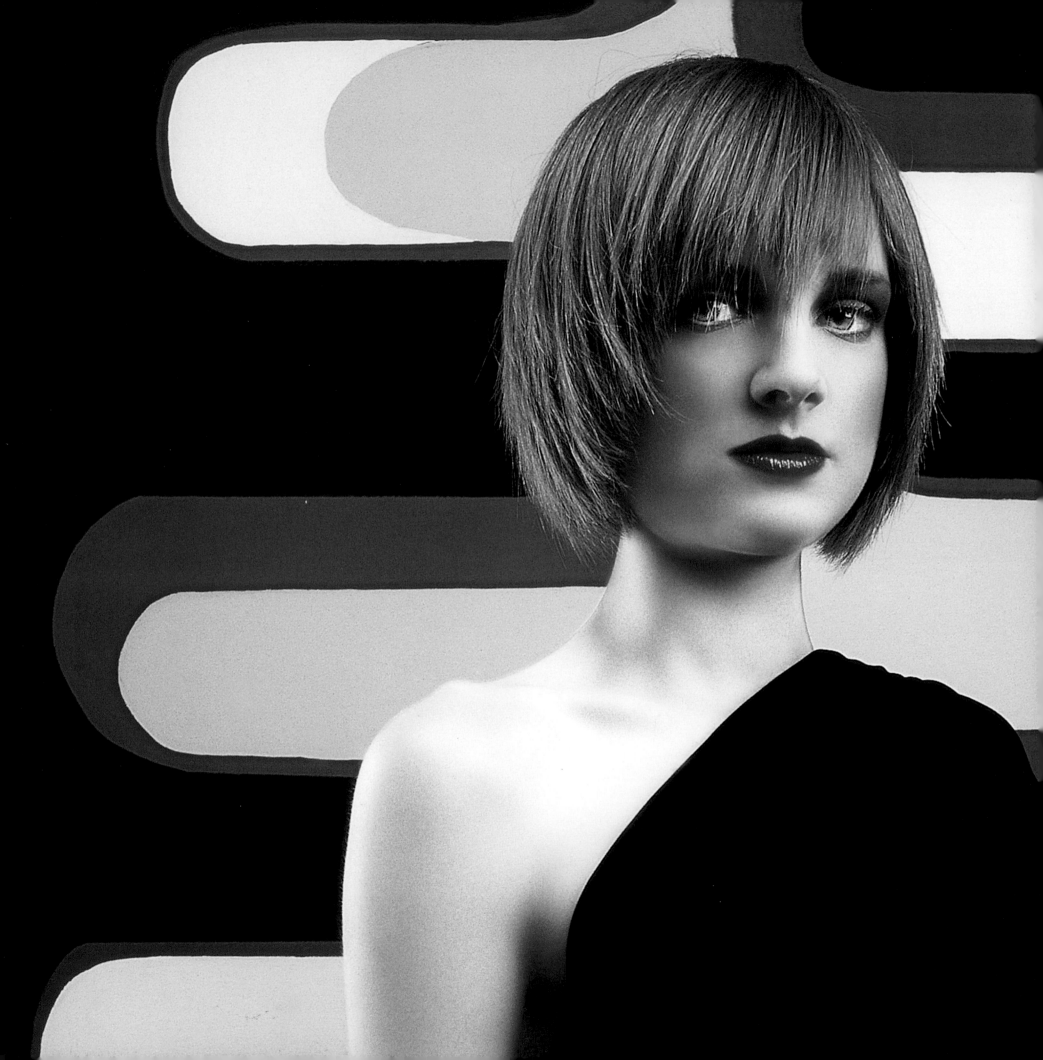

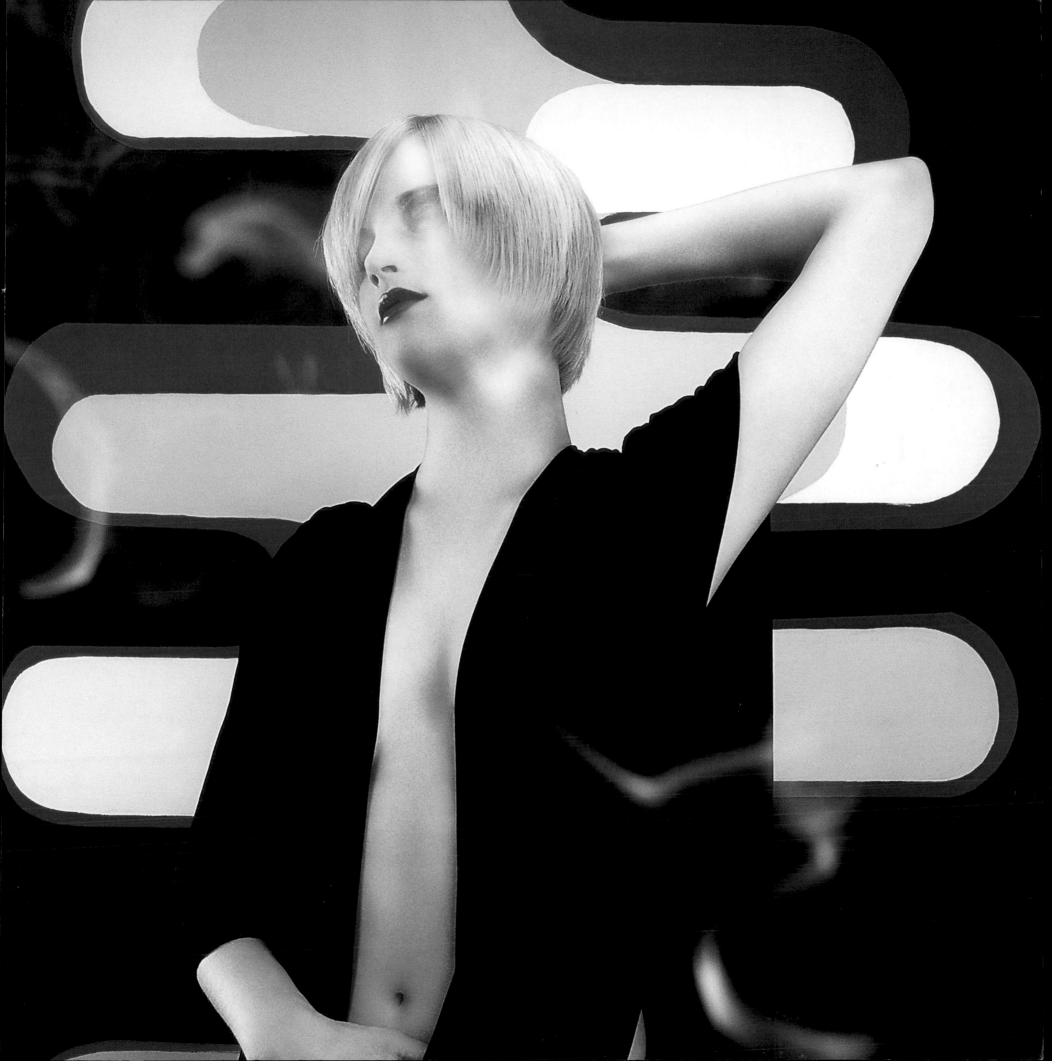

PATRIZIA GRECHT pages 140–143

Concept Partizia Grecht, Operngasse 25, 1040 Wien, Austria, www.concept-grecht.at

Hair: Patrizia Grecht
Make-up: Patrizia Grecht (p. 140, 141) Silvia Albegger (p. 142) Wolfgang Lindenhofer (p. 143)
Styling: Christina, Perfectprops (p. 140, 141) Monika Buttinger (p. 142)
Photography: Klaus Mähring (p. 140, 141, 143) Norbert Kniat (p. 142)
Models: Thom K. Agentur Visage (p.140) Nora, Agentur Stella (p. 141)

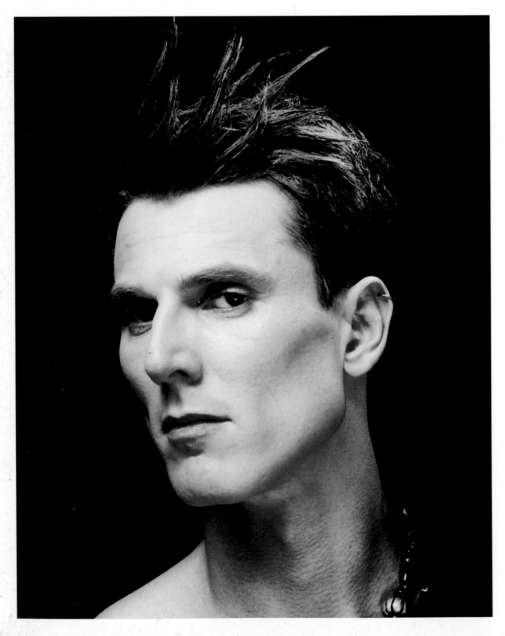

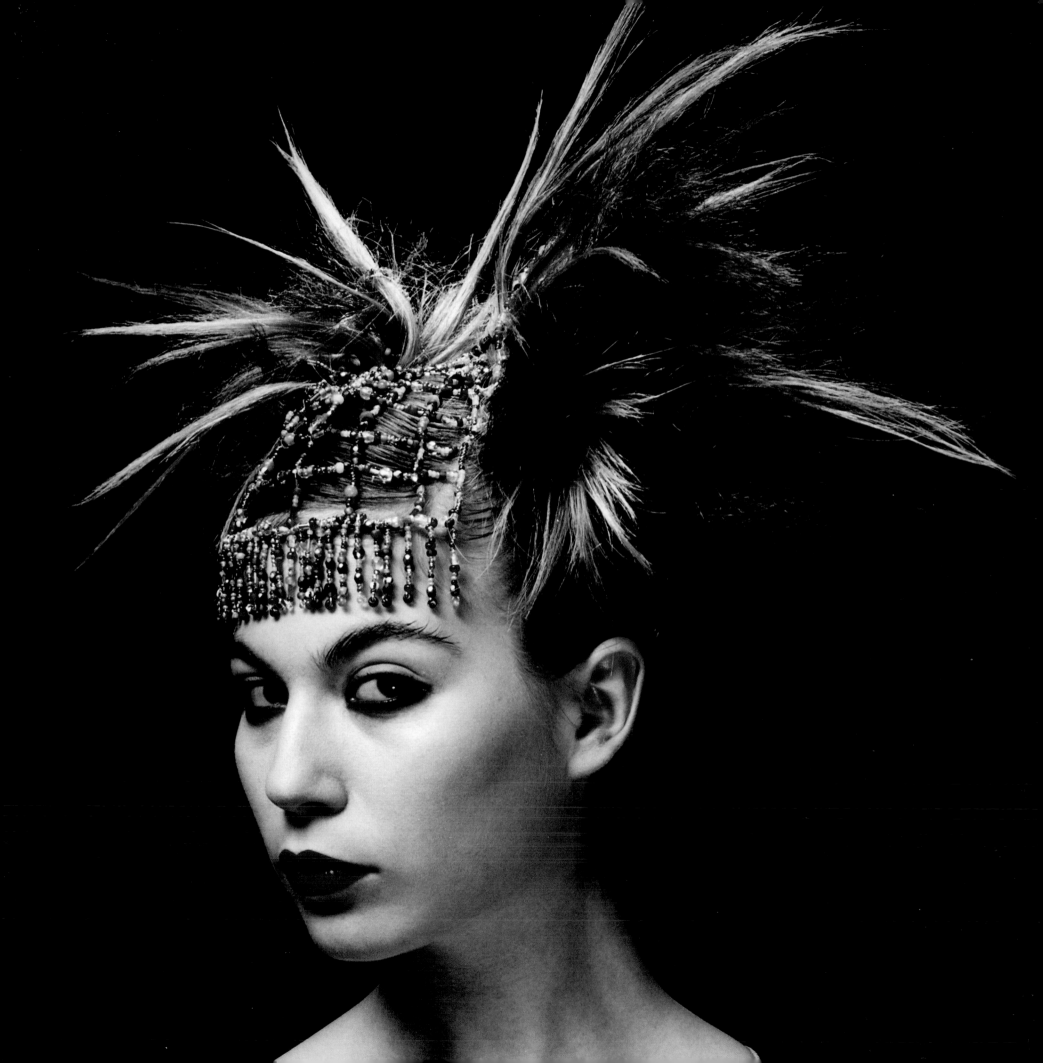

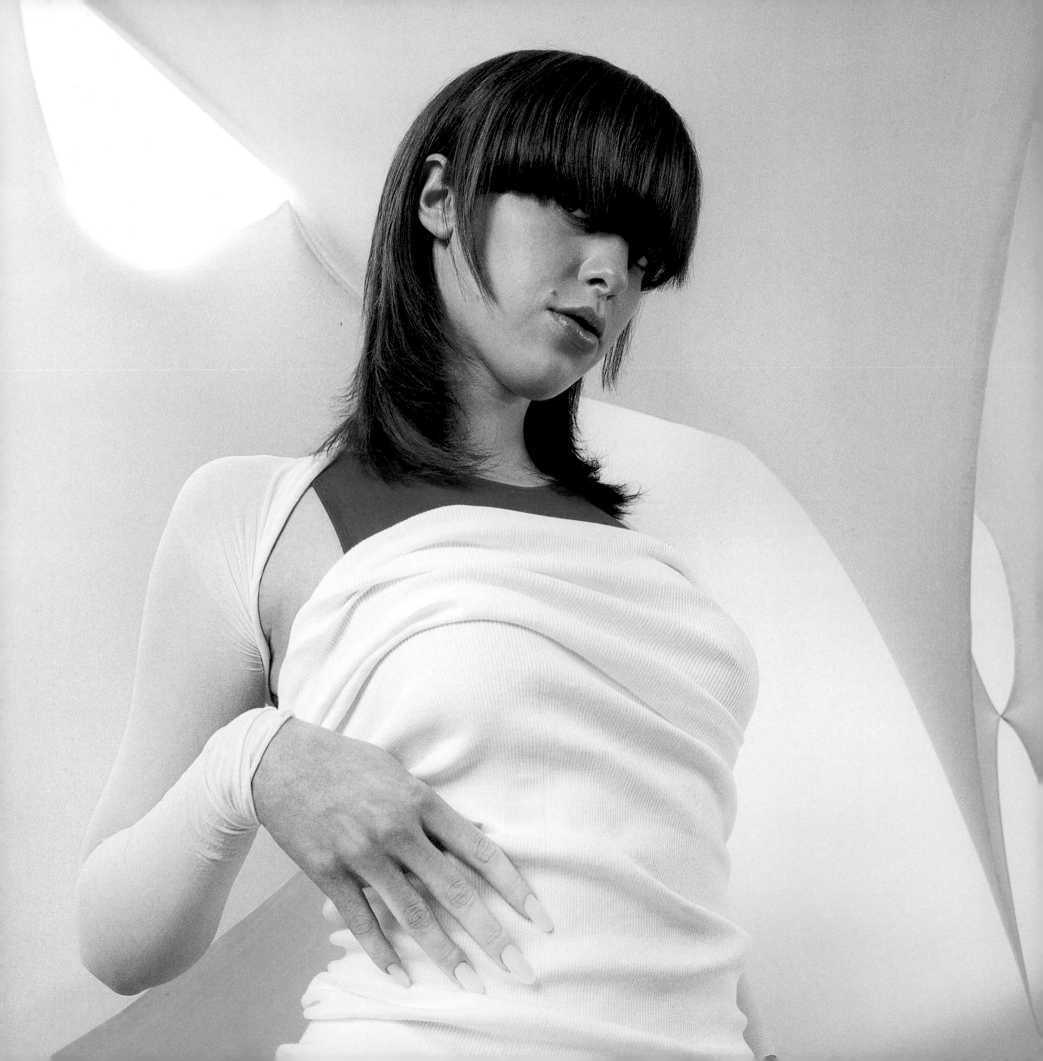

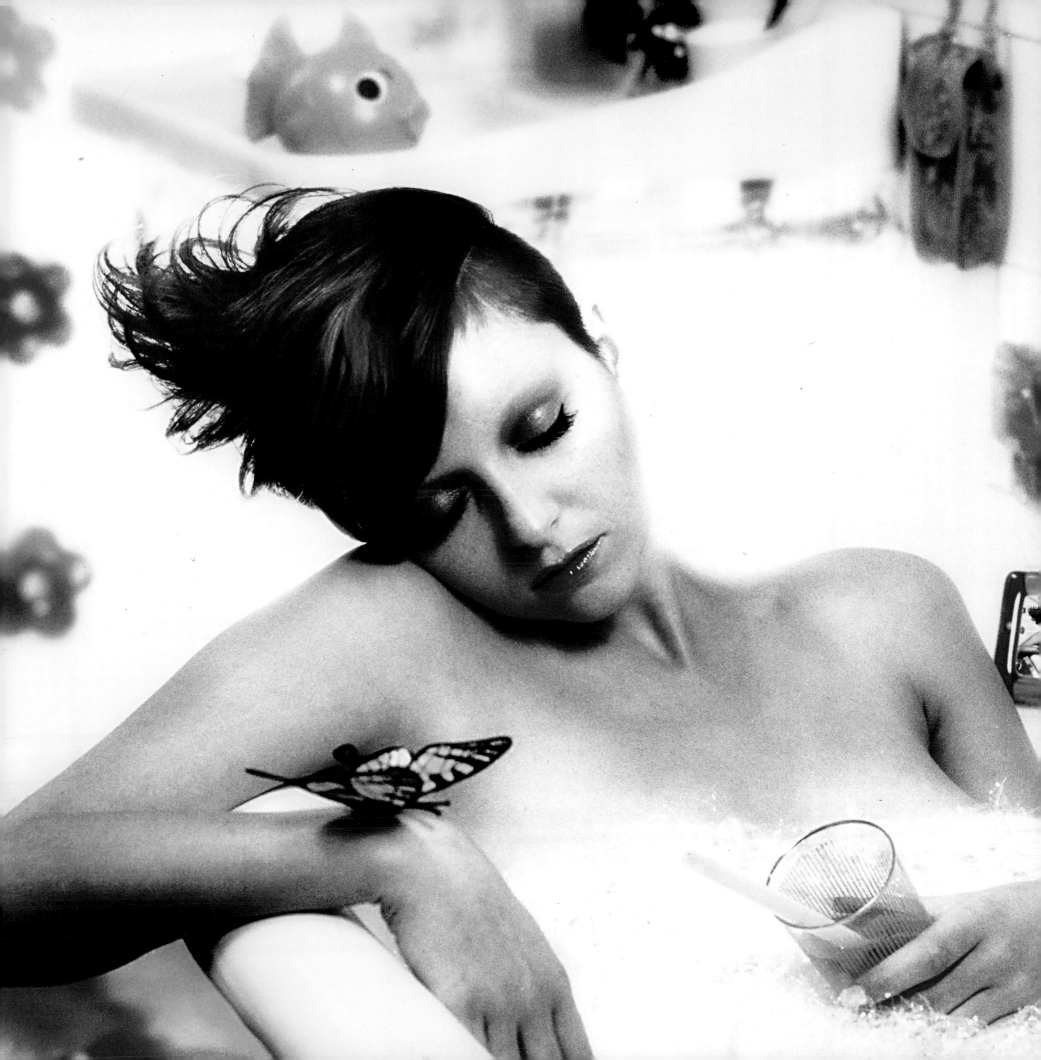

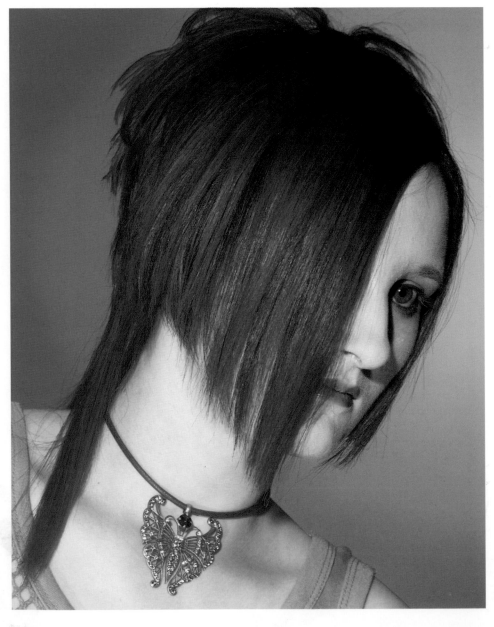

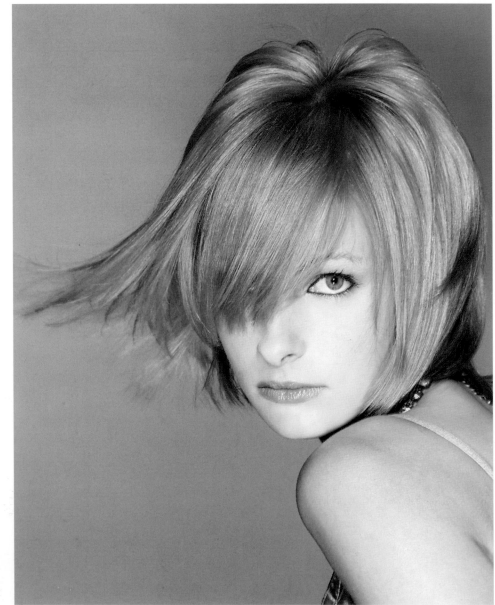

144

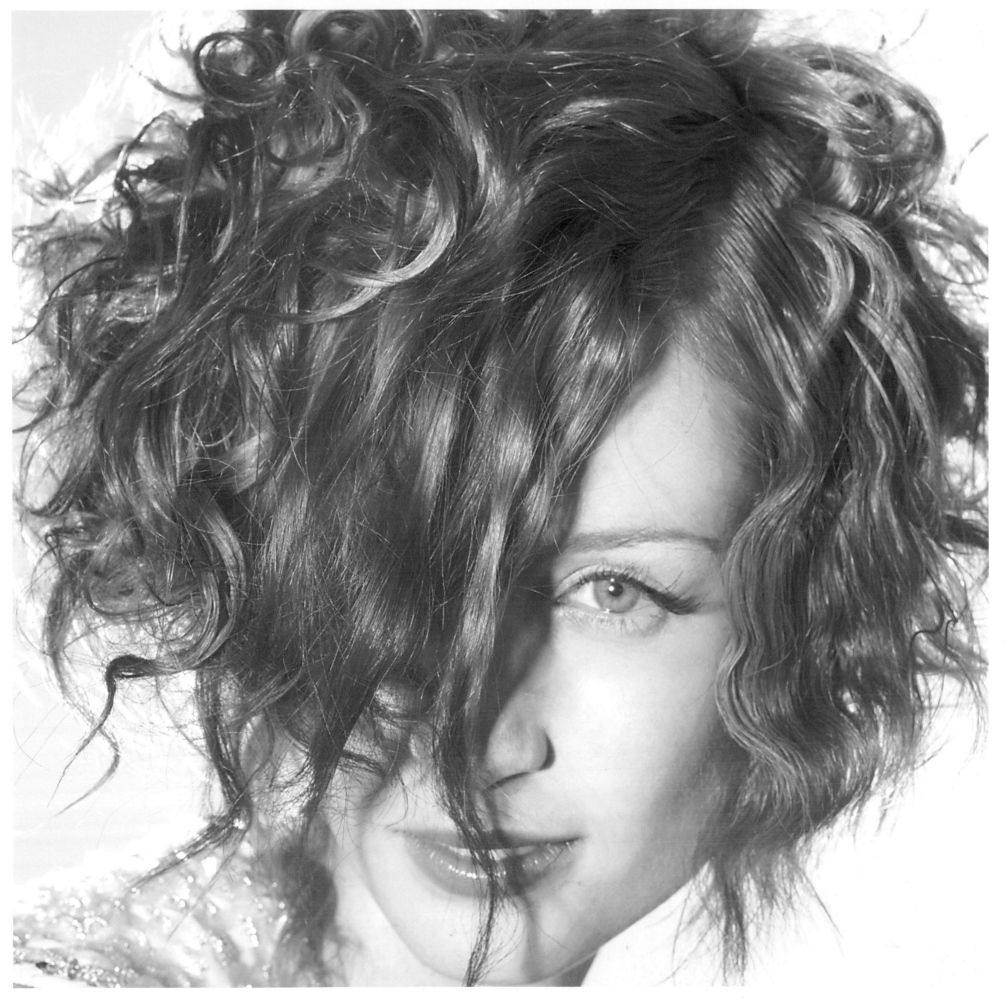

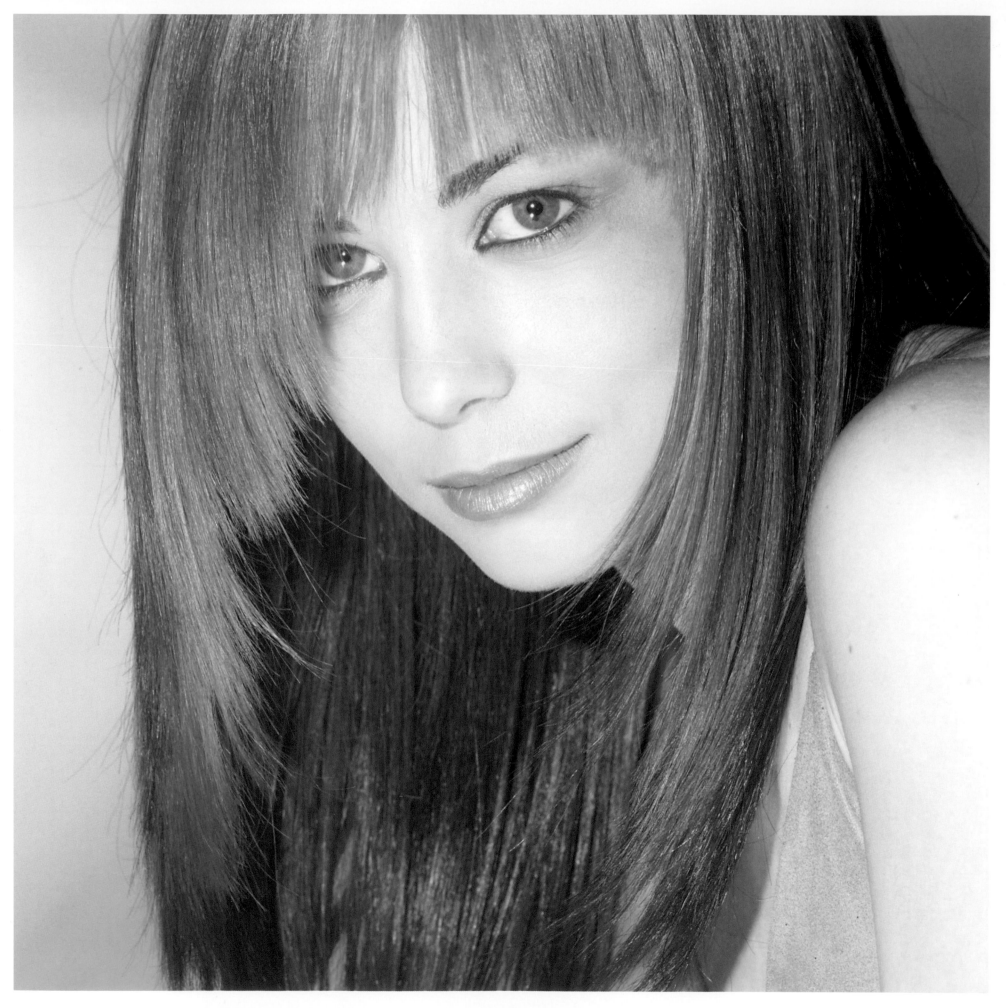

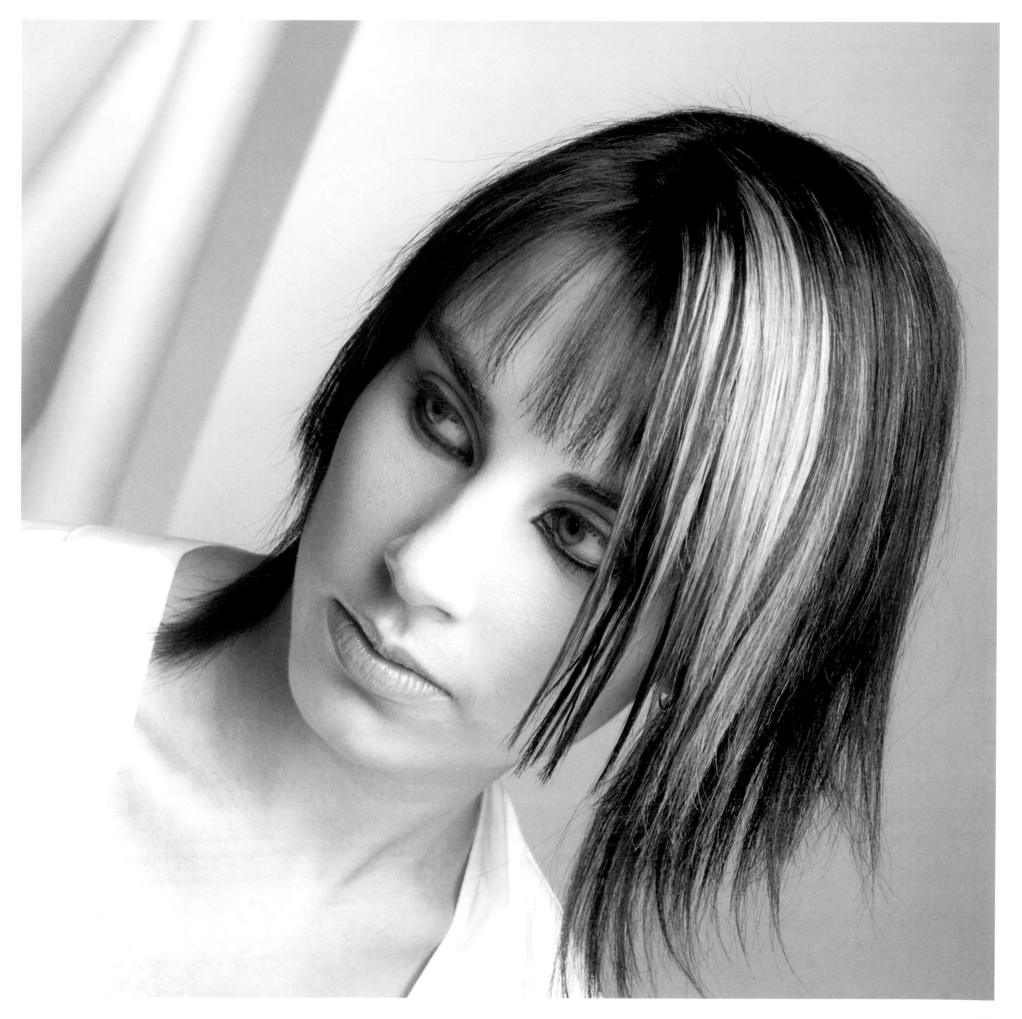

ESSENSUALS HAIRDRESSING pages 148–155

19 Doughty Street, London WC1N 2PL, United Kingdom, www.essensuals.co.uk

Hair: Essensuals Creative Team (p. 148 - 151) Sacha Mascolo-Tarbuck (p. 152, 153) Nina Beckert (p. 154, 155)
Make-up: Lucia Burghi and Sarah Walsh (p. 148 - 151) Irena Rogers (p. 154, 155)
Styling: Natalie Fajer (p. 148 - 151) Gayle Rinkoff (p. 152, 153) Lilia B. Toncheva (p. 154, 155)
Photography: Andy Morrison (p. 148, 149, 150, 151, 154, 155) Stuart Weston (p. 152, 153)
Art Director: Sacha Mascolo-Tarbuck (p. 148 - 151)

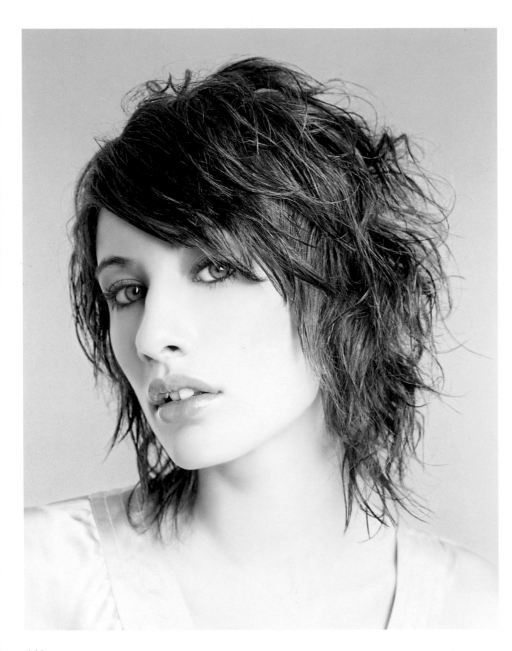

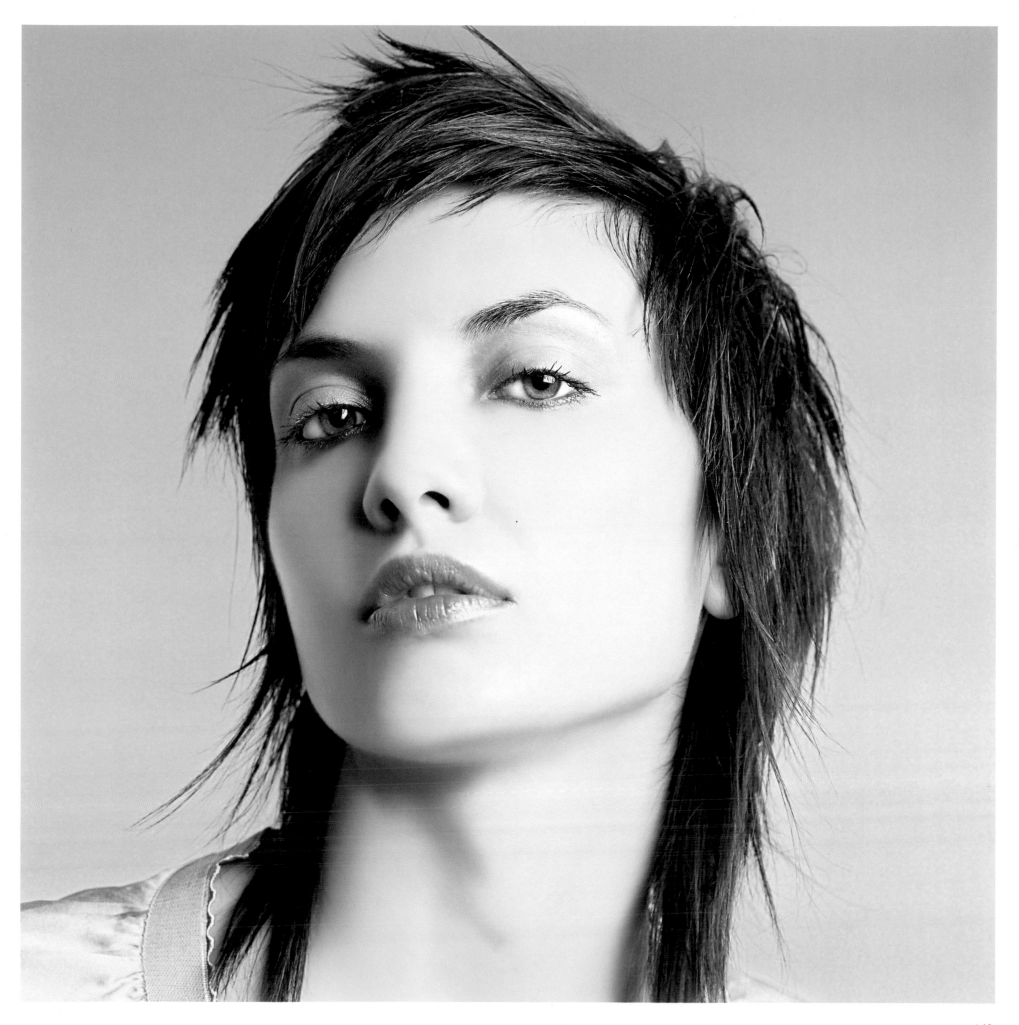

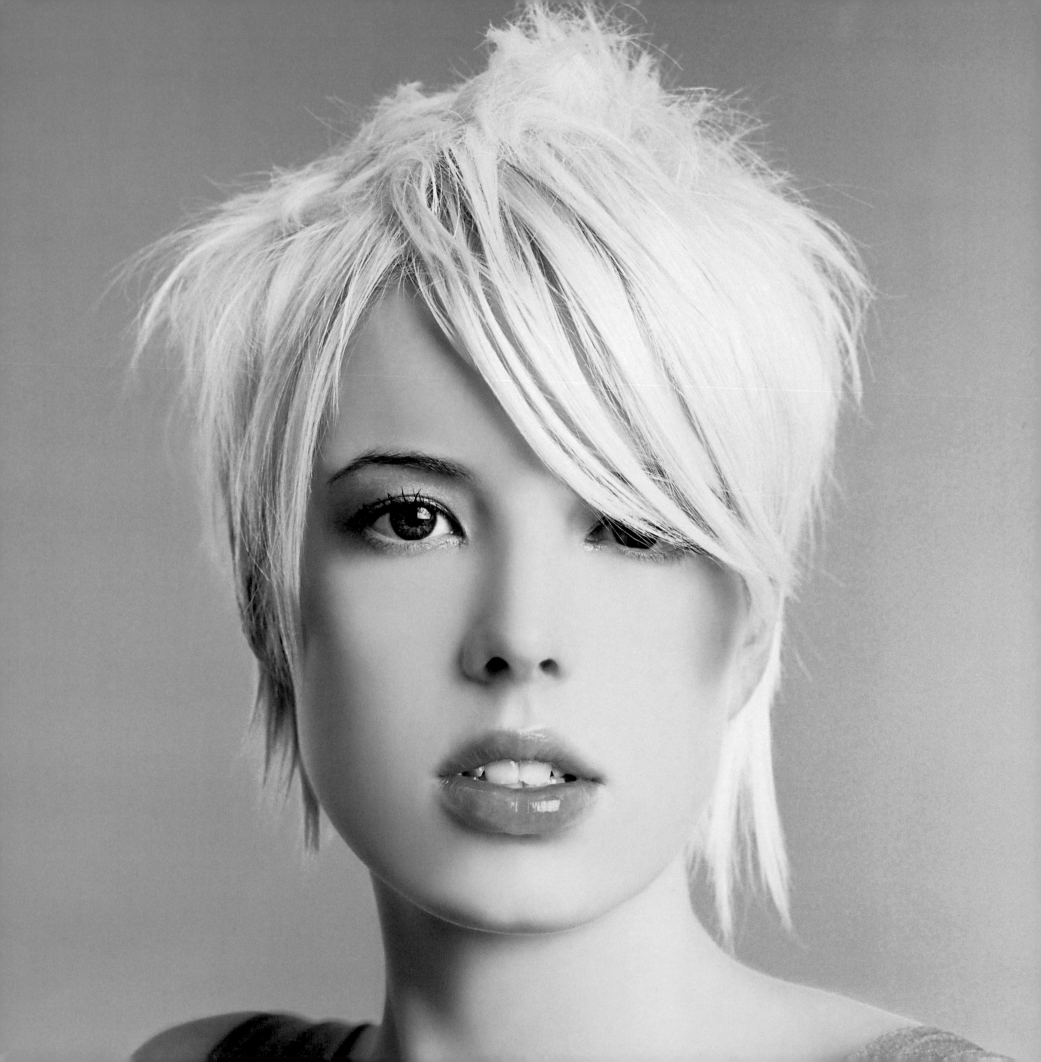

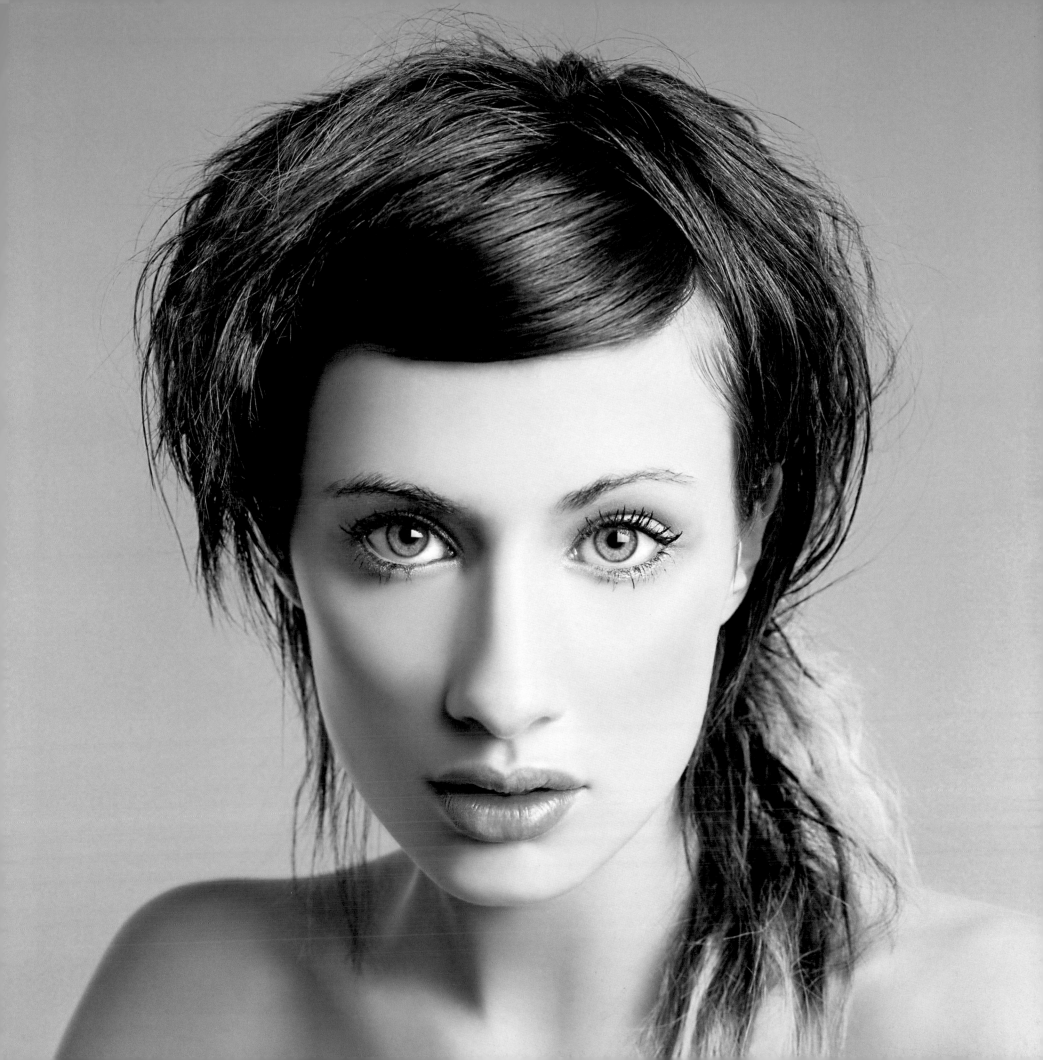

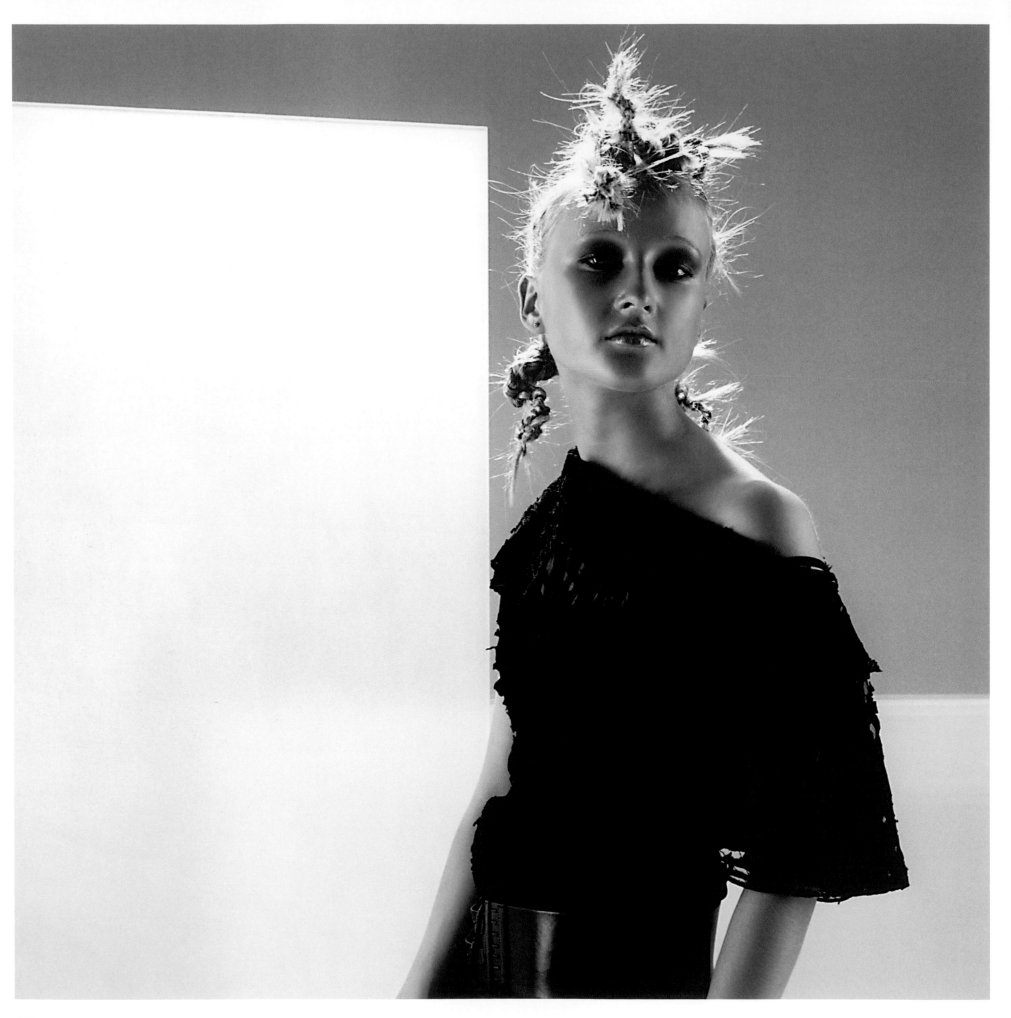

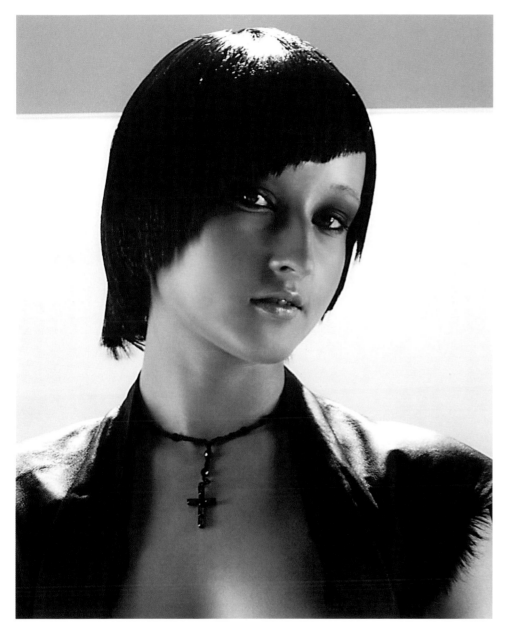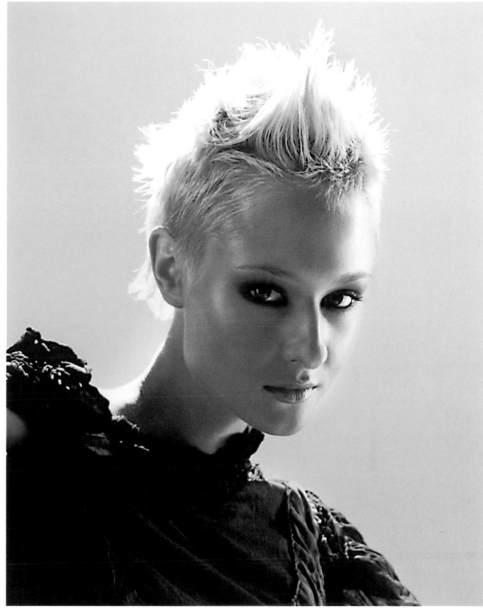

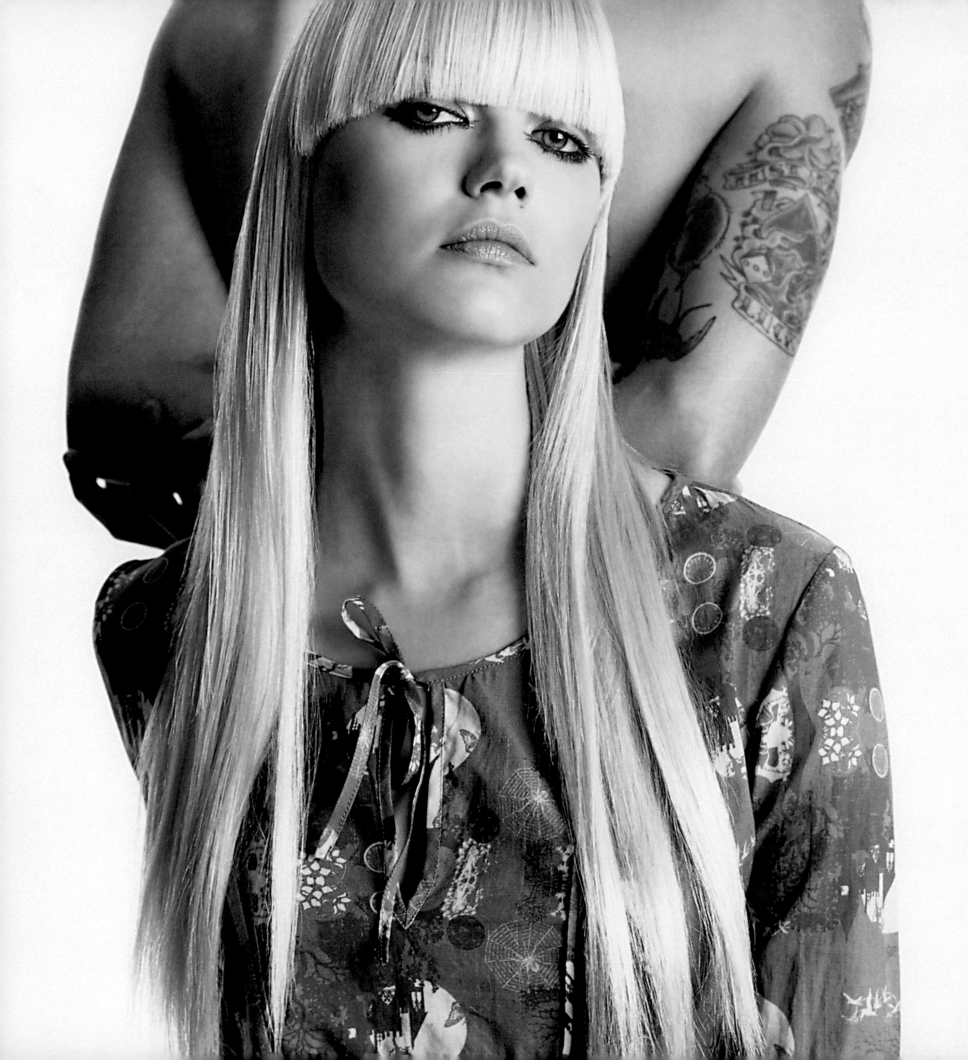

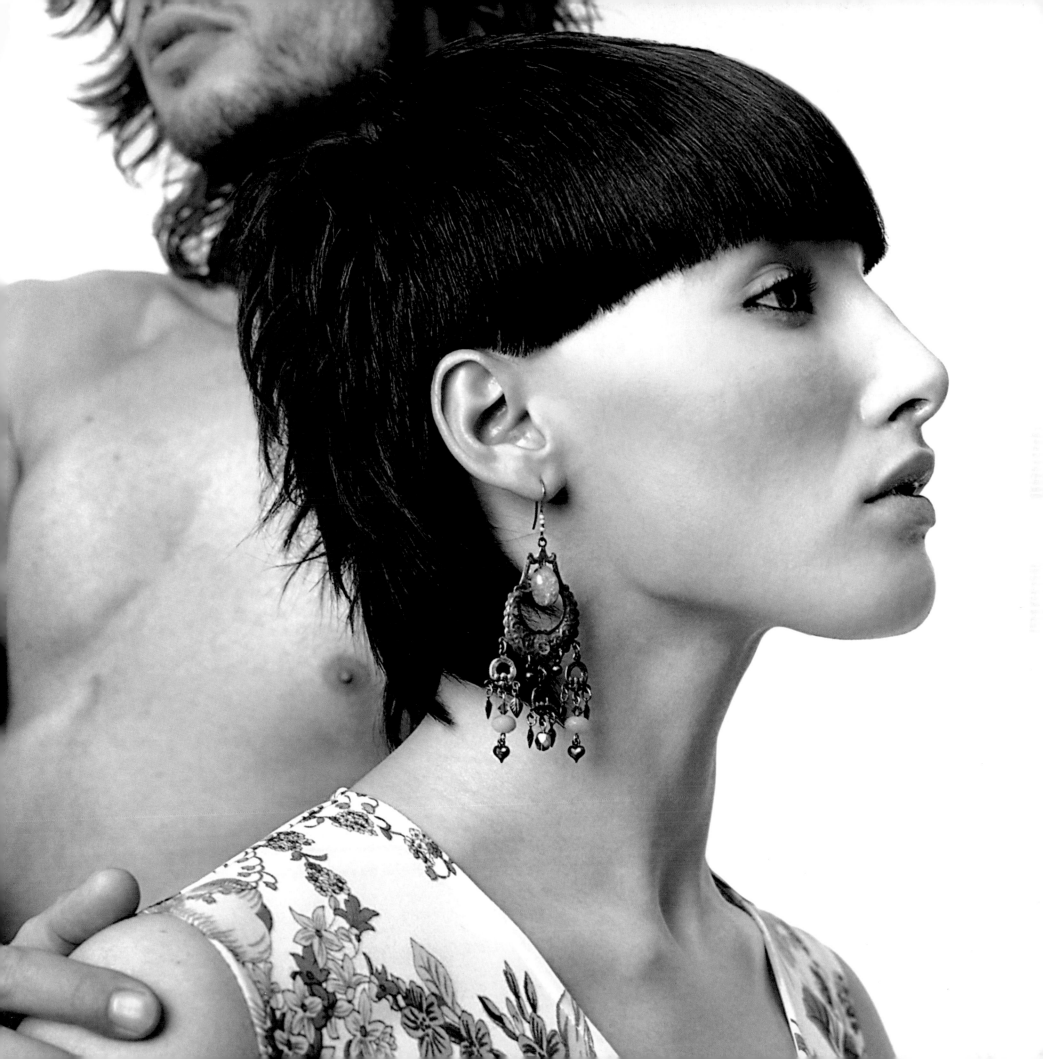

SERGIO BOSSI pages 156–157

38 rue Baron Le Roy, 75012 Paris, France, www.sergiobossi.fr

Hair: Sylver and Sophie
Salon: Sergio Bossi
Make-up: Vesna
Styling: Bruno Guiot
Photography: Stéphane Gizard

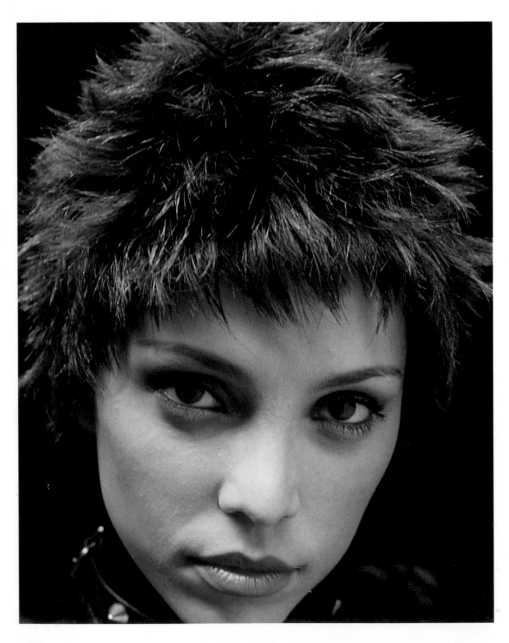

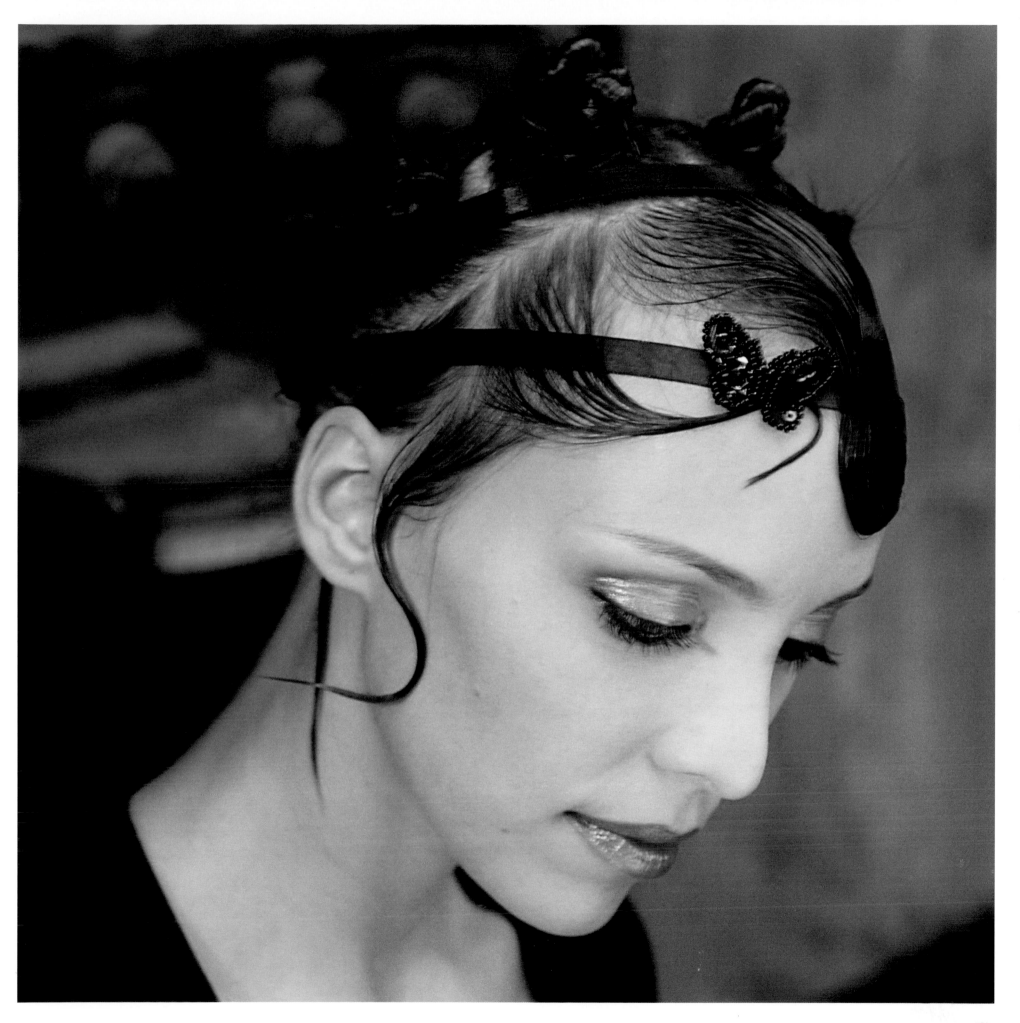

KIND INC pages 158–159

351bld blf, 3-5-1 Jingumae, Shibuya-ku, Tokyo 150-0001, Japan, www.hair-kind.co.jp

Hair: Kind Inc
Salon: Kind Inc

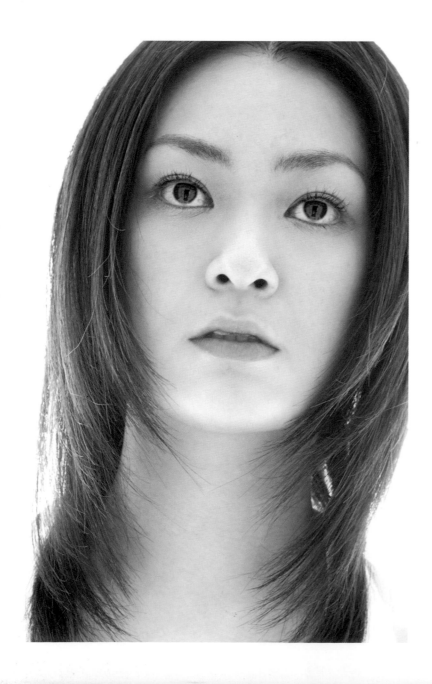

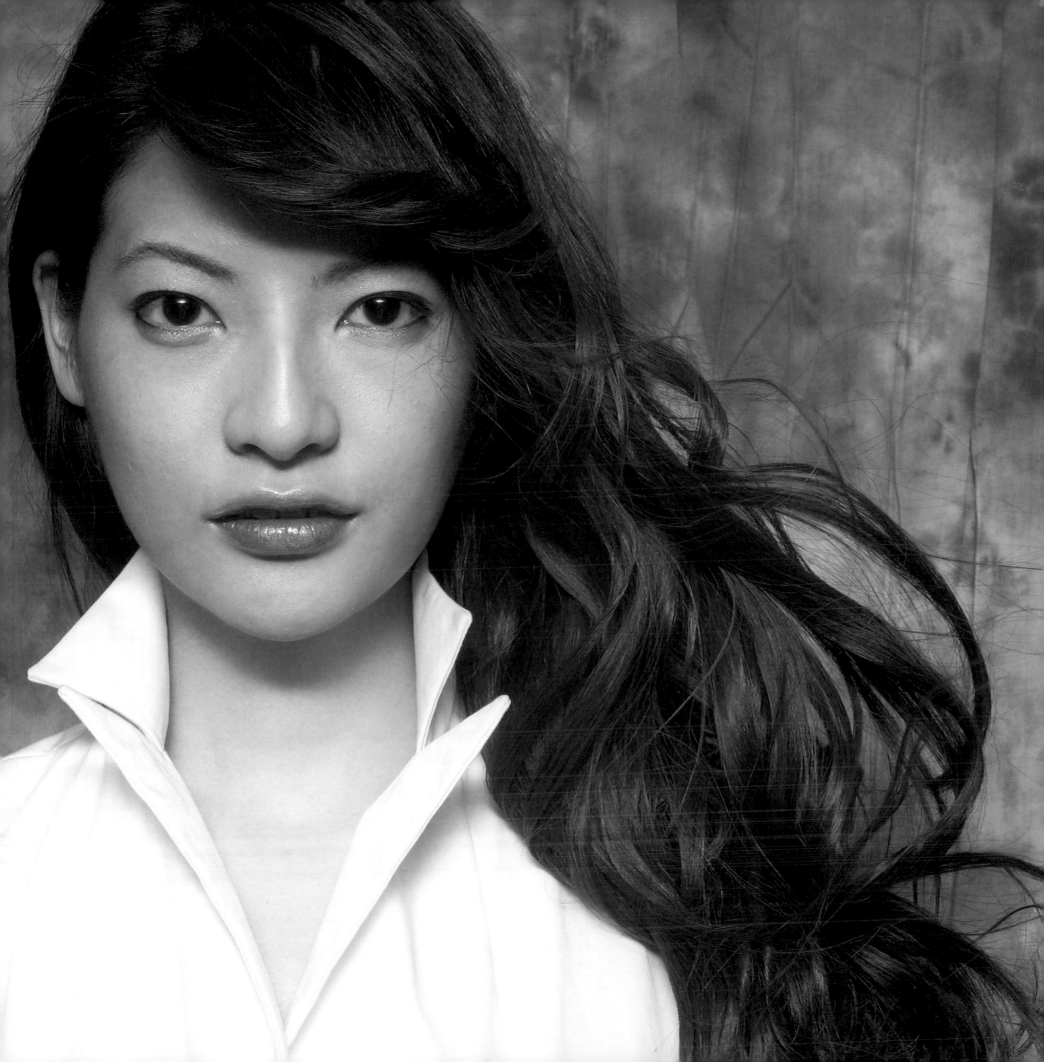

BUOY pages 160–169

Skeye Garden, Majestic Tower, 100 Willis Street, Wellington, New Zealand, www.buoy.co.nz

Hair: Derek Elvy
Salon: Buoy
Make-up: Michelle Perry (p. 161, 162, 163, 167, 168, 169) Claudine Stace (p. 164 - 166)
Styling: Laura Ming Wong
Photography: Meek Zuiderwyk
Post Production: Andy Salisbury
Models: Sally Anne Moffat and Sonia Burn @The Agencie
Products: Sebastian International

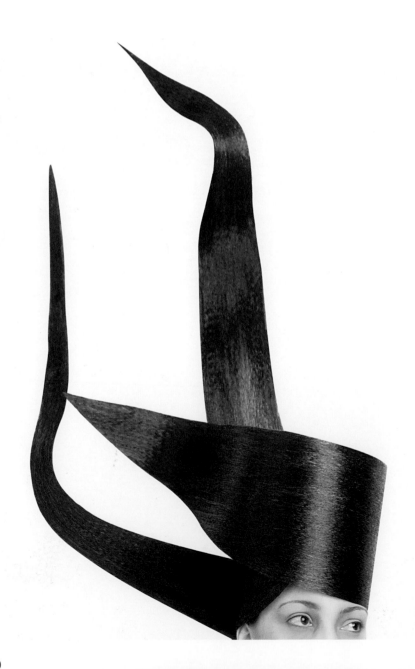

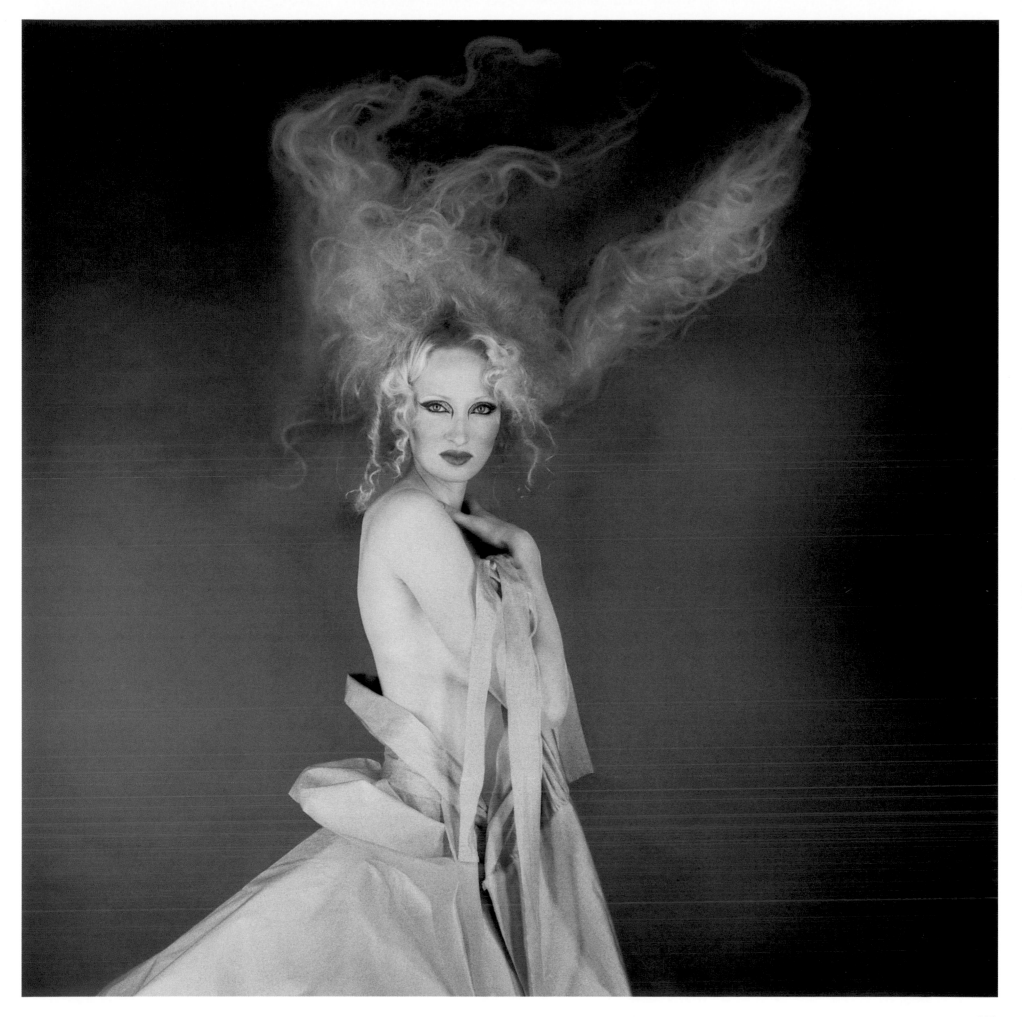

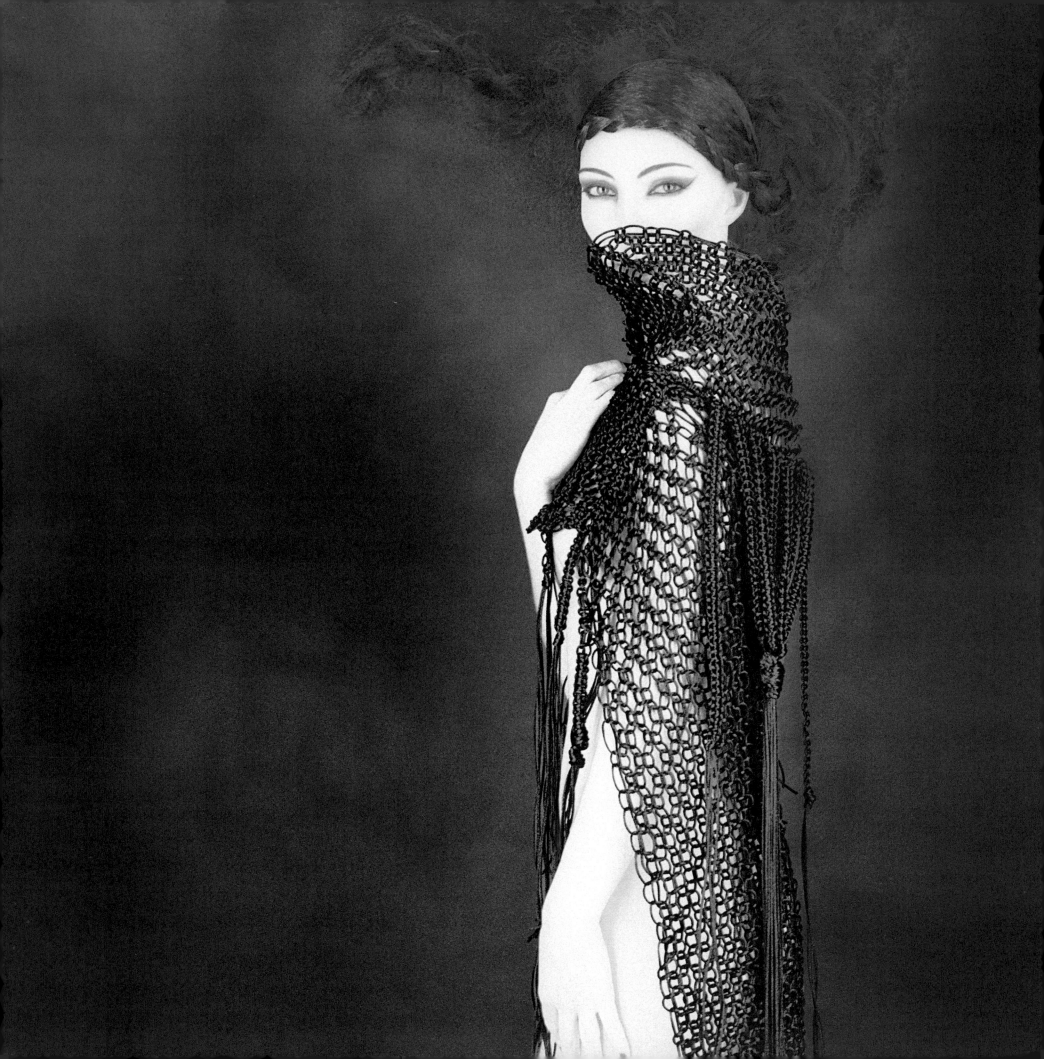

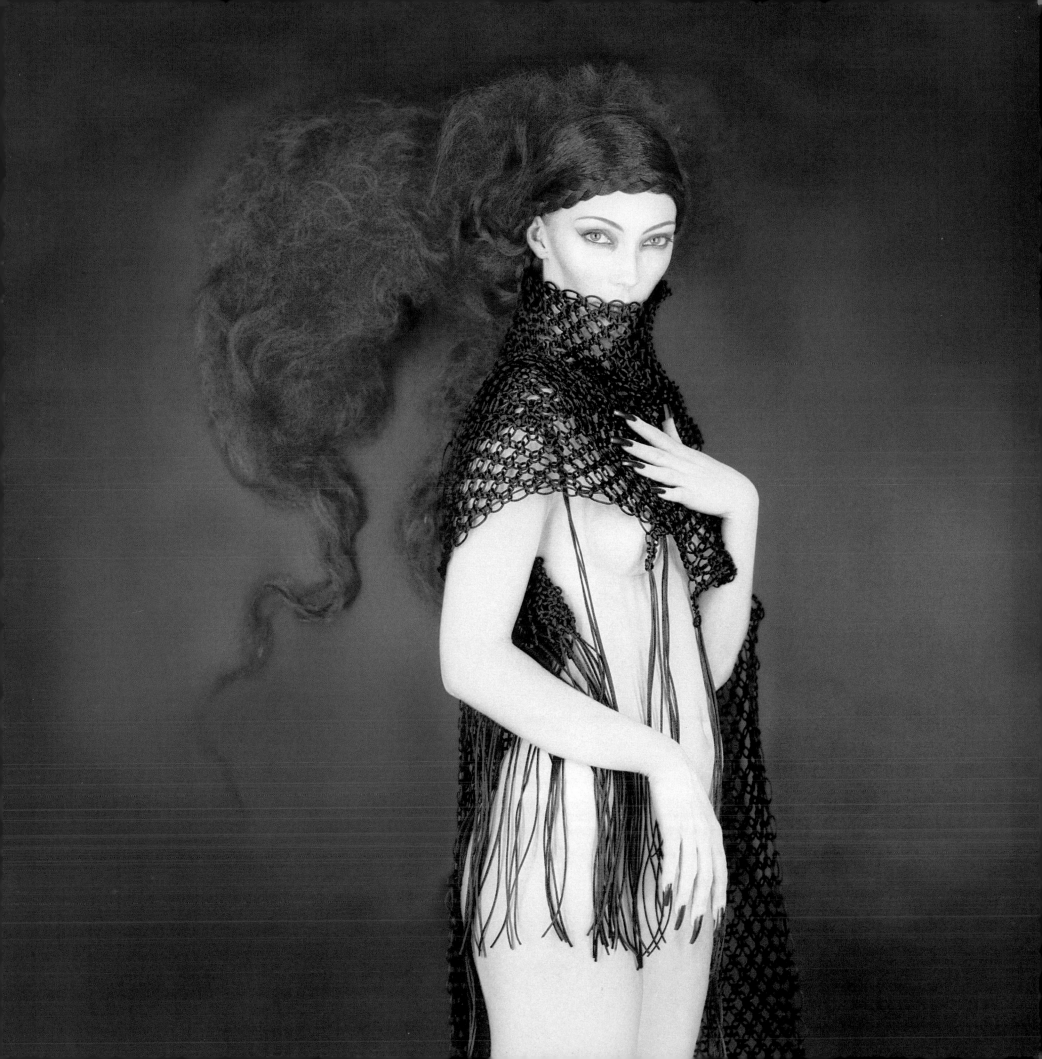

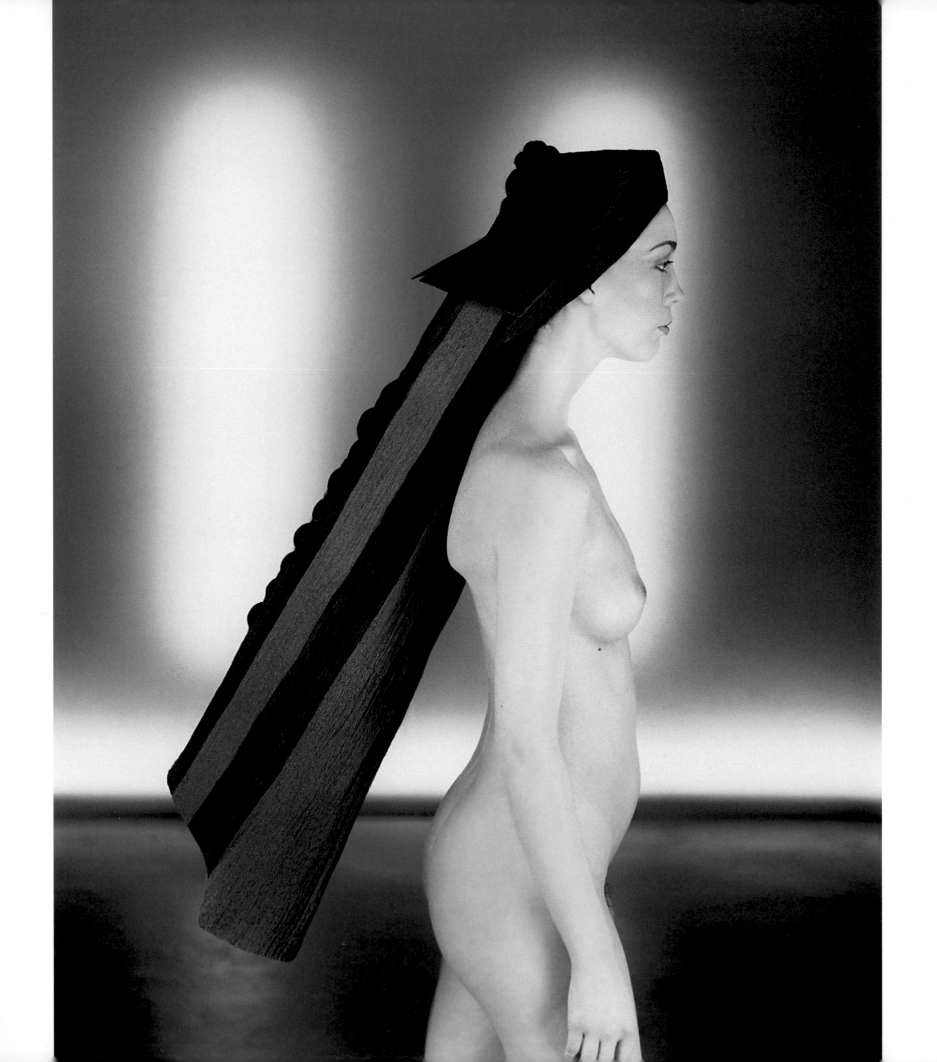

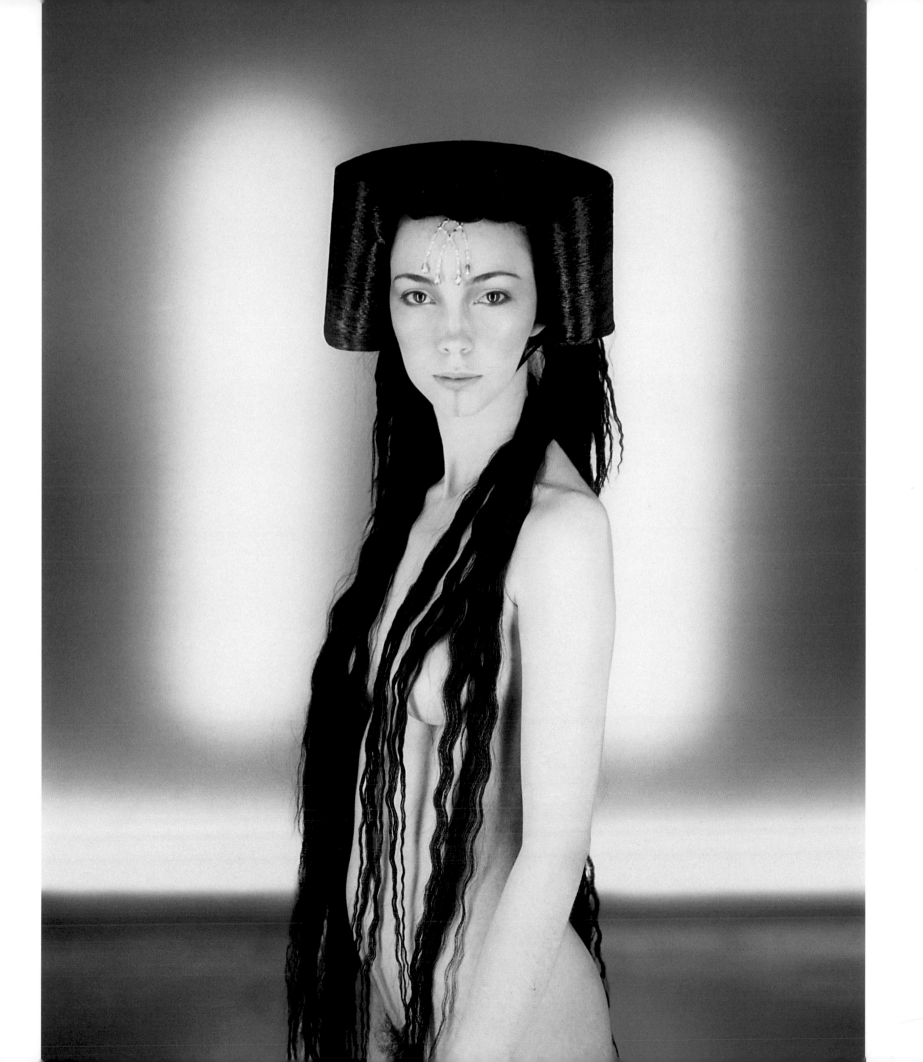

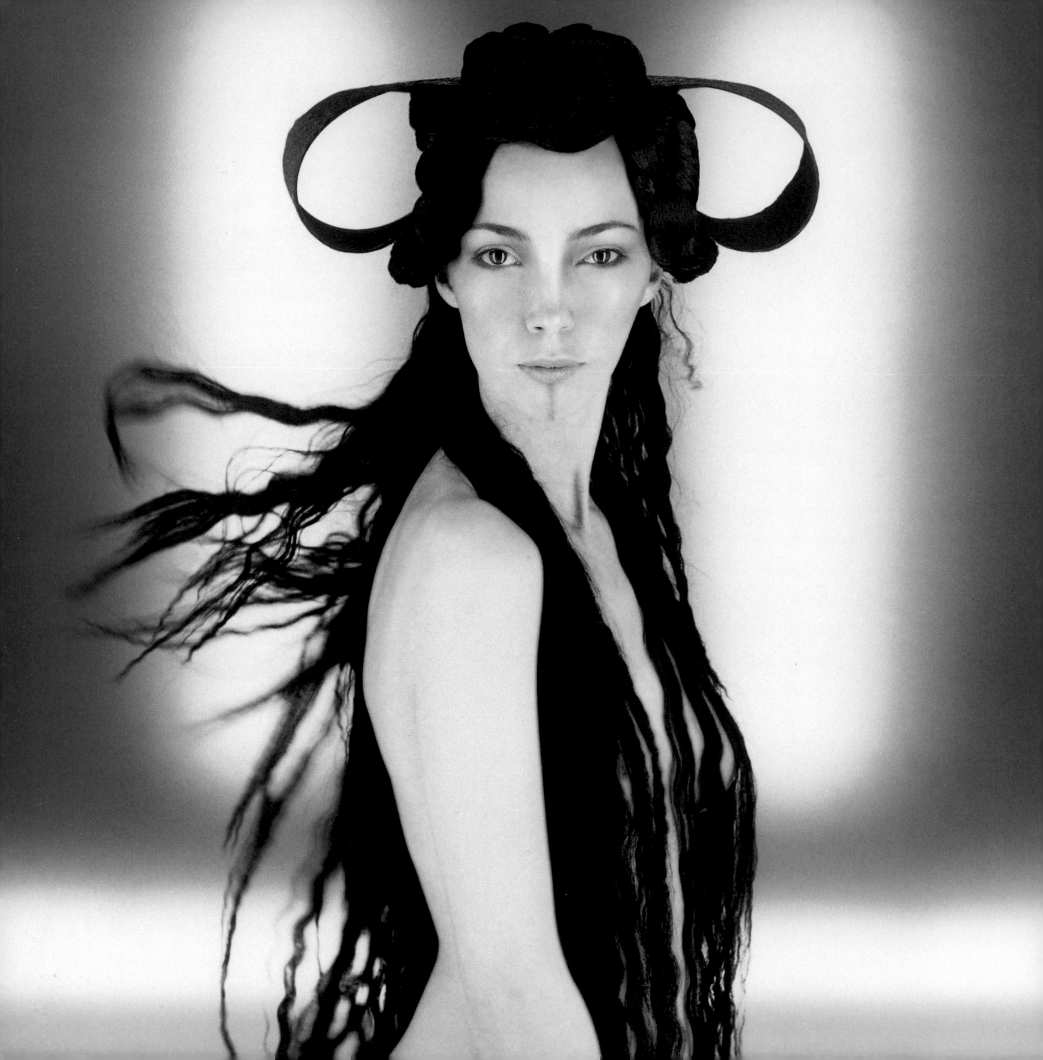

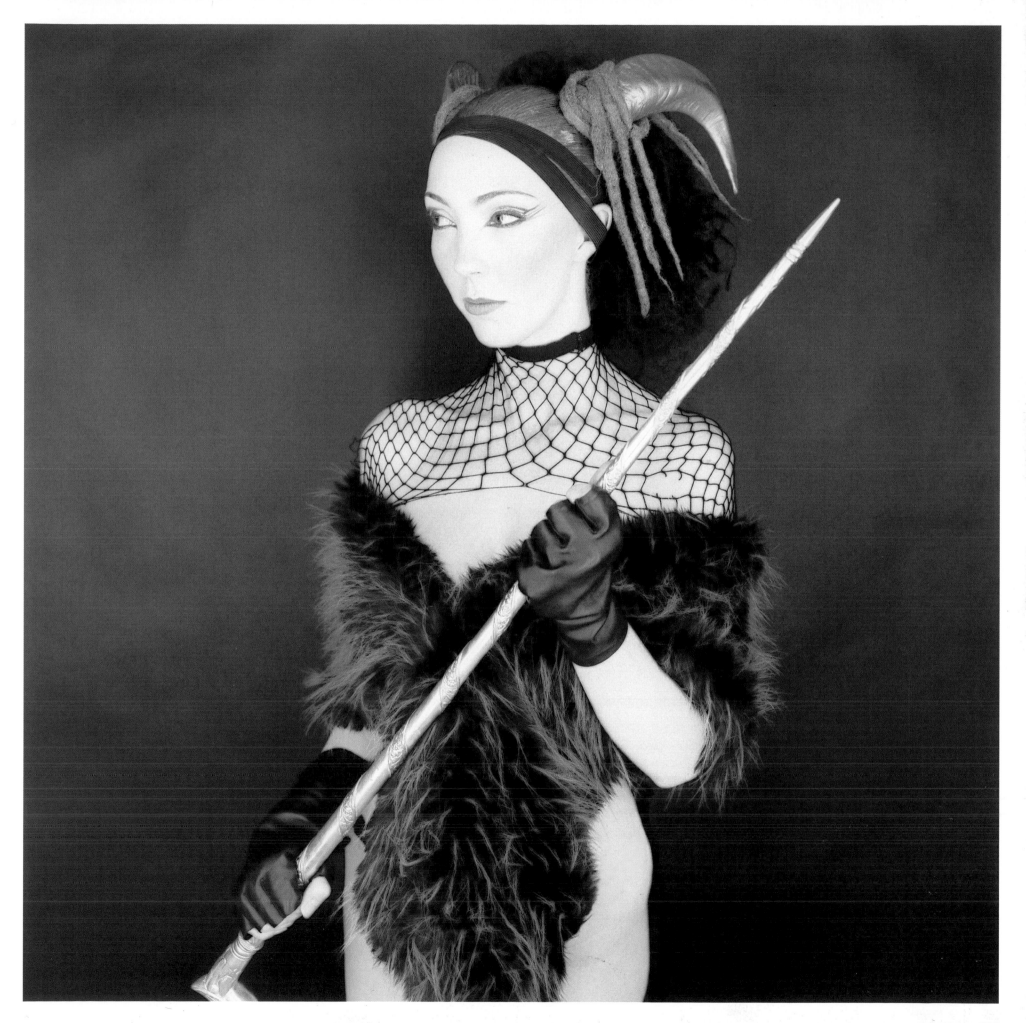

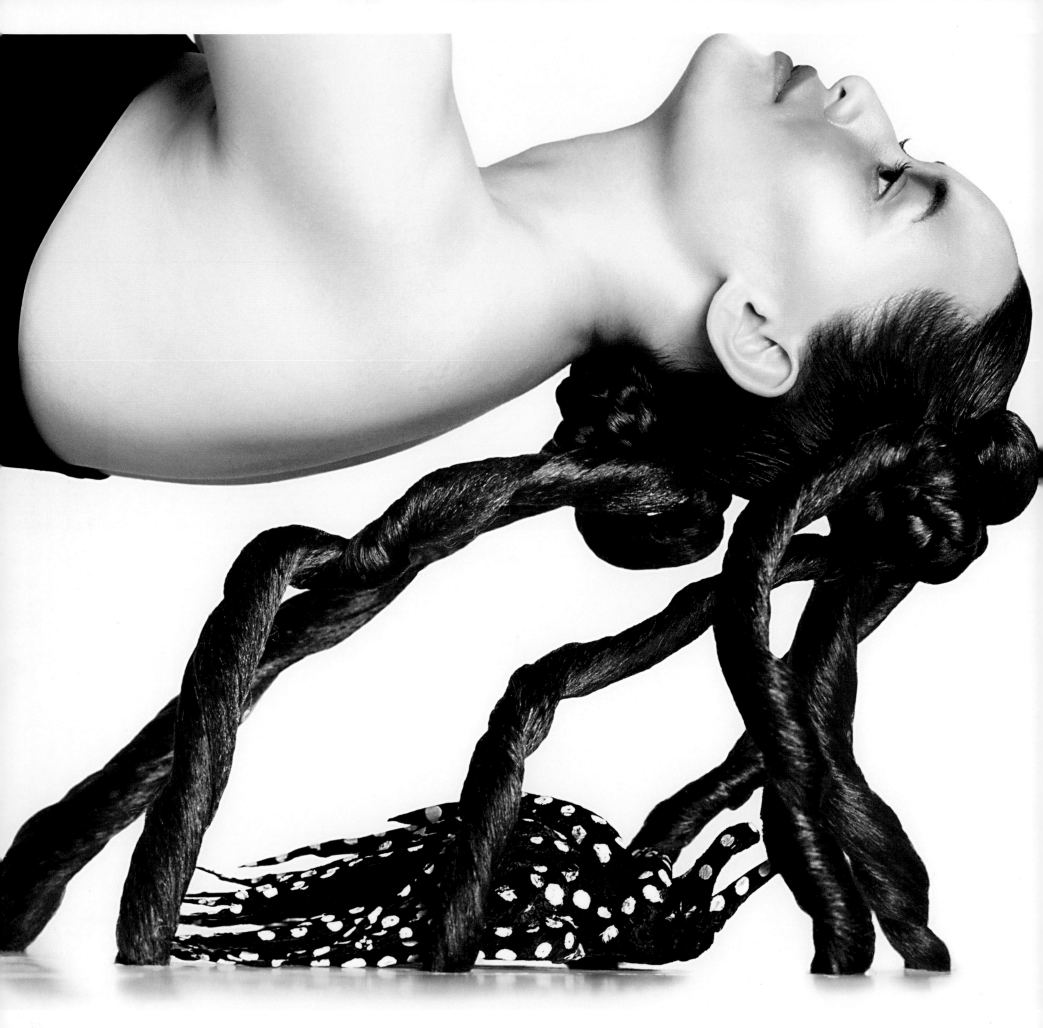

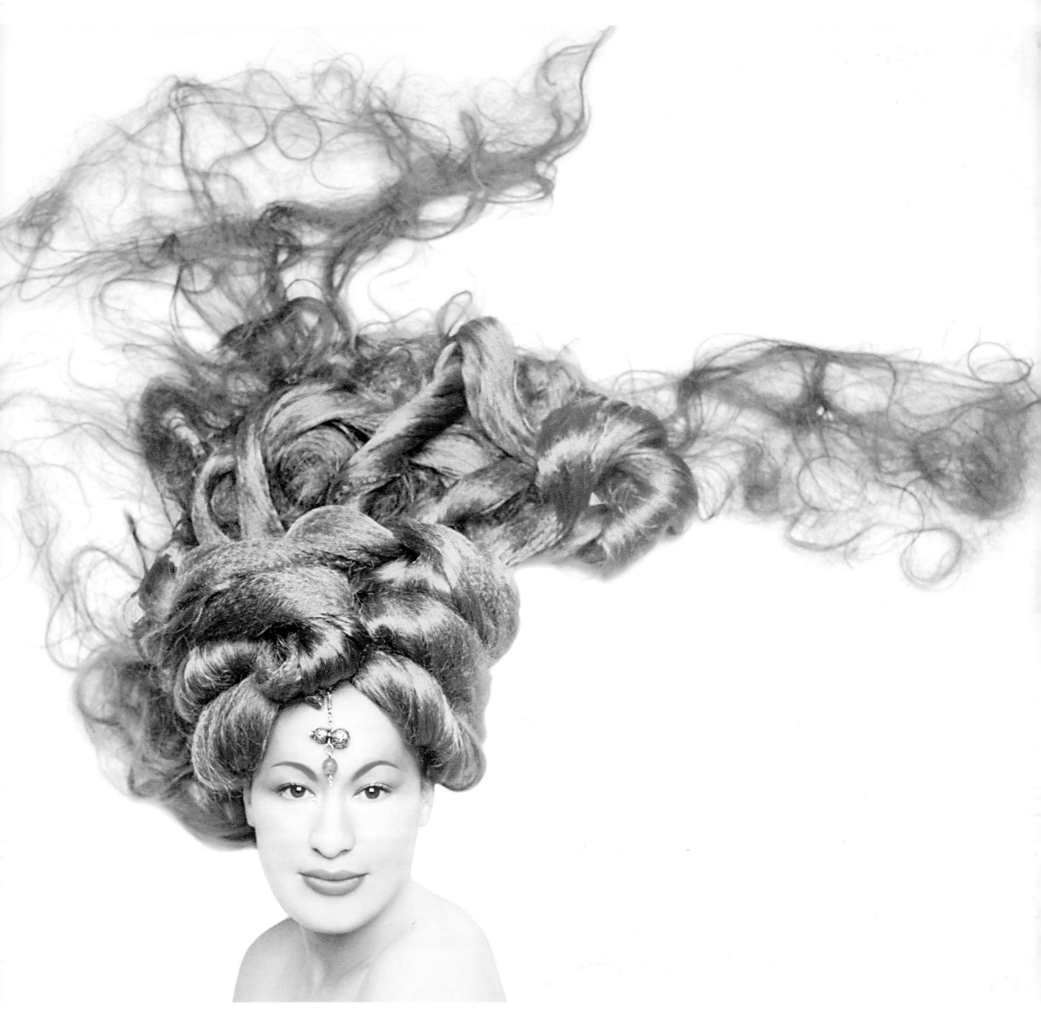

TWISTAR LTD. pages 170–173
189 Ridell Road, Glendowie, Auckland, New Zealand

Hair: Jo May, Durham Hair, Auckland
Make-up: Kathy Lang
Photography: Kelly Loveridge, ECT Photography
Products: Schwarzkopf, Osis product range, Twistar for Professional

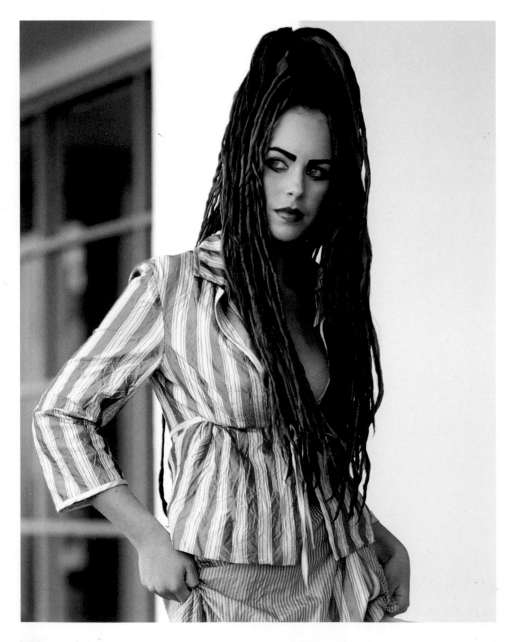

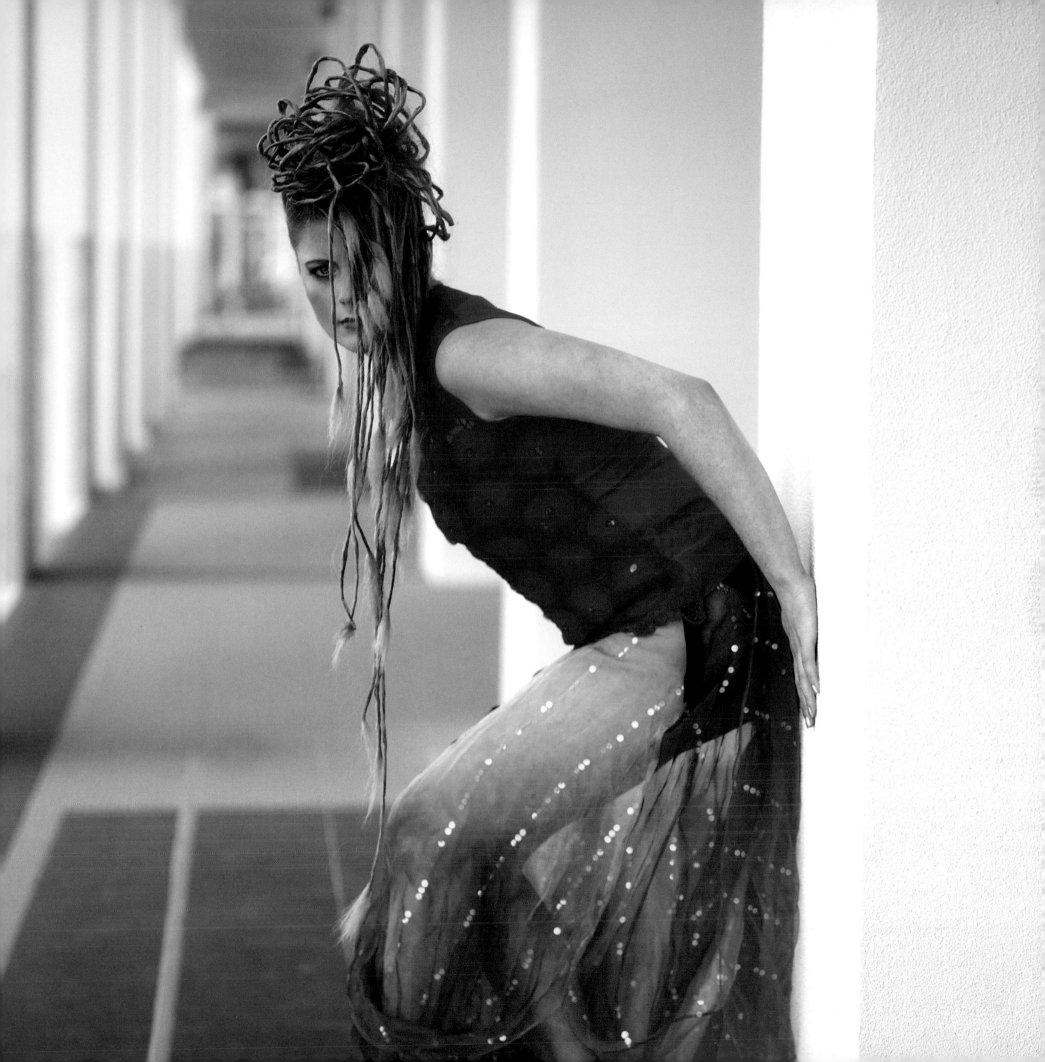

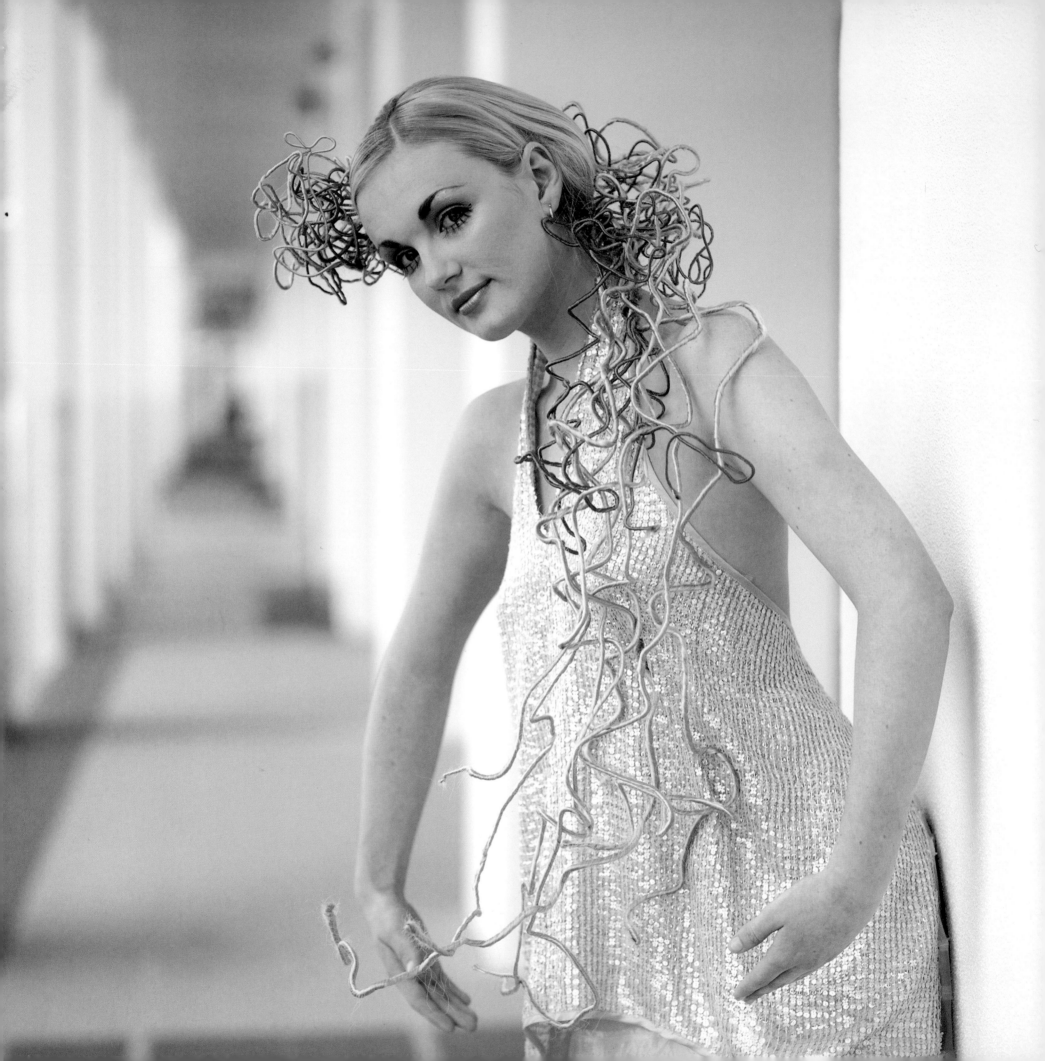

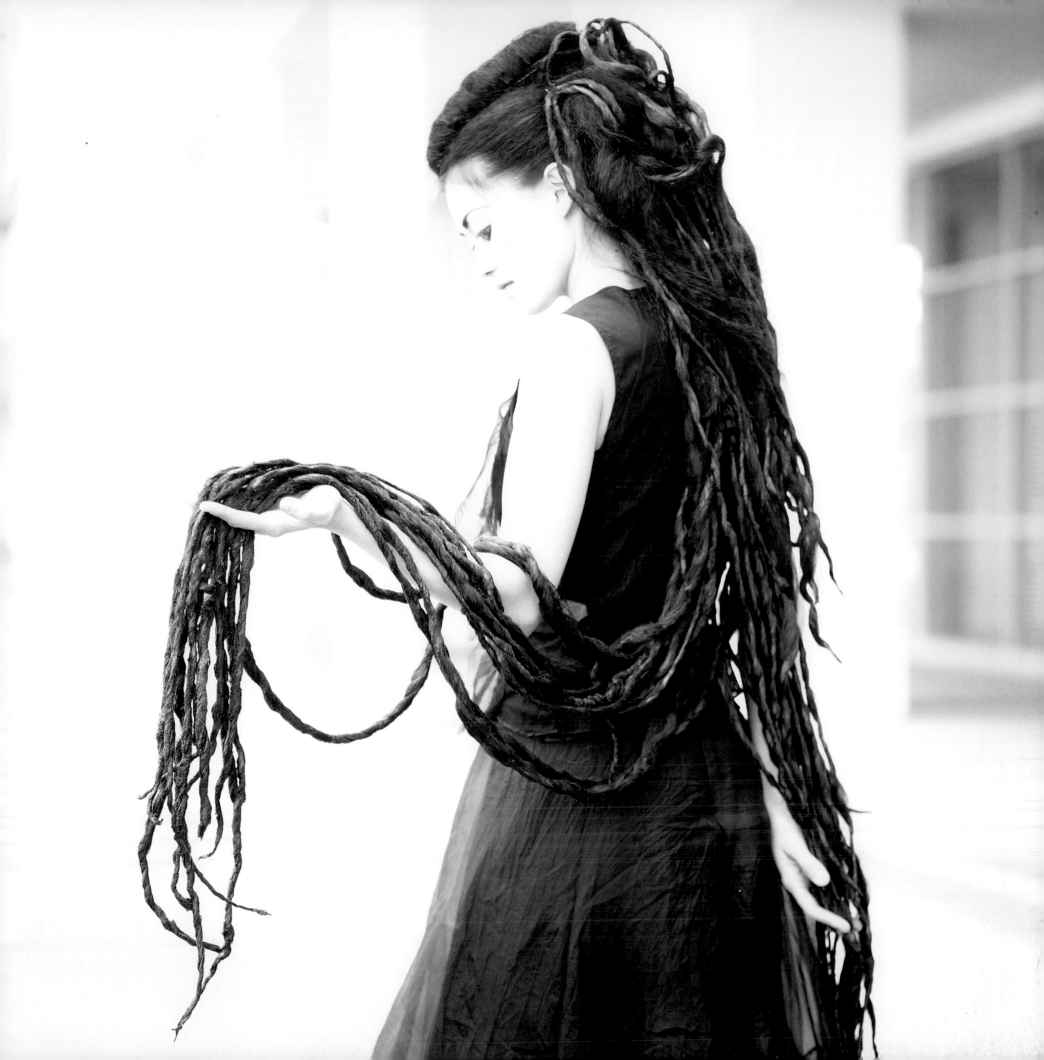

RUDY HADISUWARNO pages 174–177

Rudy Hadisuwarno Organisation, Puri Pesanggrahan IV/NR 7, Bukit Cinere Indah, Jakarta 16514, Indonesia

Hair: Rudy Hadisuwarno Team Art, Gunawan Hadisuwarno and Sonny Soesanto for Rudy Hadisuwarno Team Art
Make-up: Rudy Hadisuwarno Team Art and Sonny Soesanto for Rudy Hadisuwarno Team Art
Styling: Rika from Rudy Hadisuwarno Team Art
Photography: Gerard Adhiwidjaja
Model Agency: Morzell International, We Production, Model Ola: Collection from The Book of Styles 2003
Model Nisa: Collection from Seminar Trend 2003 Bandung
Products: Rudy Hadisuwarno Cosmetics

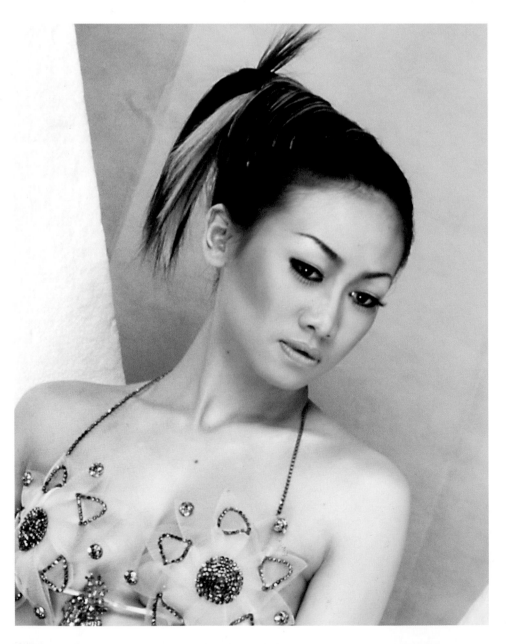

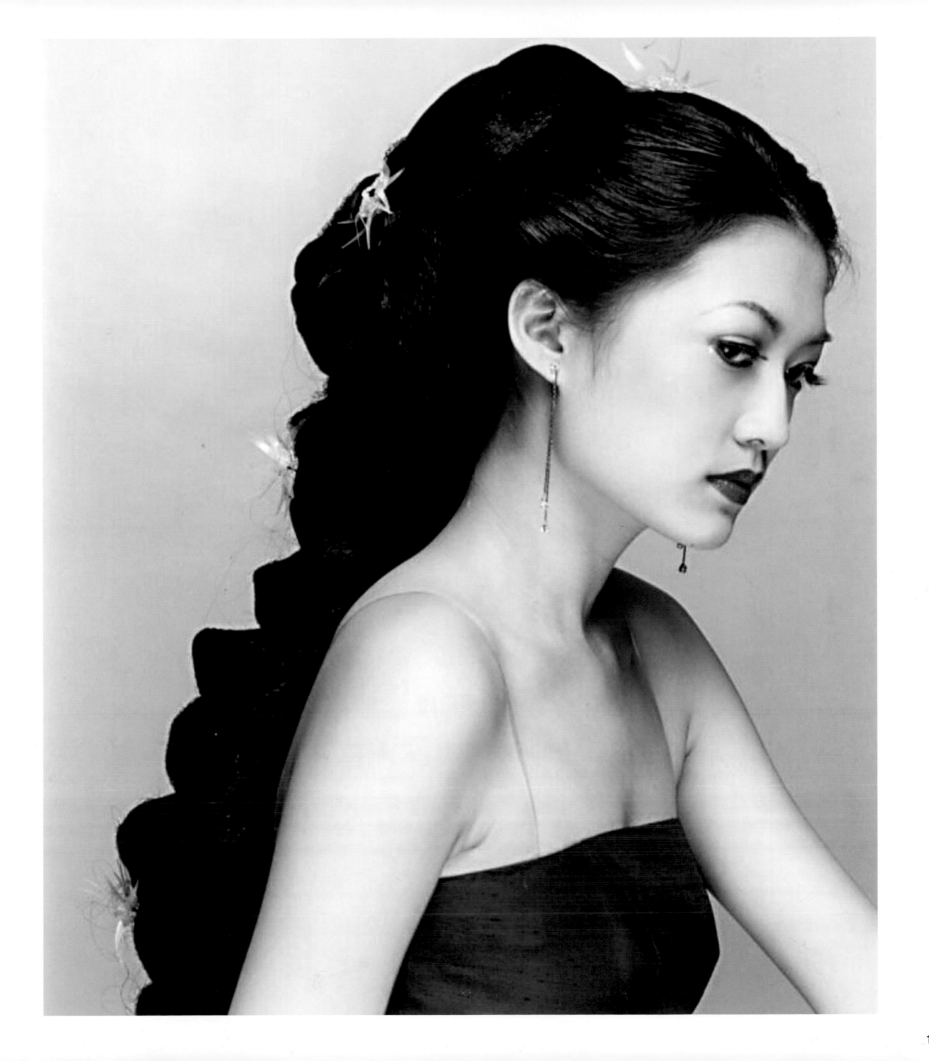

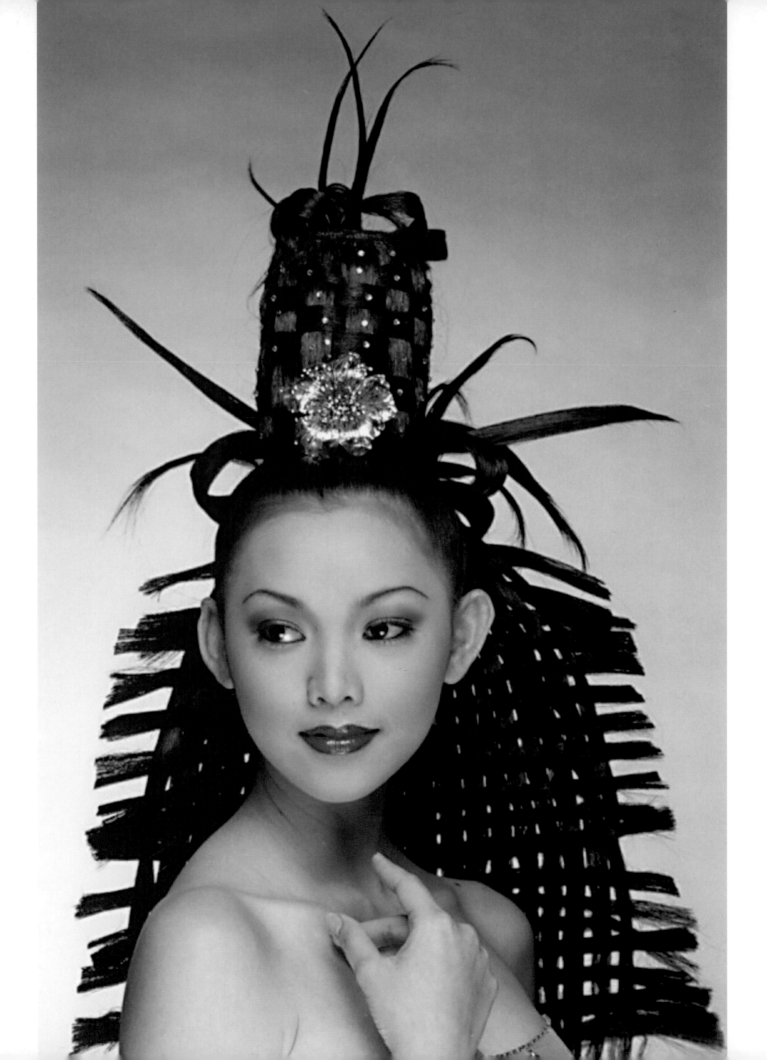

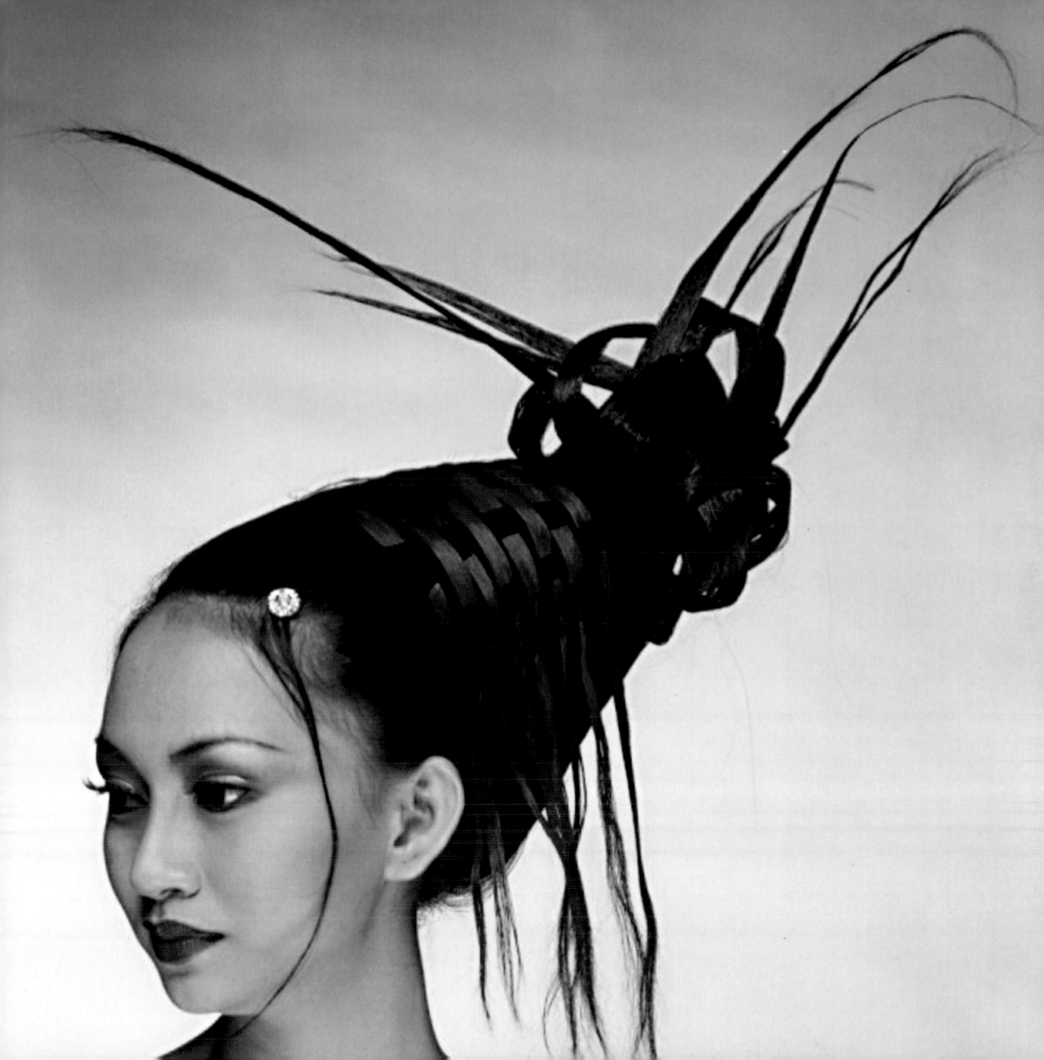

CARLOS GÁLICO pages 178–179

P° Eduardo Dato N 2, 28010 Madrid, Spain, www.carlosgalico.com

Hair: Carlos Gálico
Make-up: Carlos Gálico
Photography: Carlos Gálico

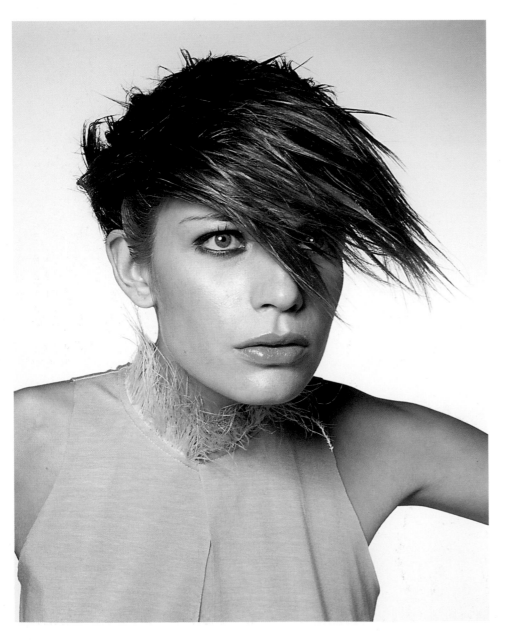
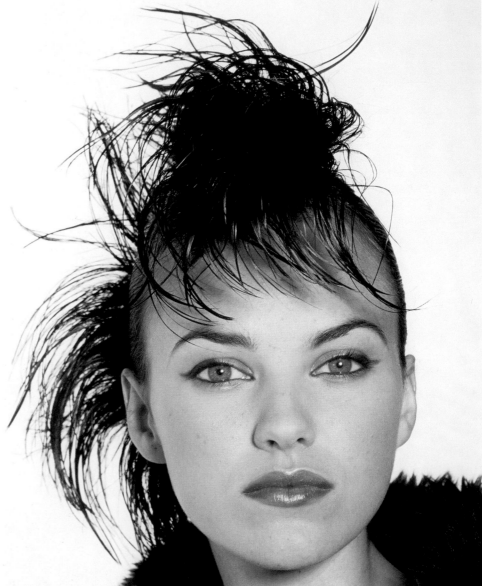

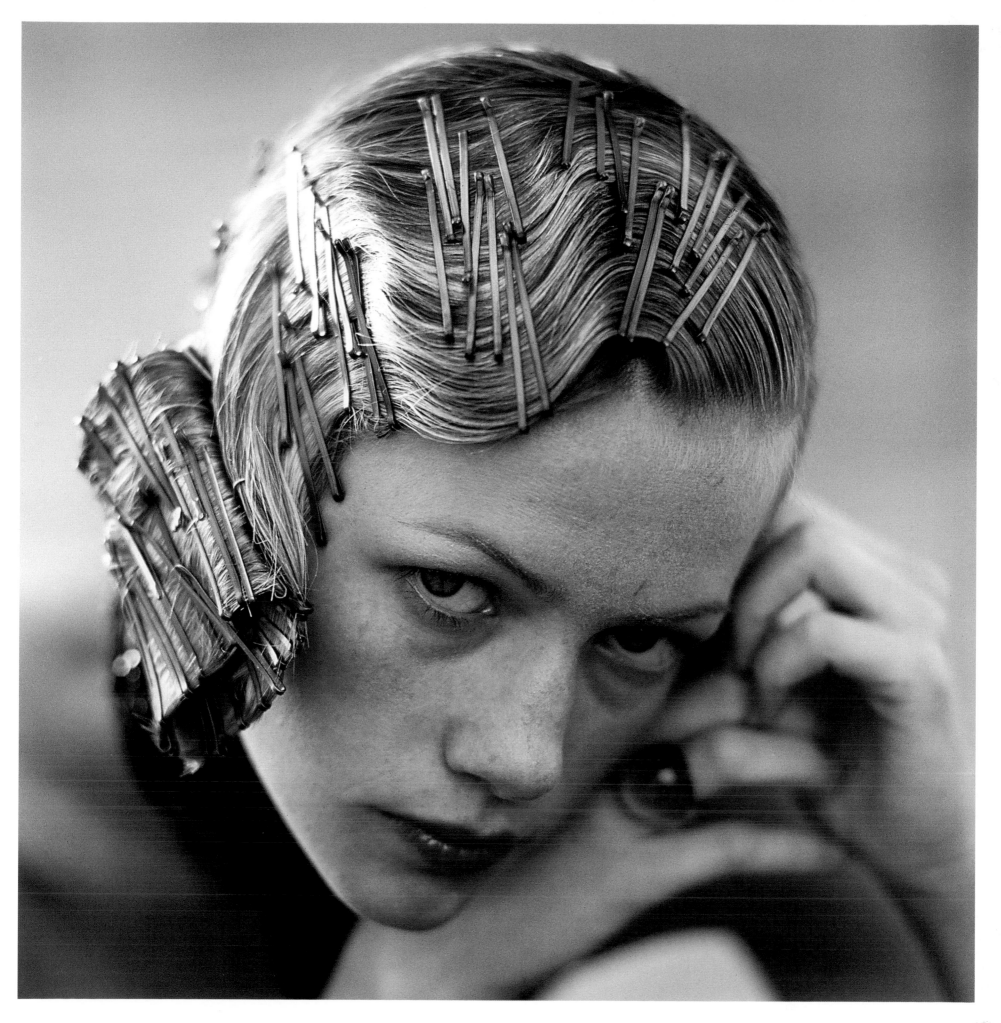

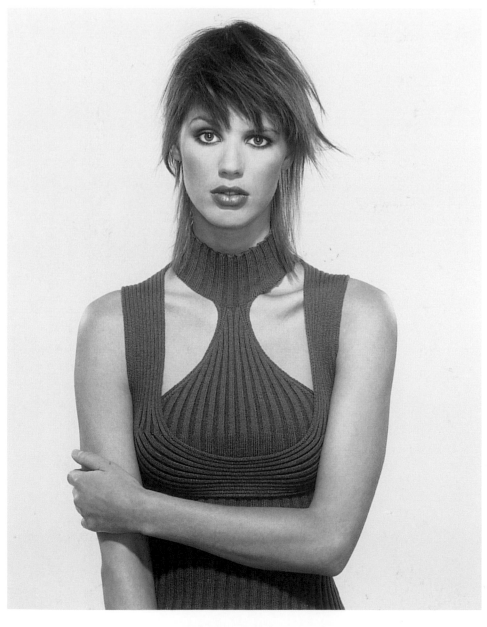
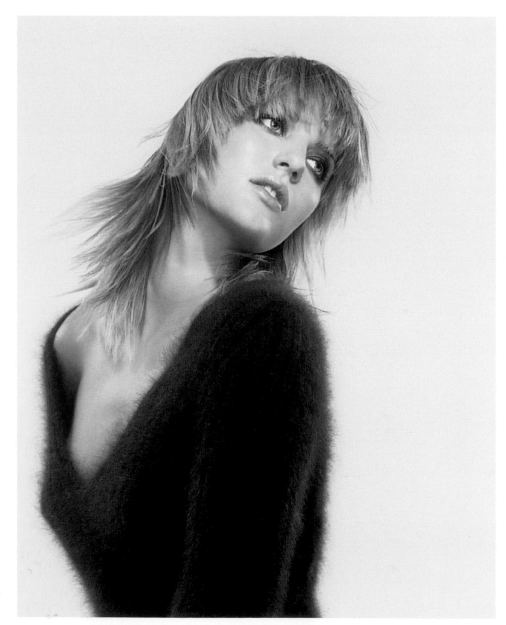

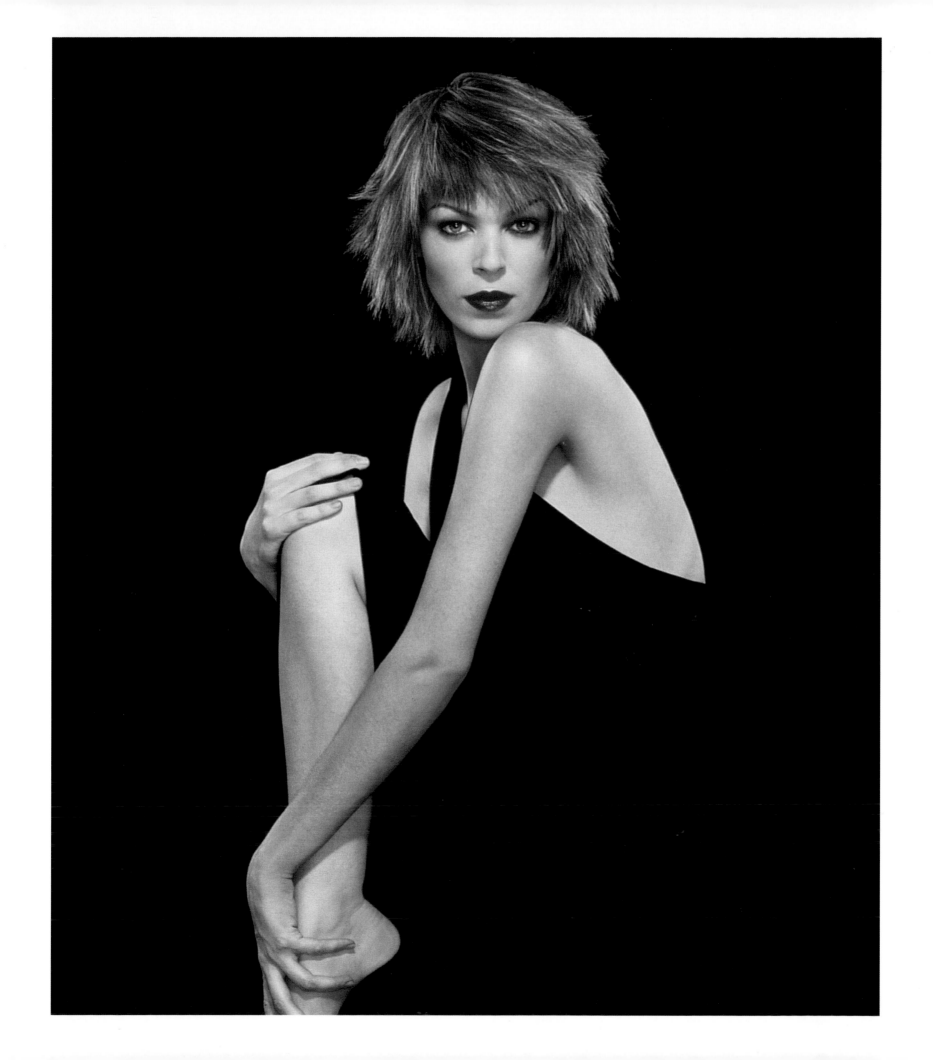

Hair: Stylist Kapanov Team
Salon: Stylist Kapanov
Make-up: Gulia Angelova, Roumen Tchakurov
Photography: Raditch Banev
Model Agency: Vizages
Products: Framesi, Kemon

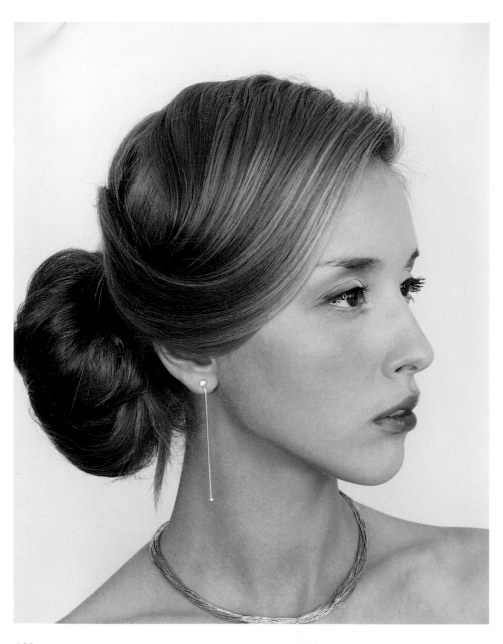

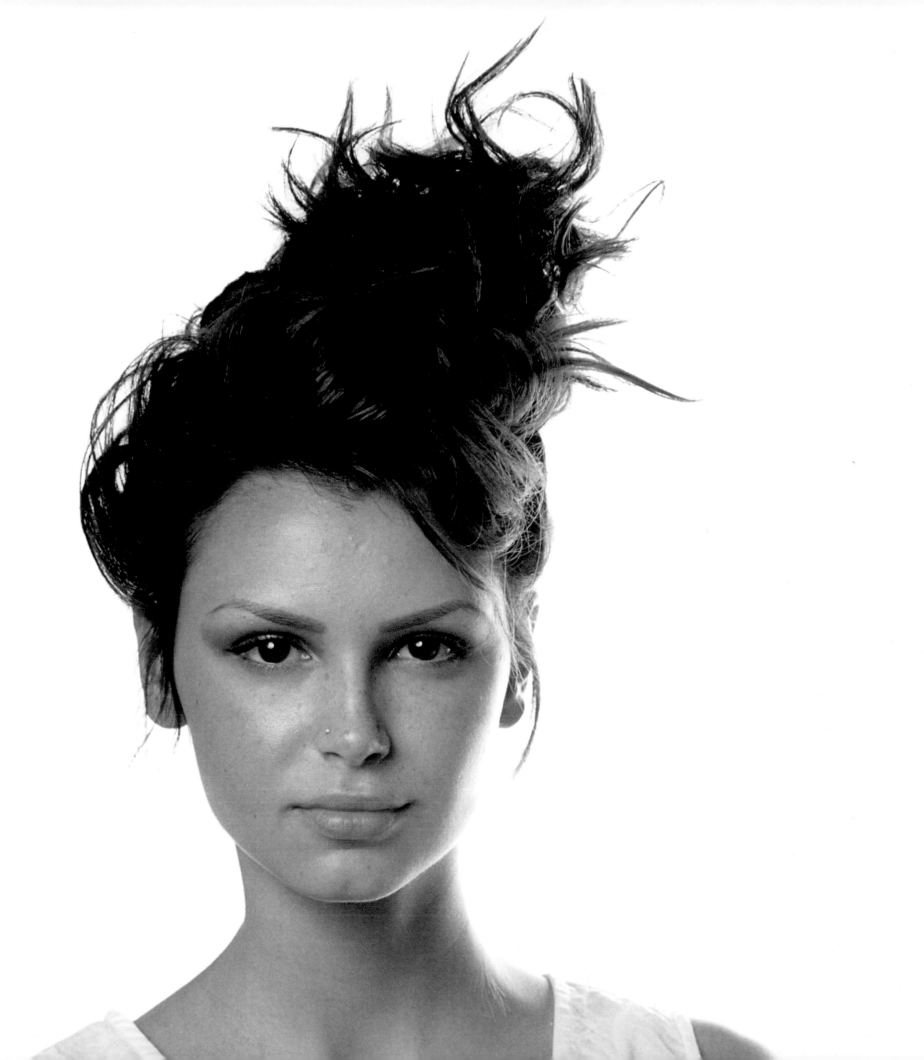

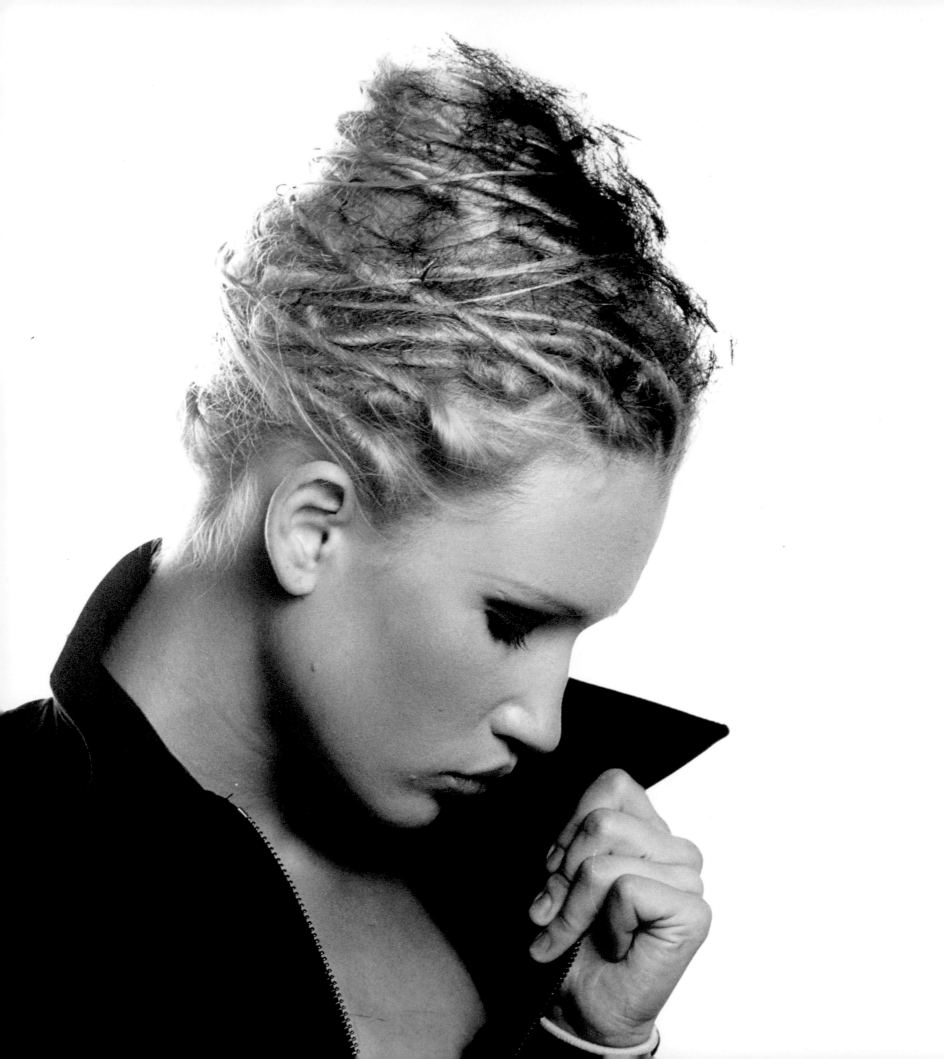

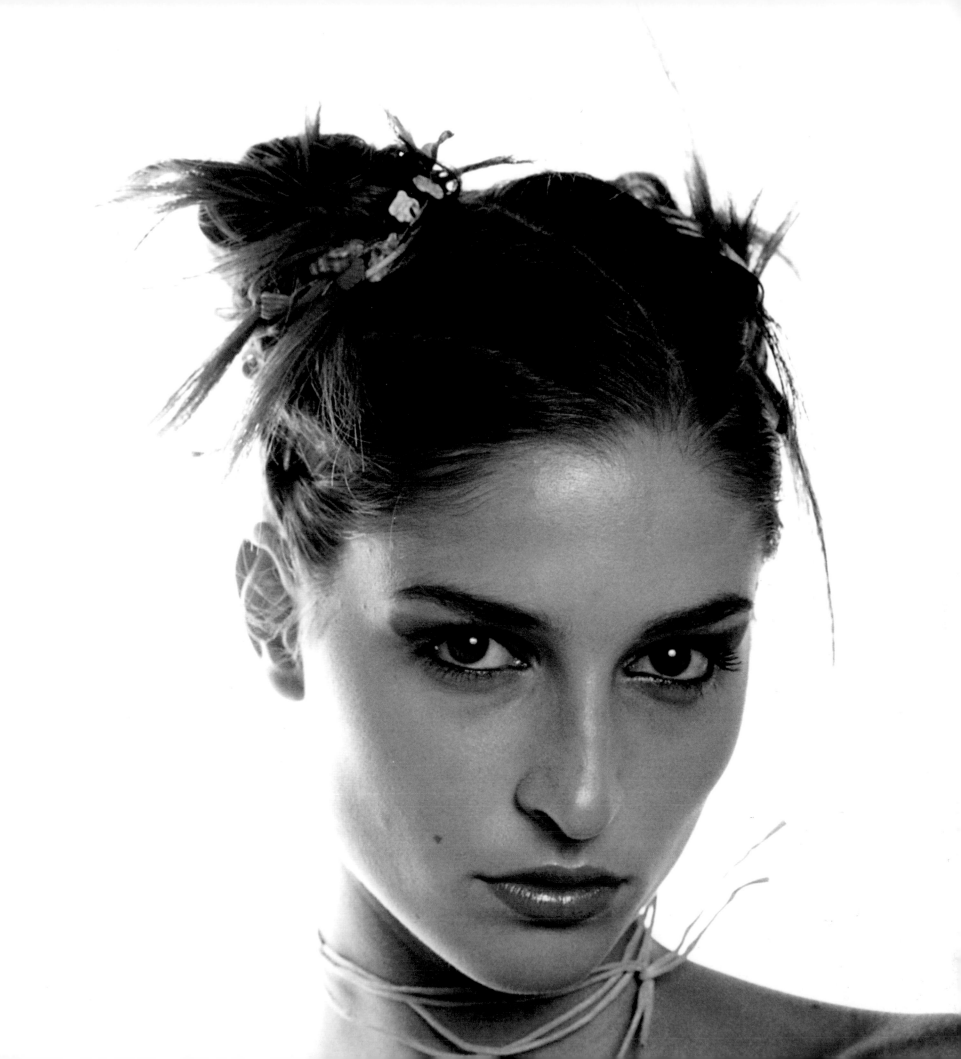

KLAUS PETER OCHS pages 186–191

KPOchs, Orber Straße 30, 60386 Frankfurt am Main, Germany, www.kp-ochs.com

Hair: Klaus Peter Ochs Artistic Team with Corina Böhm and Jean-Michel Faretra
Make-up: Gundrun Müller, Jasmin Heinz (p. 190, 191)
Styling: Hendrik Schaulin, Xenia Bous (p. 190, 191)
Photography: Axel Zajaczek (p. 186, 187)
Products: Wella

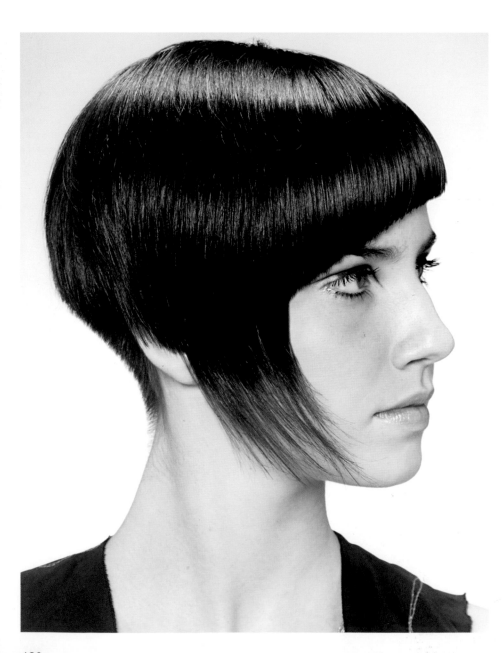

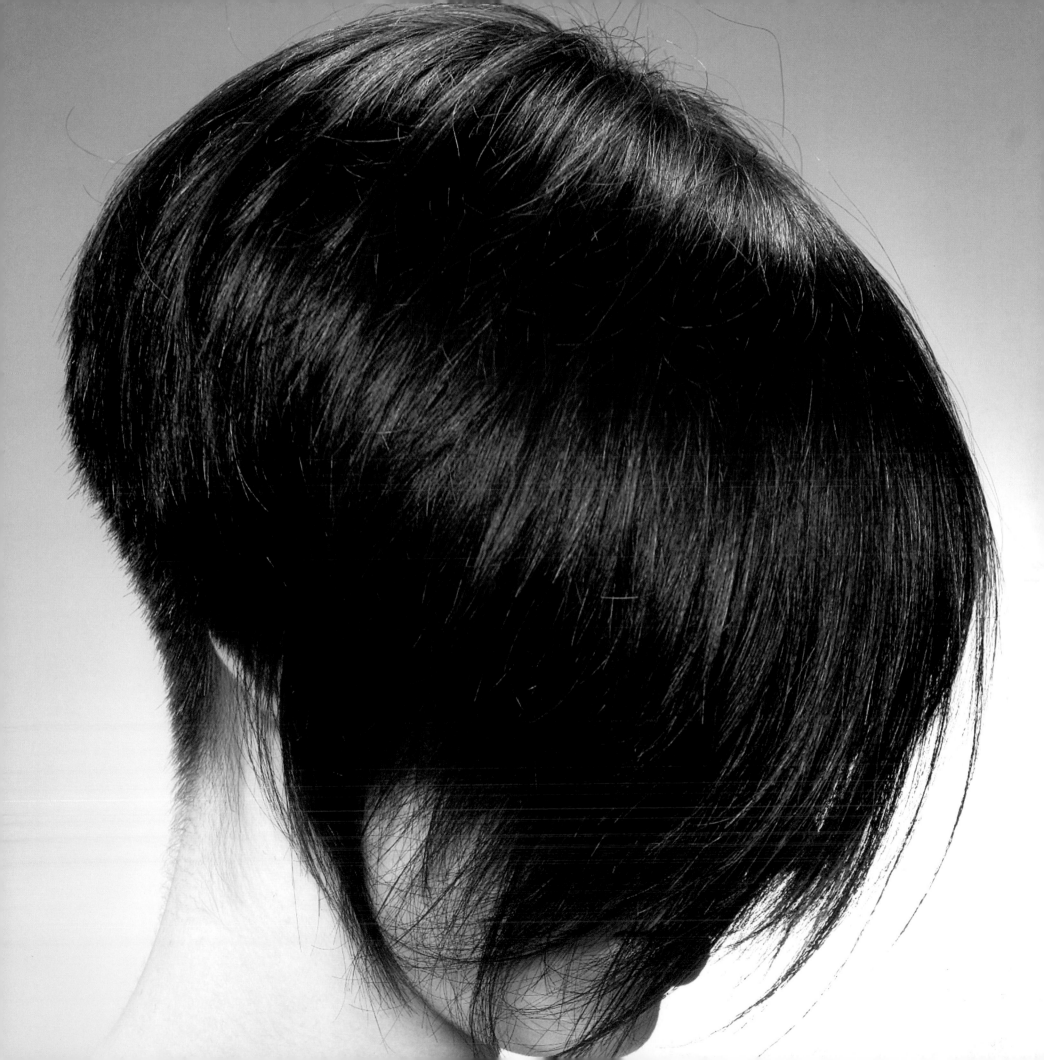

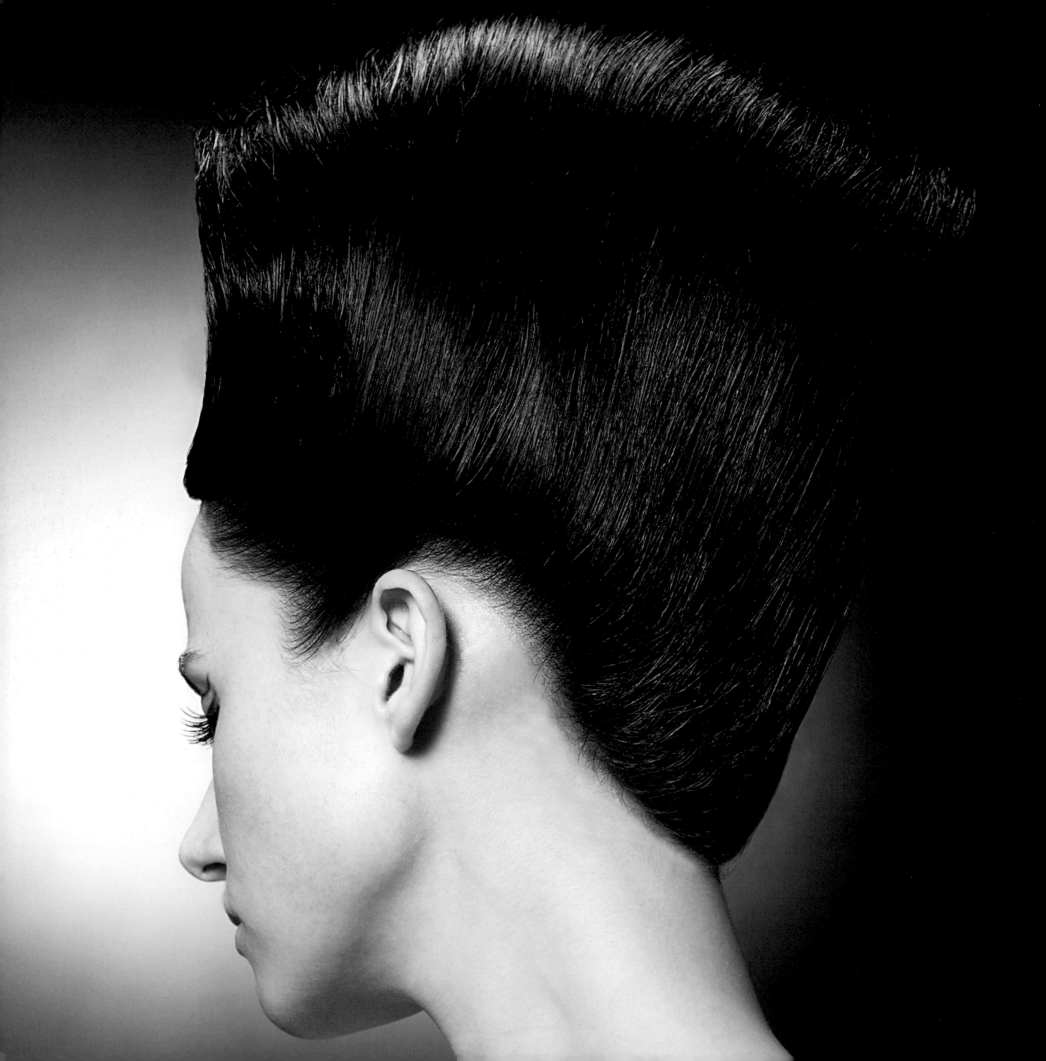

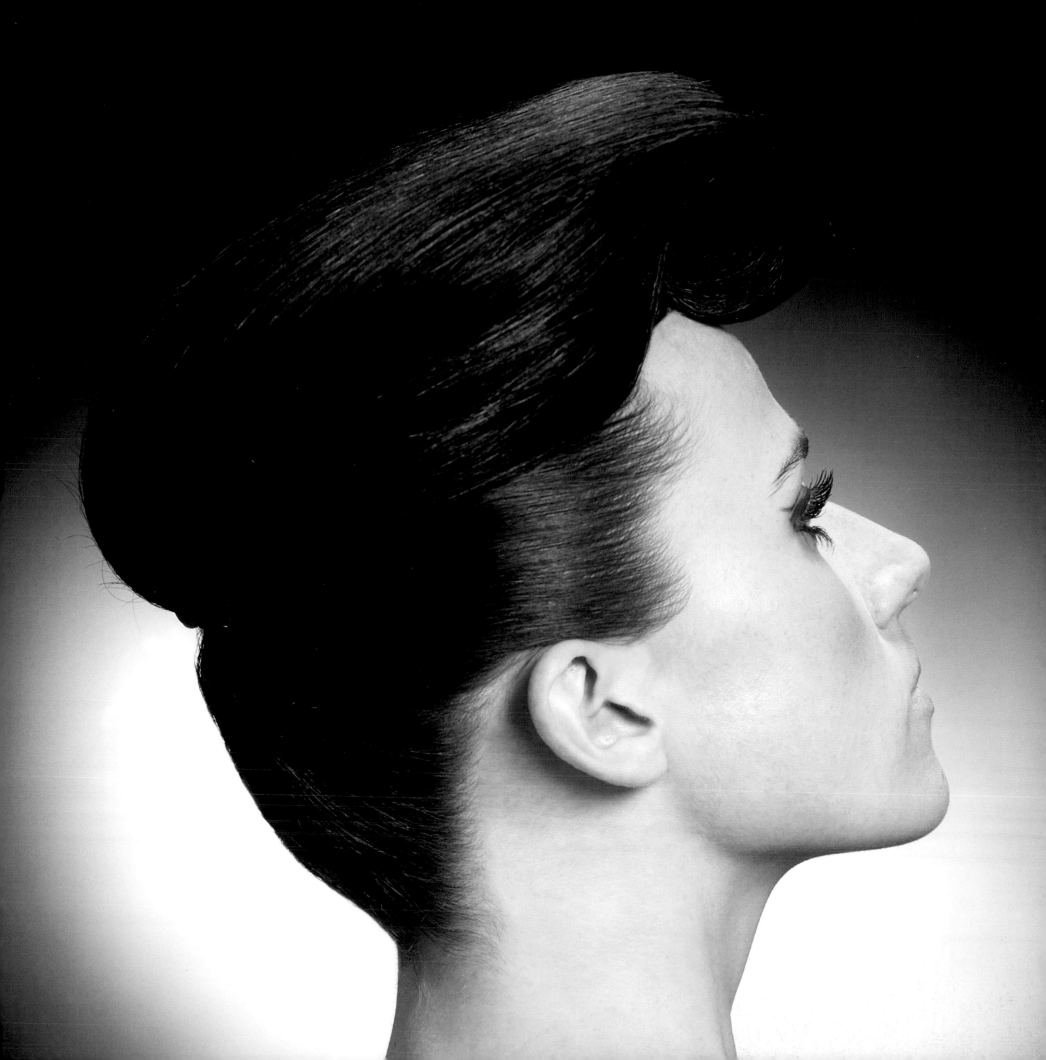

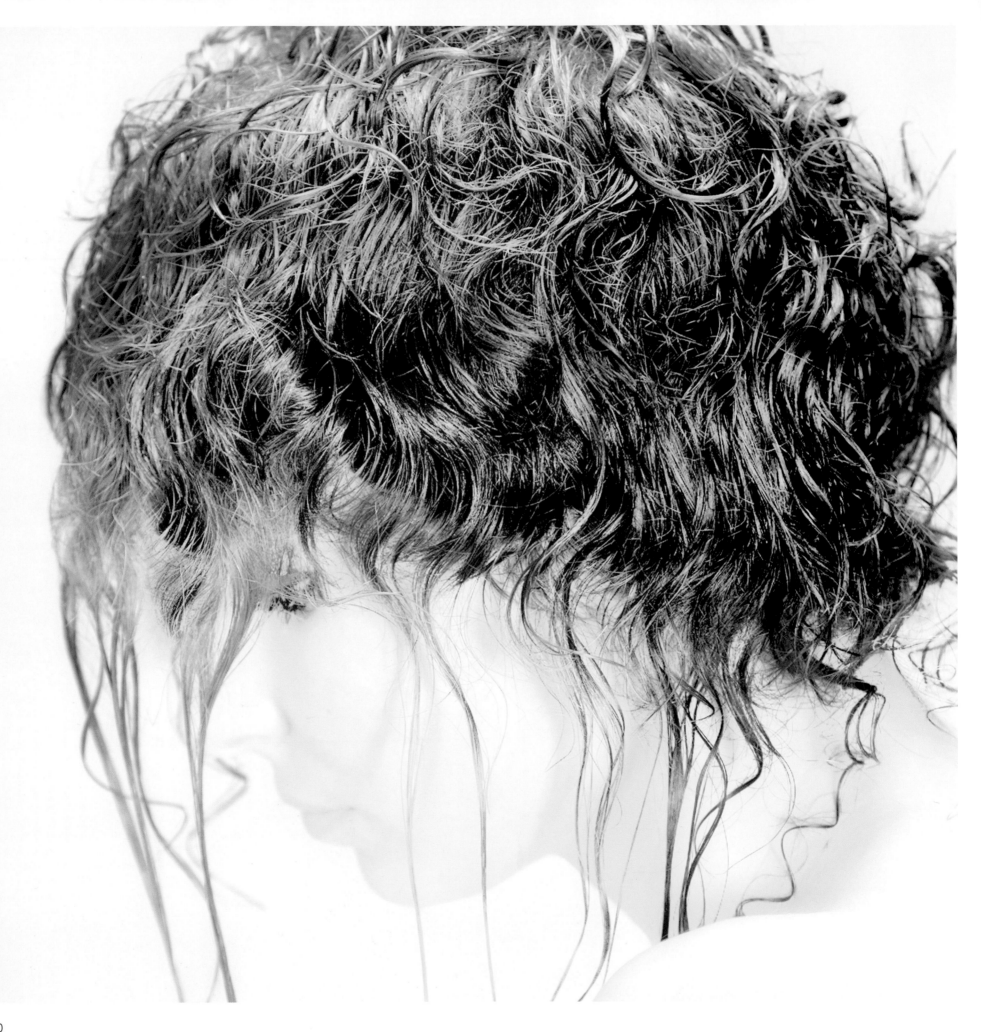

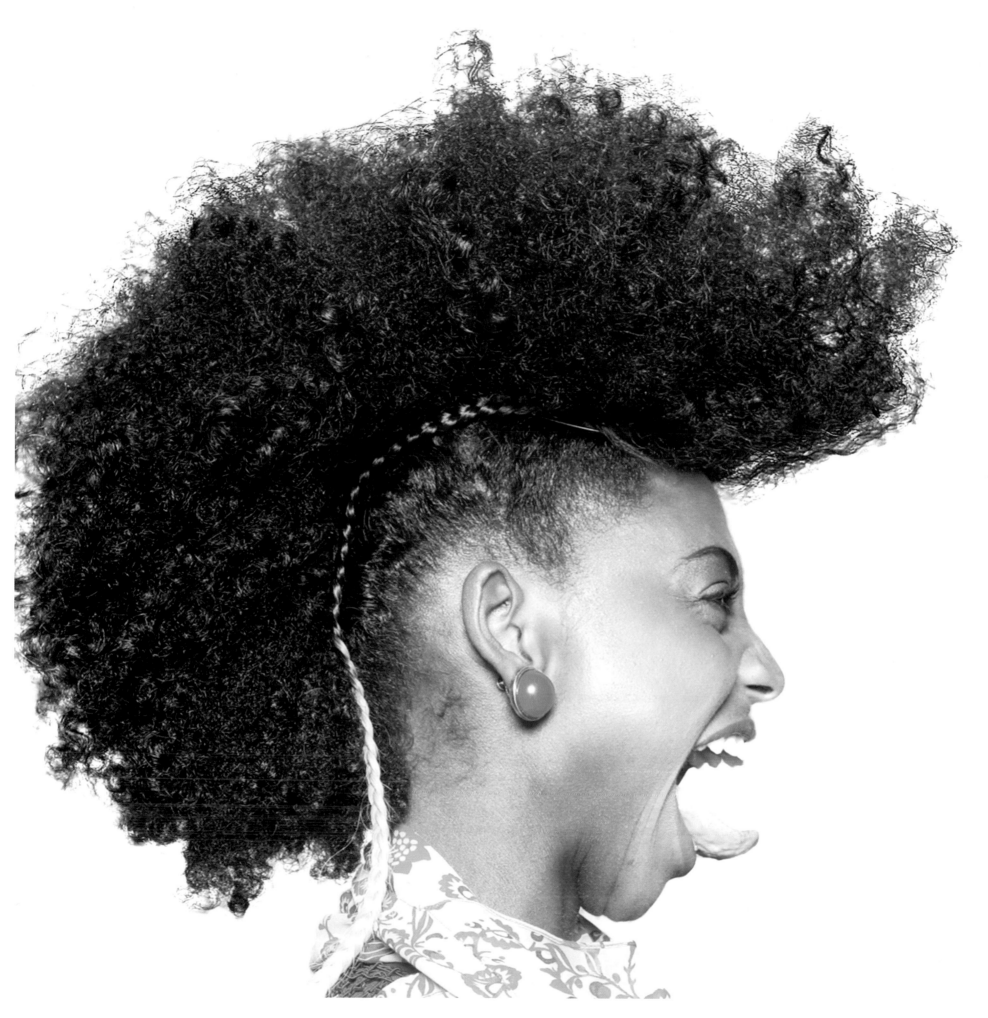

H2 SCANDINAVIA AS pages 192–193

Thomas Angellsgt 5, 7011 Trondheim, Norway, www.h2.no

Hair: Hannah Røskaft, H2 London
Make-up: Orion Stylist
Photography: Orion

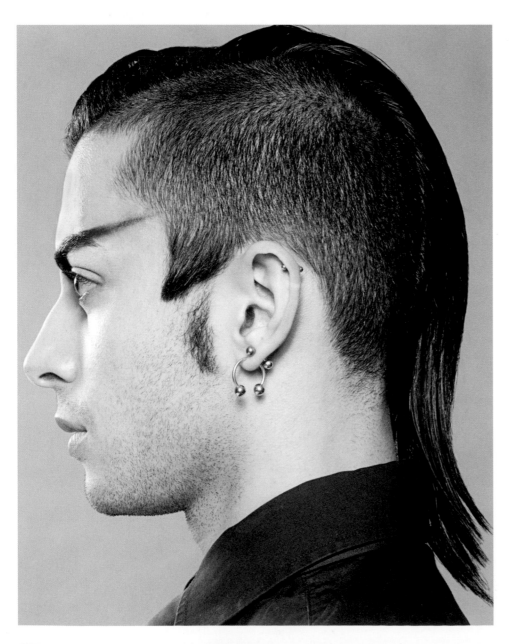

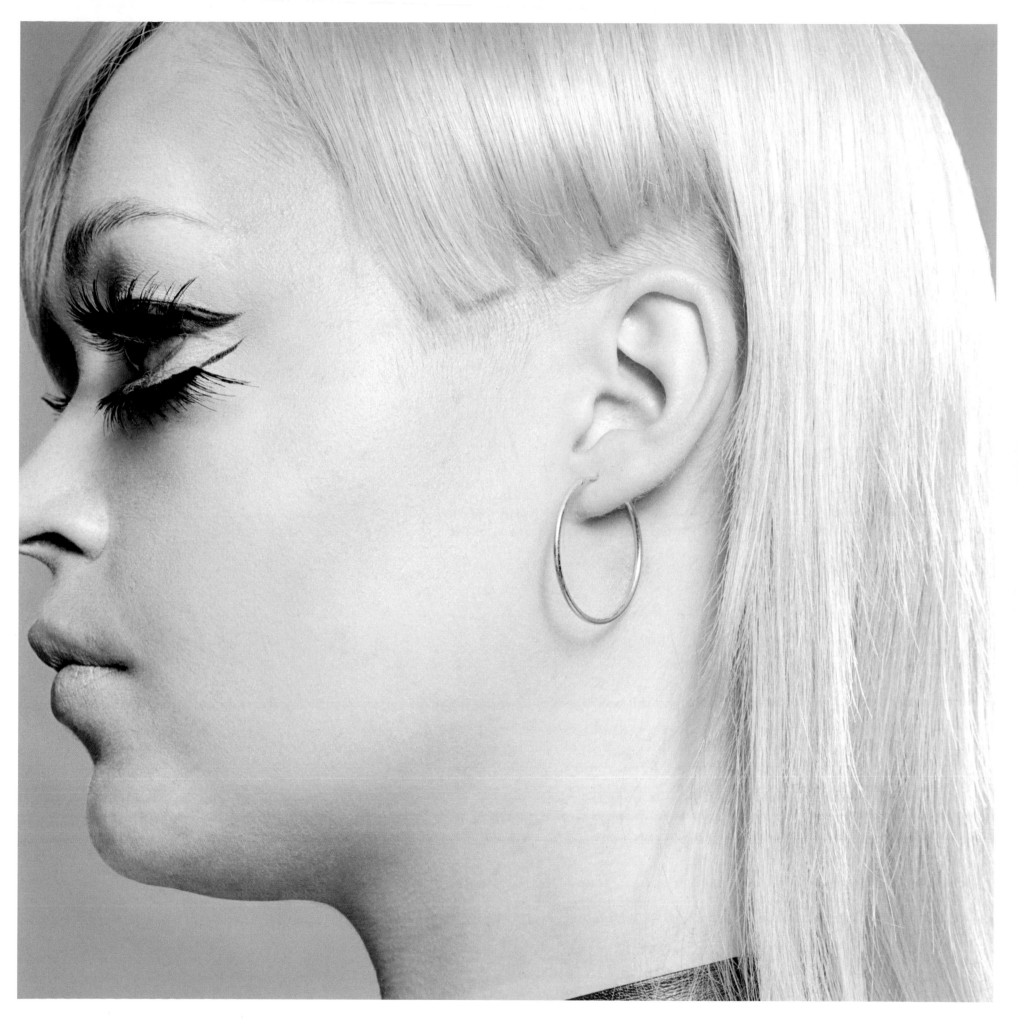

NEDJETTI pages 194–195

Hair by Nedjetti, 1583 Leslie St, suite 3, Hillside NJ 07205 , USA, 646.236.6726, www.nedjetti.com, nedjetti@nedjettishouseofpeace.com

Hair: Nedjetti
Make-up: Danessa Myricks
Photography: Jo Lance (p. 194) Corey Hayes (p. 195)
Models: Hallie, Click Agency (p. 194) Olivia Redmond, M&T Agency (p. 194) Nekesha, Ikon Agency (p. 195)
Products: Aveda, Redken, Aura Lavender, Zotos Ultrablond

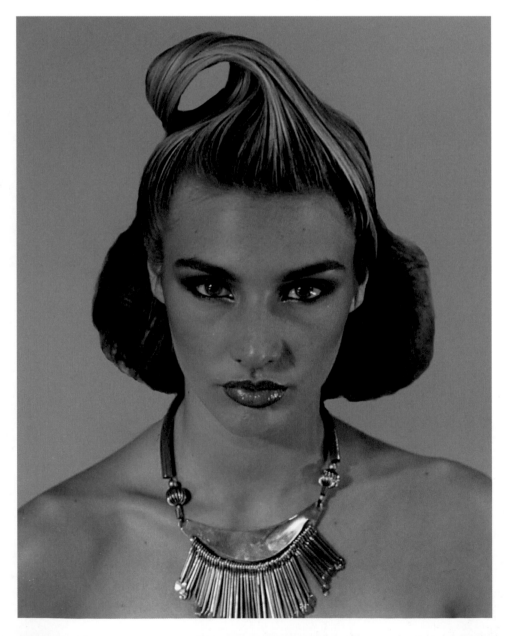

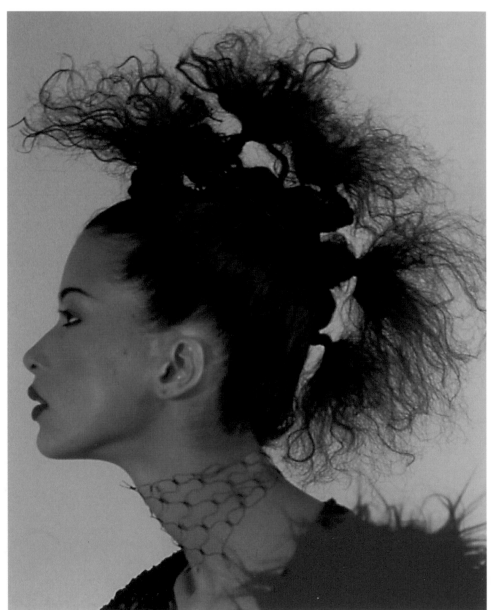

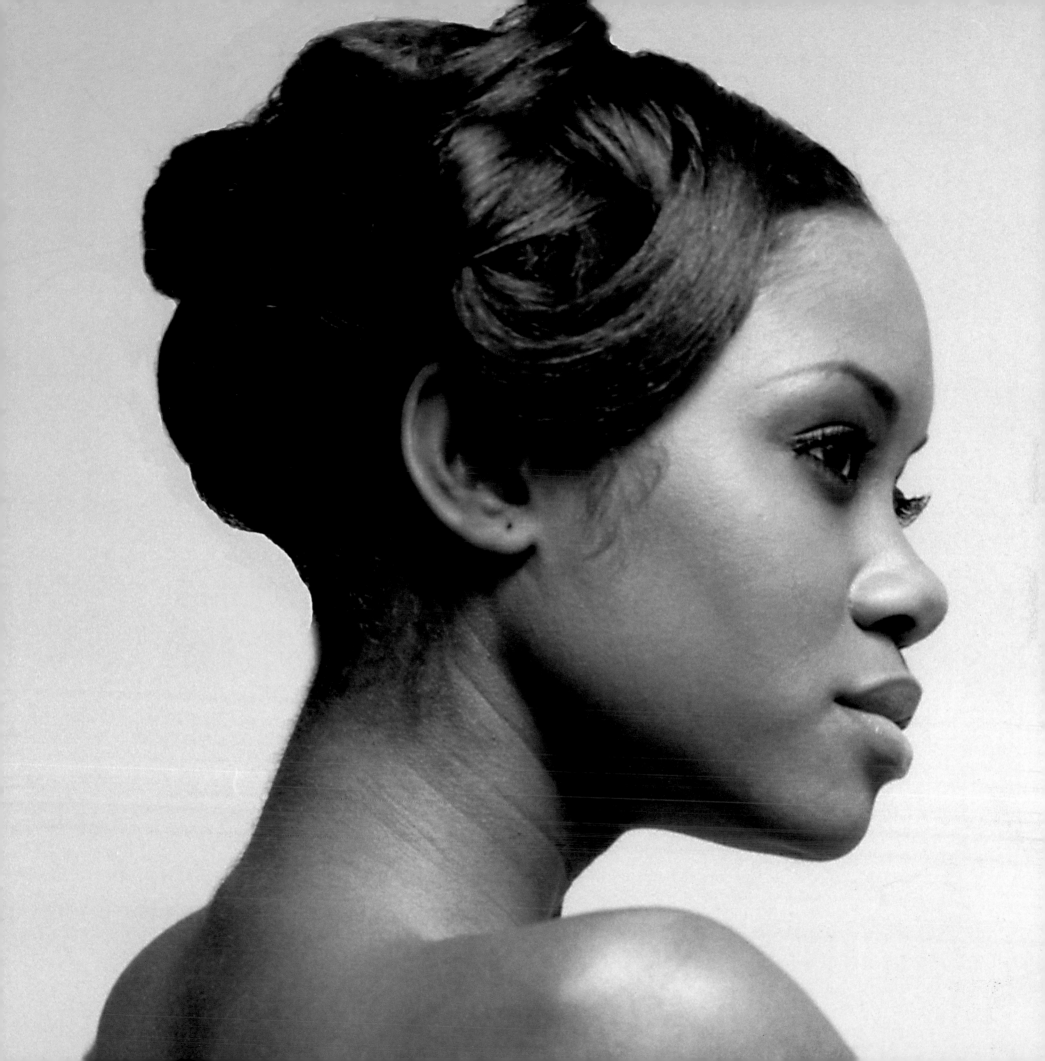

DAMIEN CARNEY pages 196–197

International editorial hairdresser, London, United Kingdom, damienPcarney@aol.com

Hair: Damien Carney
Photography: Damien Carney

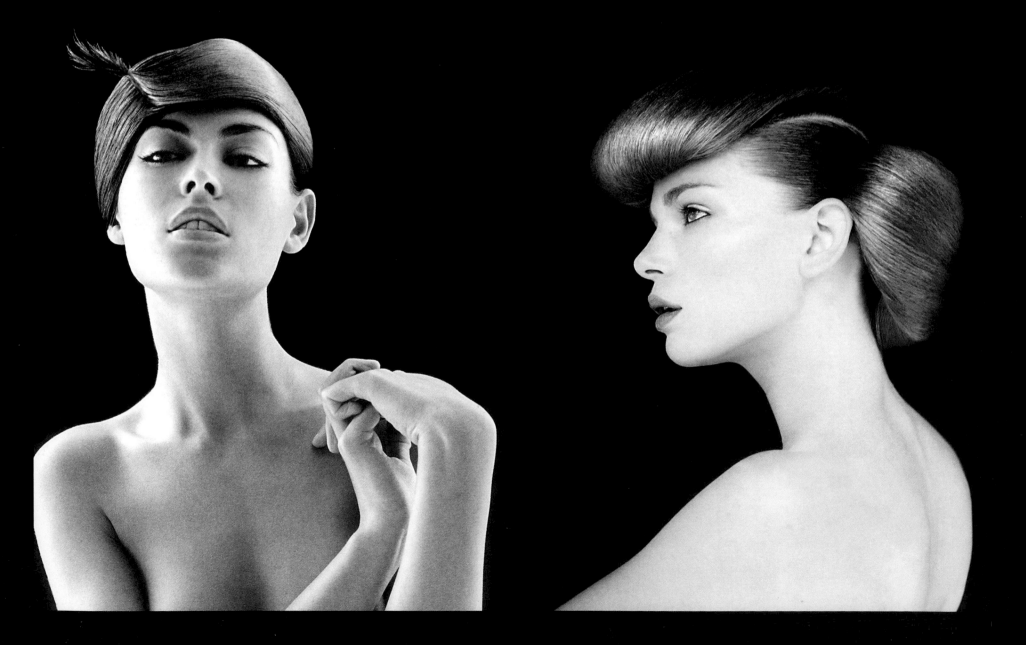

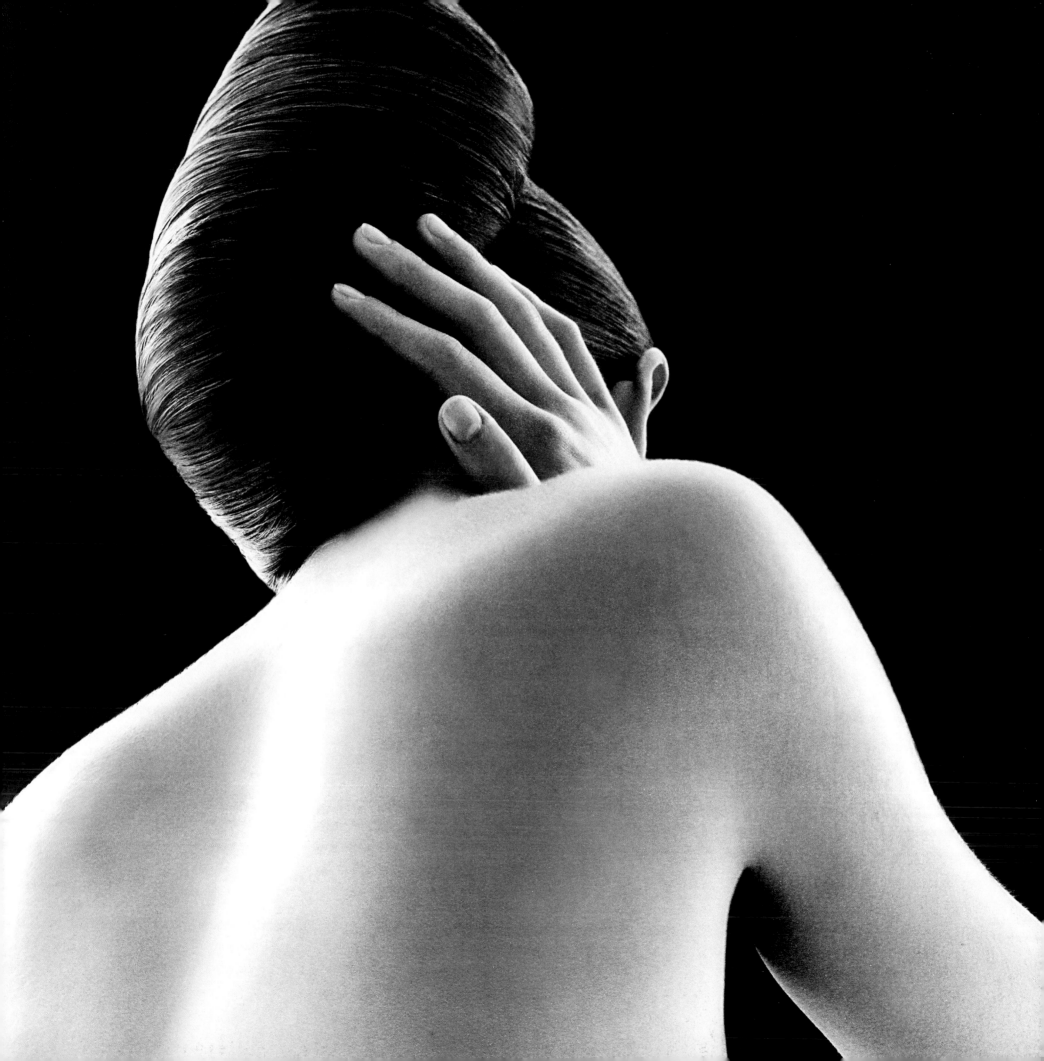

GRACE HAIRDRESSING pages 198–201

64 Ghuznee, St. Wellington, New Zealand

Hair: Brendan Digby-Smith
Salon: Grace Hairdressing
Photography: Meek Zuiderwyk
Model: Sarah Garlic, The Agencie
Products: L'Oréal

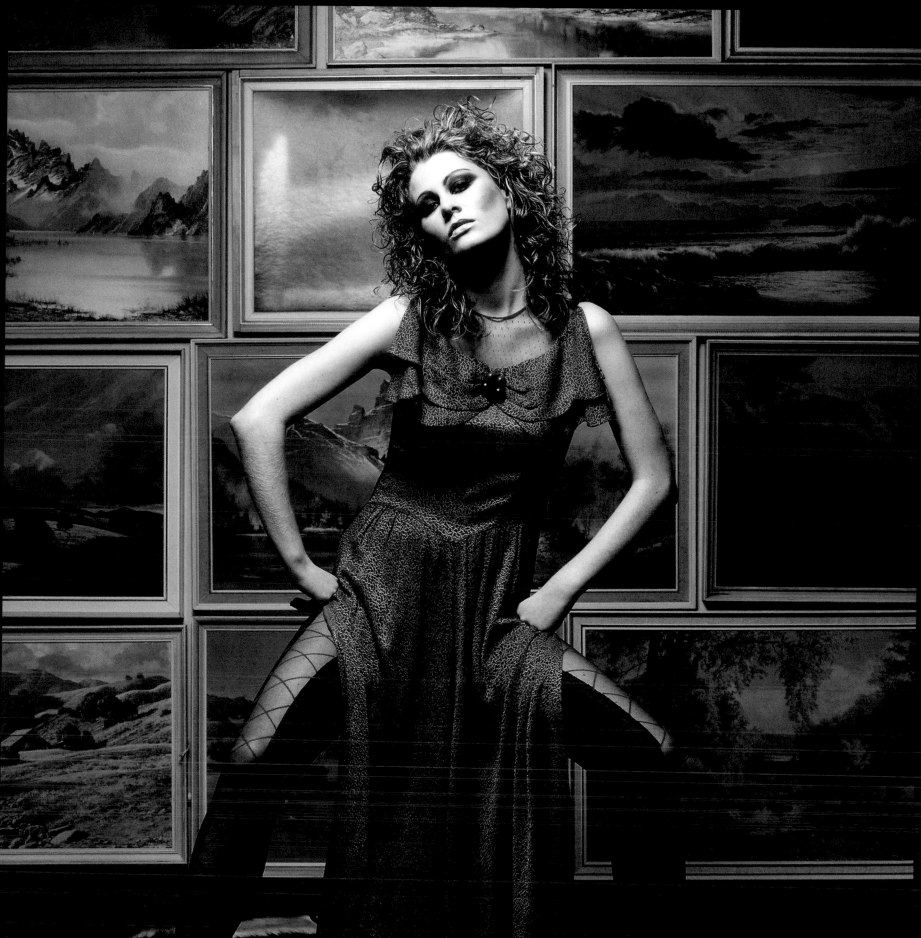

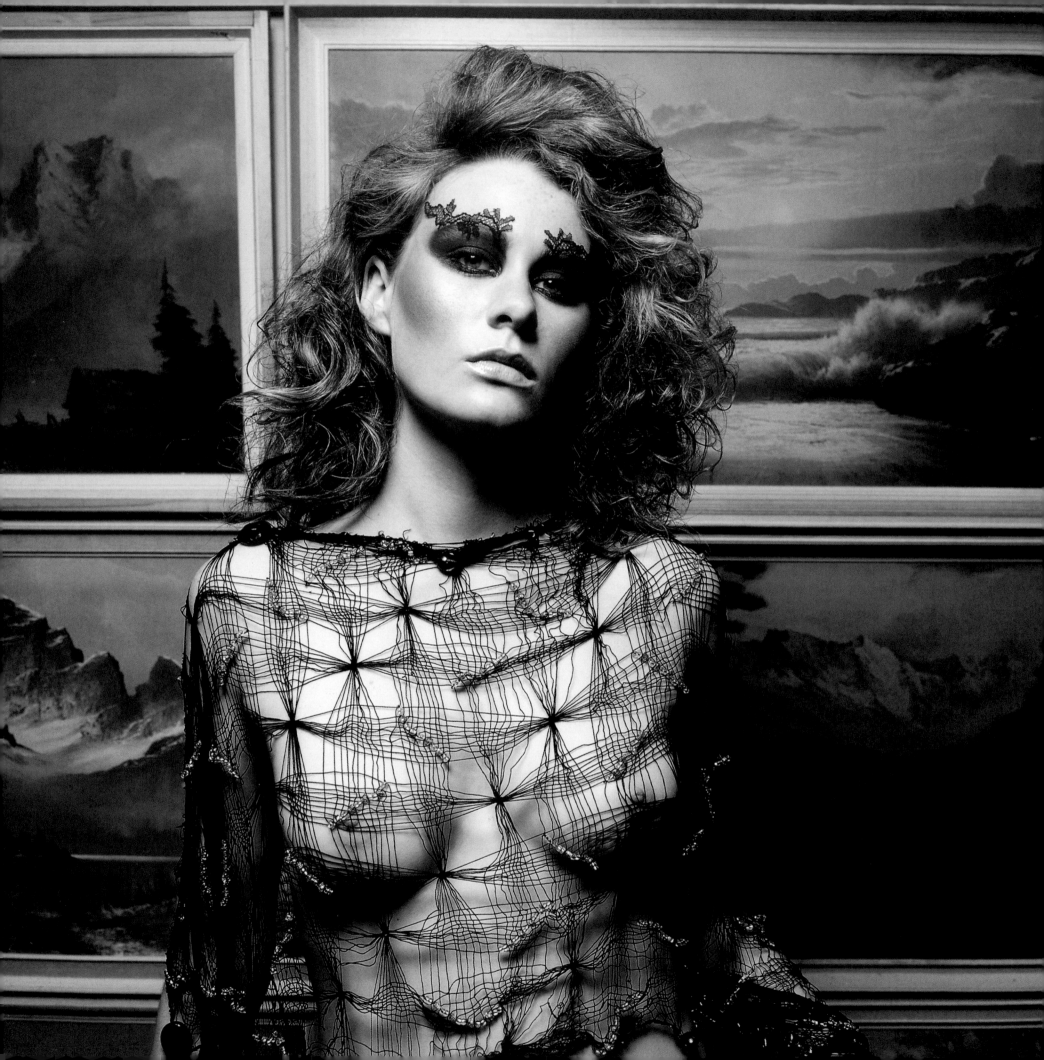

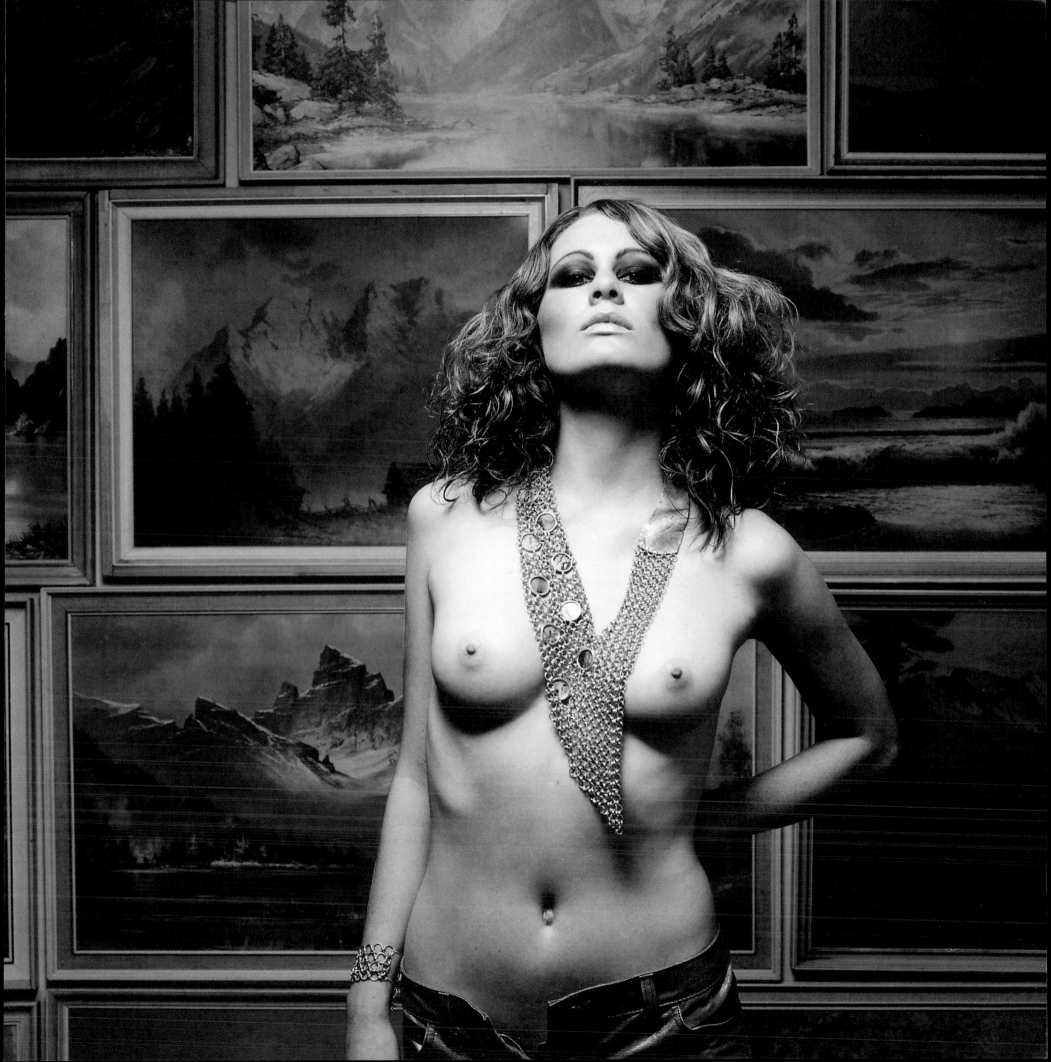

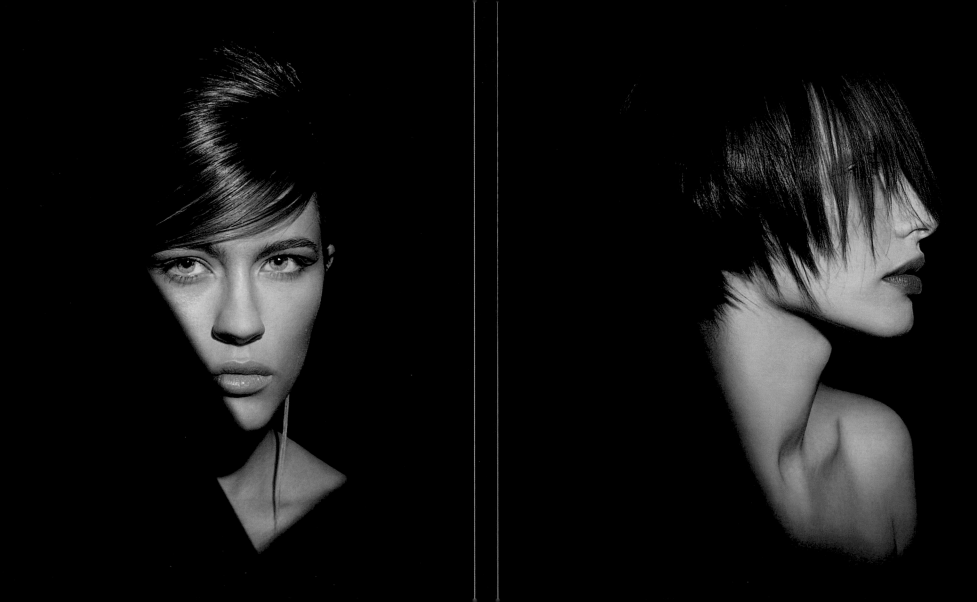

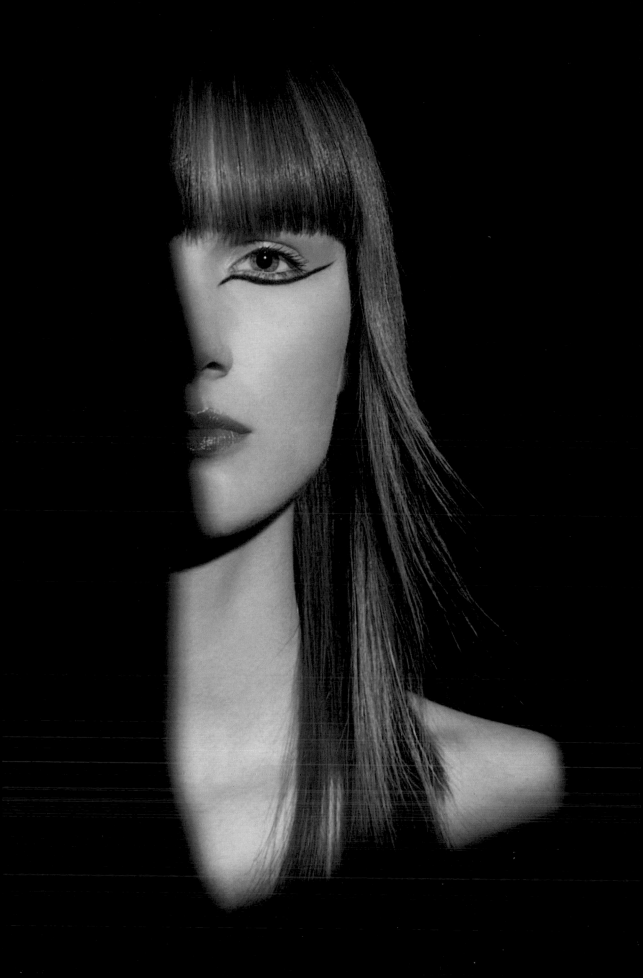

CHARLIE TAYLOR pages 204–207

Charlie Taylor Hair, Health & Beauty, 20-28 South Methven Street, Perth, United Kingdom, www.charlie-taylor.co.uk

Hair: Charlie Taylor
Salon: Charlie Taylor Hair Health & Beauty
Make-up: Cheryl Phelps-Gardiner
Styling: Holly Campbell-Mitchell
Photography: Trevor Leighton
Products: Schwarzkopf

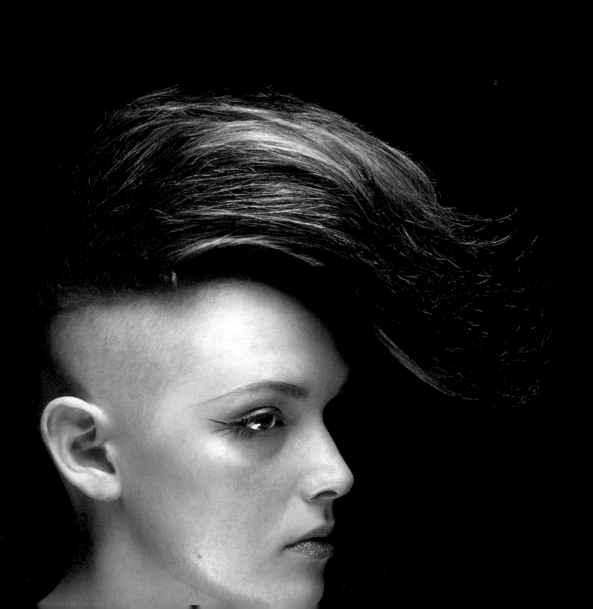

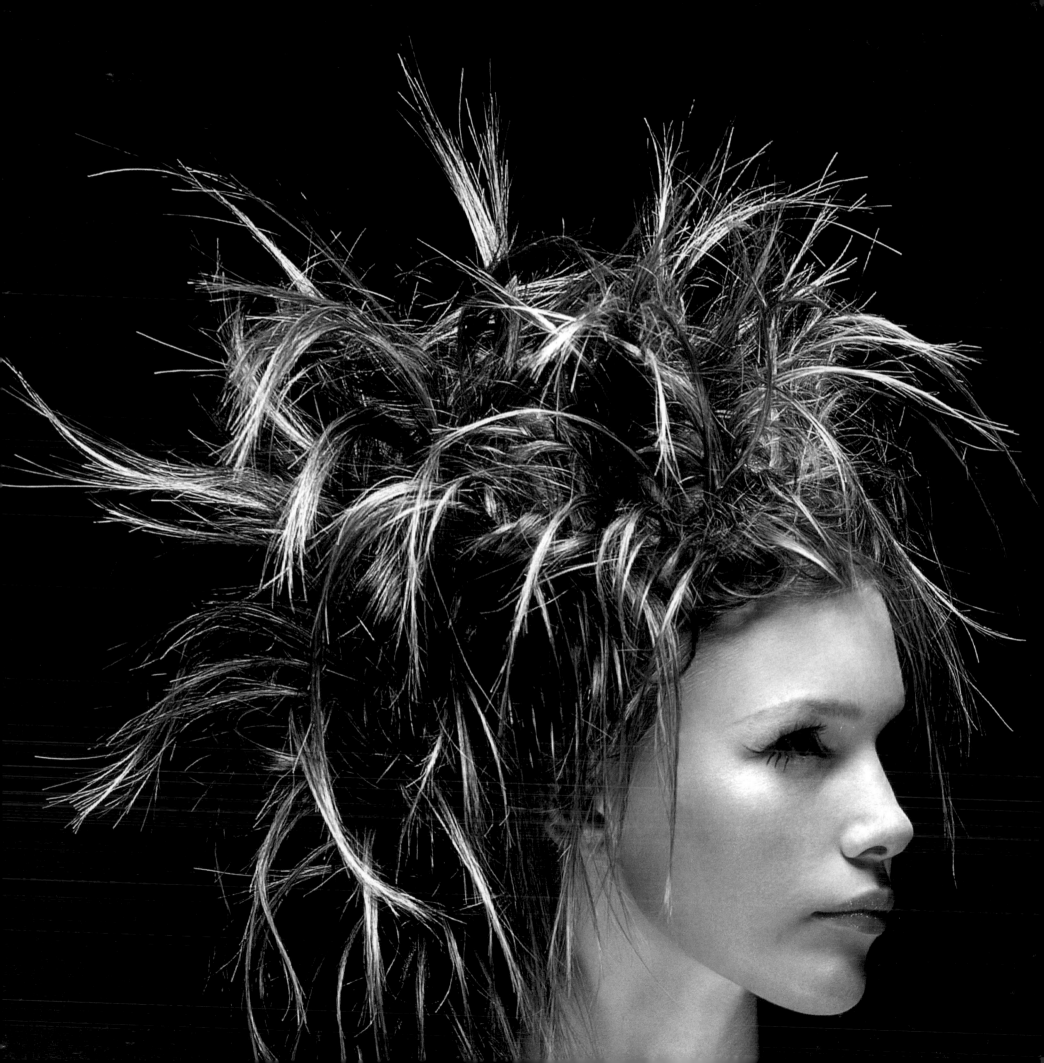

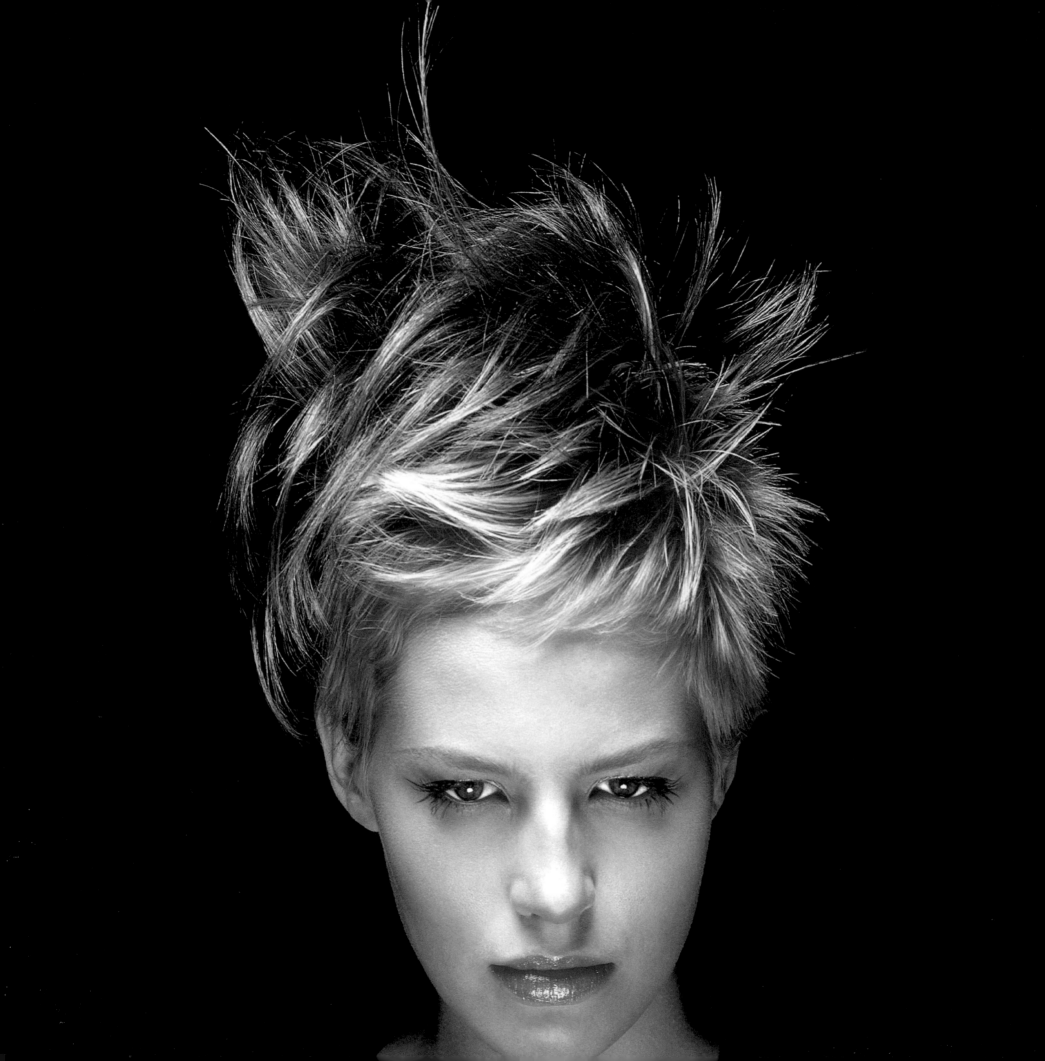

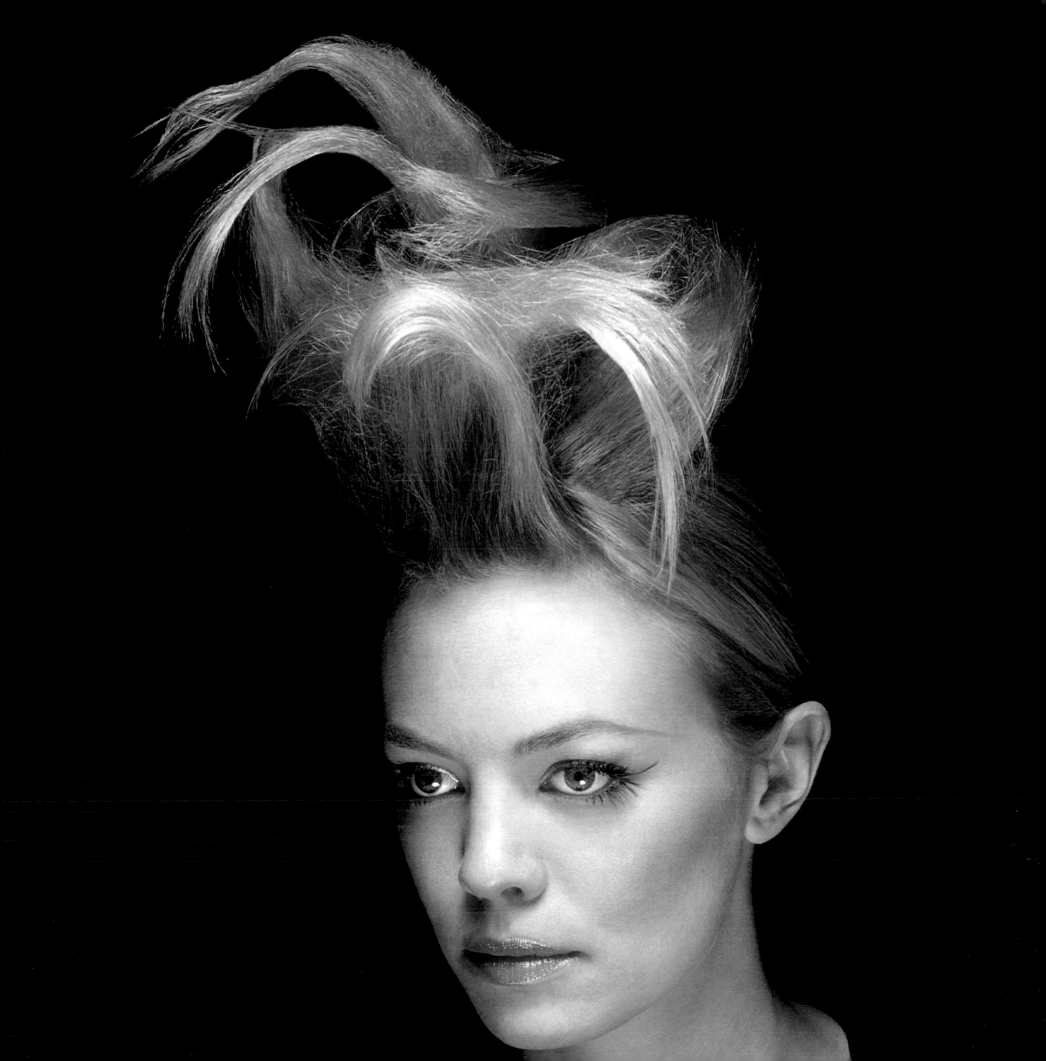

CLAUDE TARANTINO pages 208–213

Résidence Le Villandry, rue Francois Lapierre, 57120 Rombas, France

Hair: Claude Tarantino
Make-up: Wendy
Styling: Jeunes createur
Photography: Jules Egger, Jaqueline Roche
Products: L'Oréal Professionnel Paris

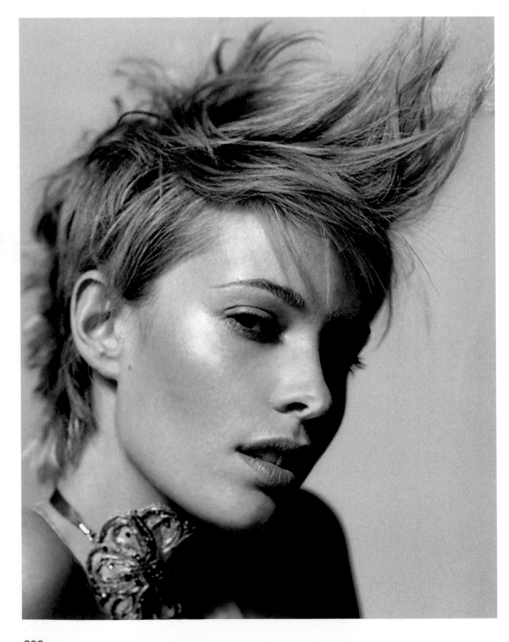

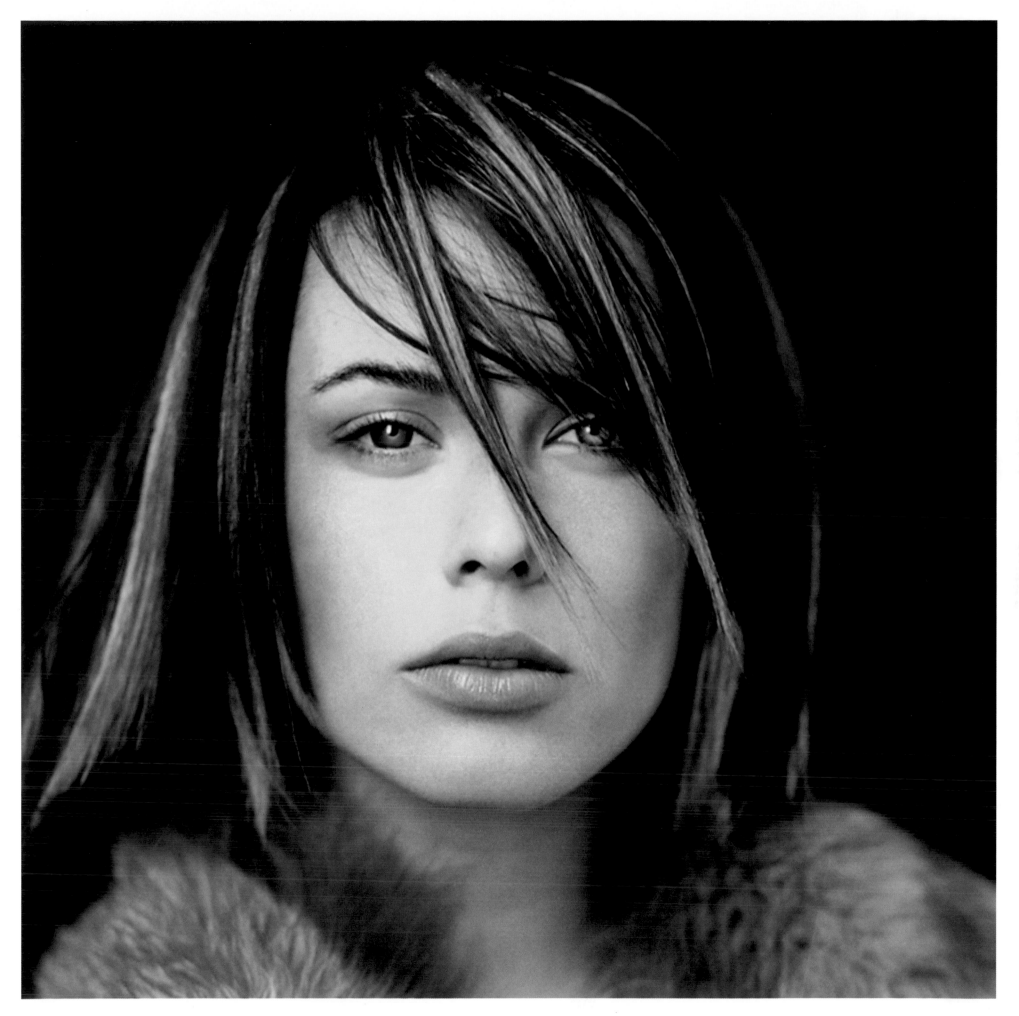

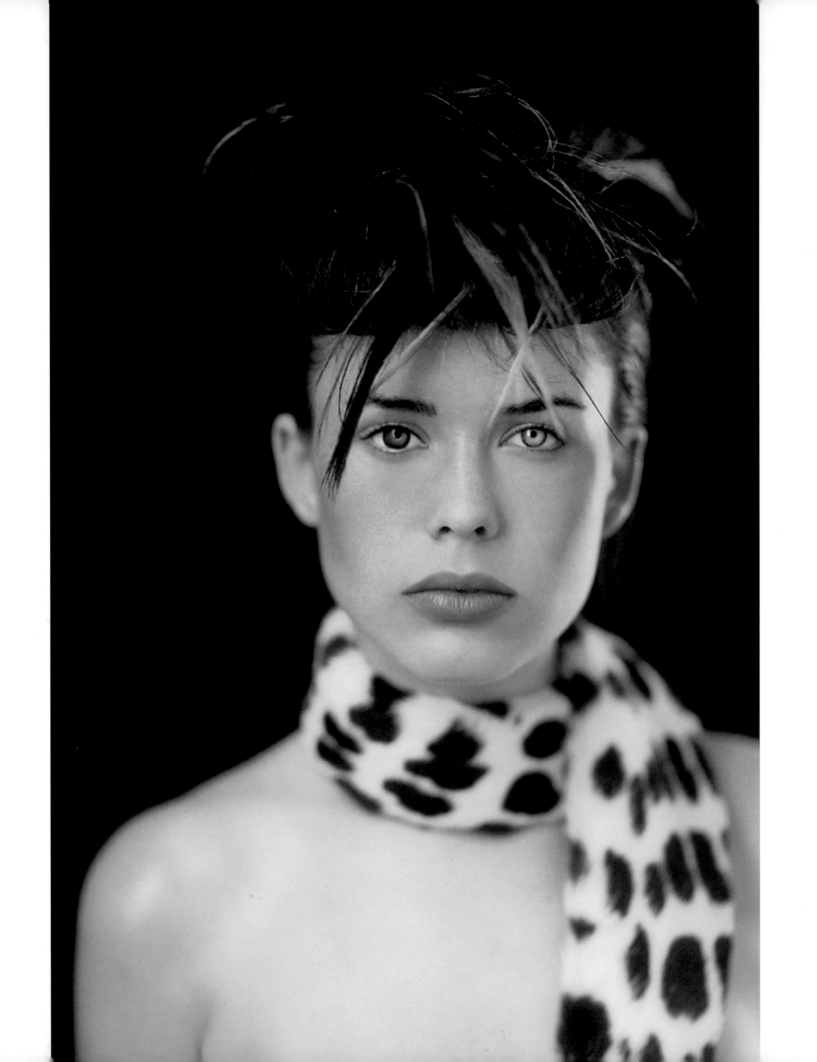

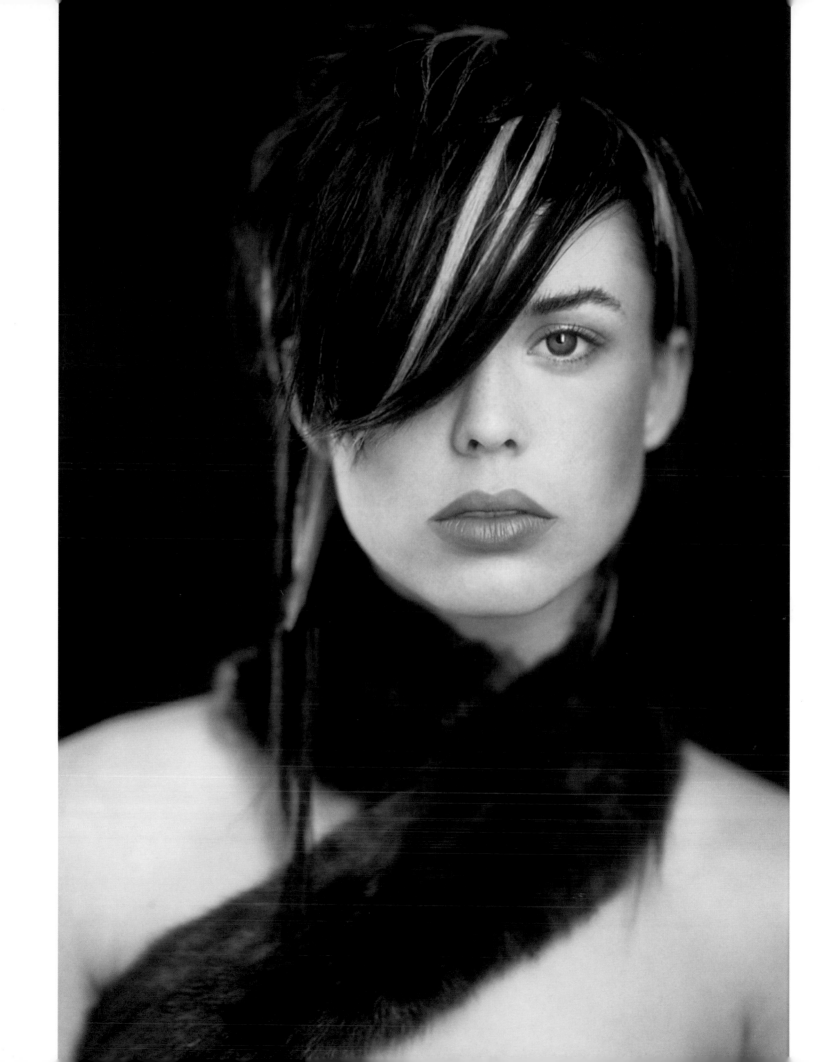

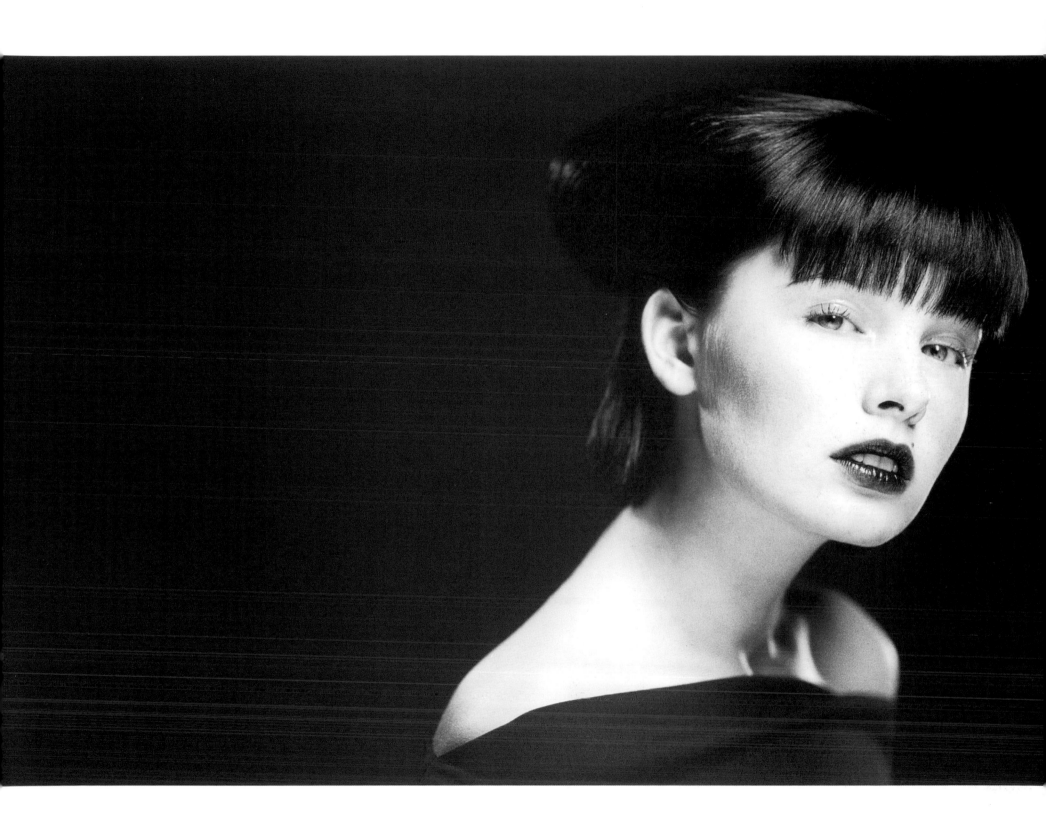

Hair: Victor Ortega
Salon: Emphasis Salon
Make-Up: Victor Ortega
Photography: Jun Barrameda
Model: Graceyann Apuad
Products: Schwarzkopf

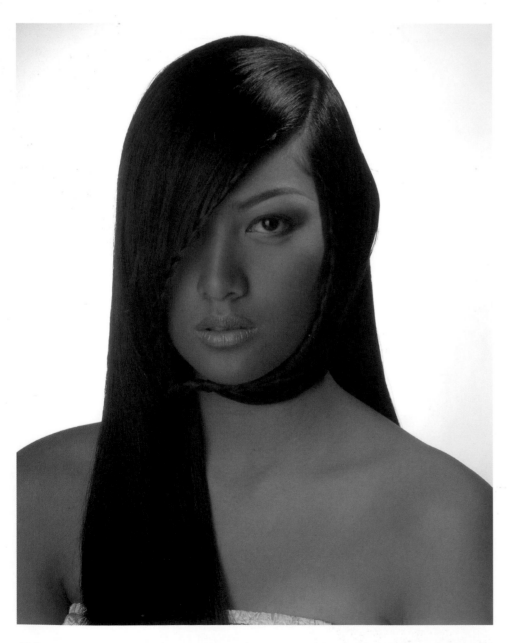

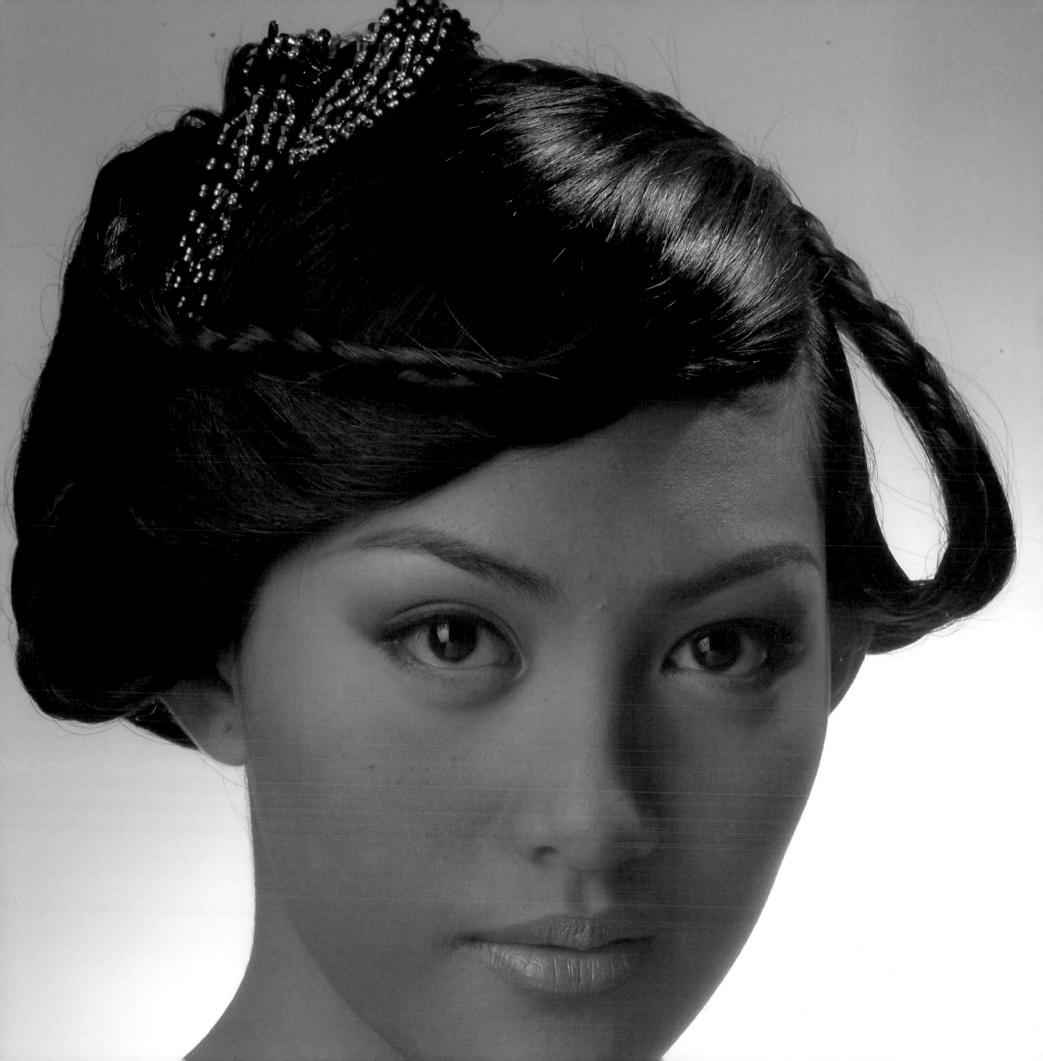

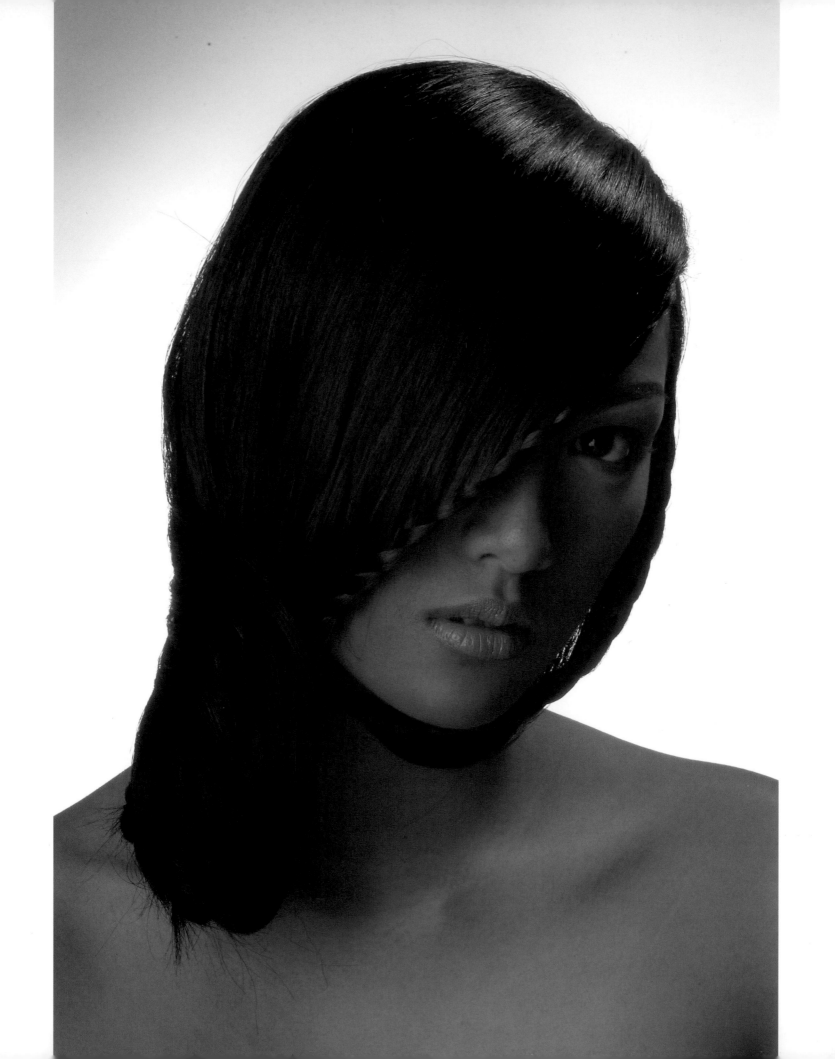

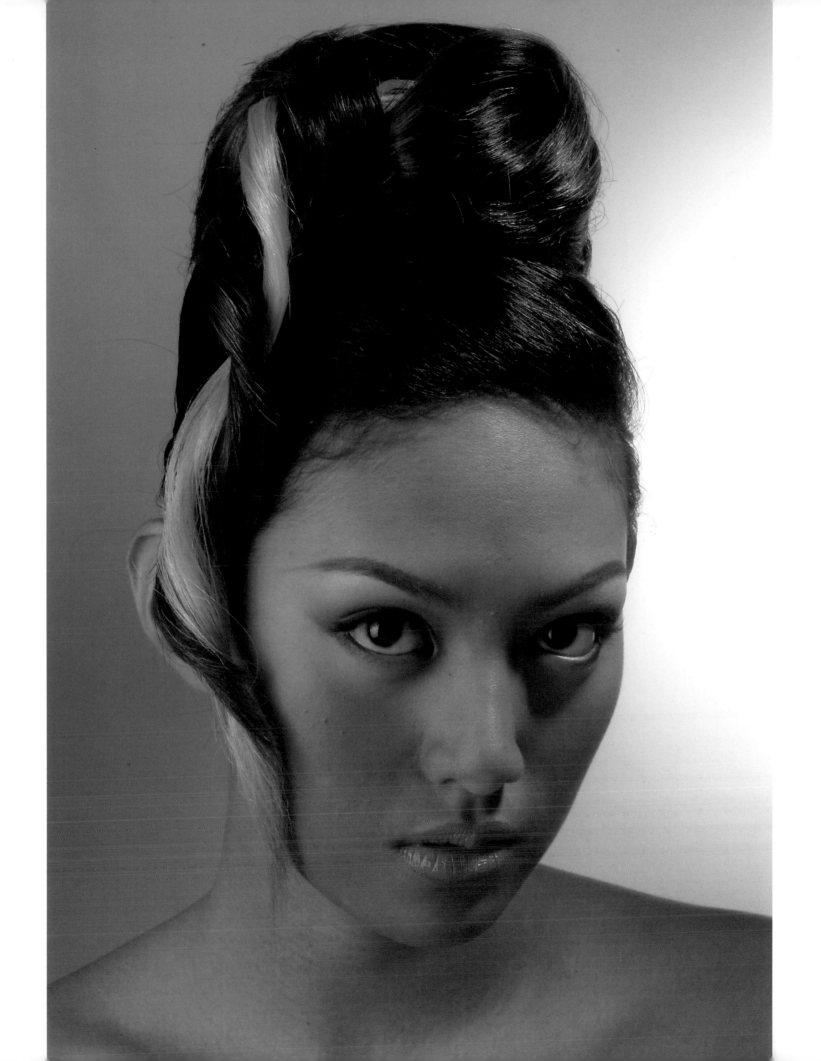

RAW HAIR pages 218–223

95 Oxford Street, Darlinghurst NSW 2010, Australia

Hair: James Pearce (p. 218, 219) Anthony Nader for Raw Hair (p. 220 - 223)
Salon: Raw Hair

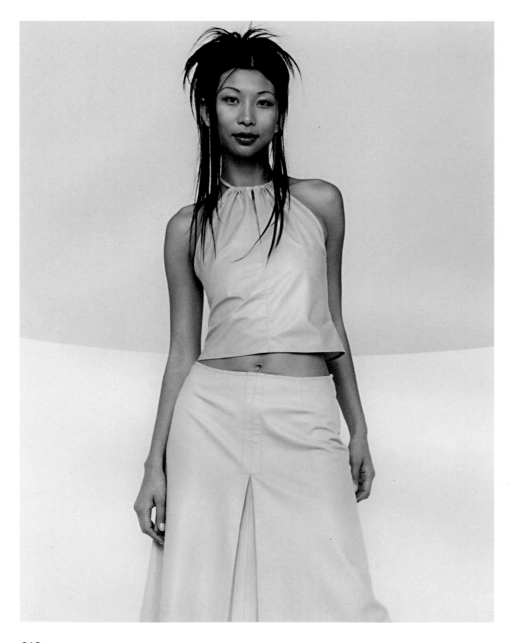

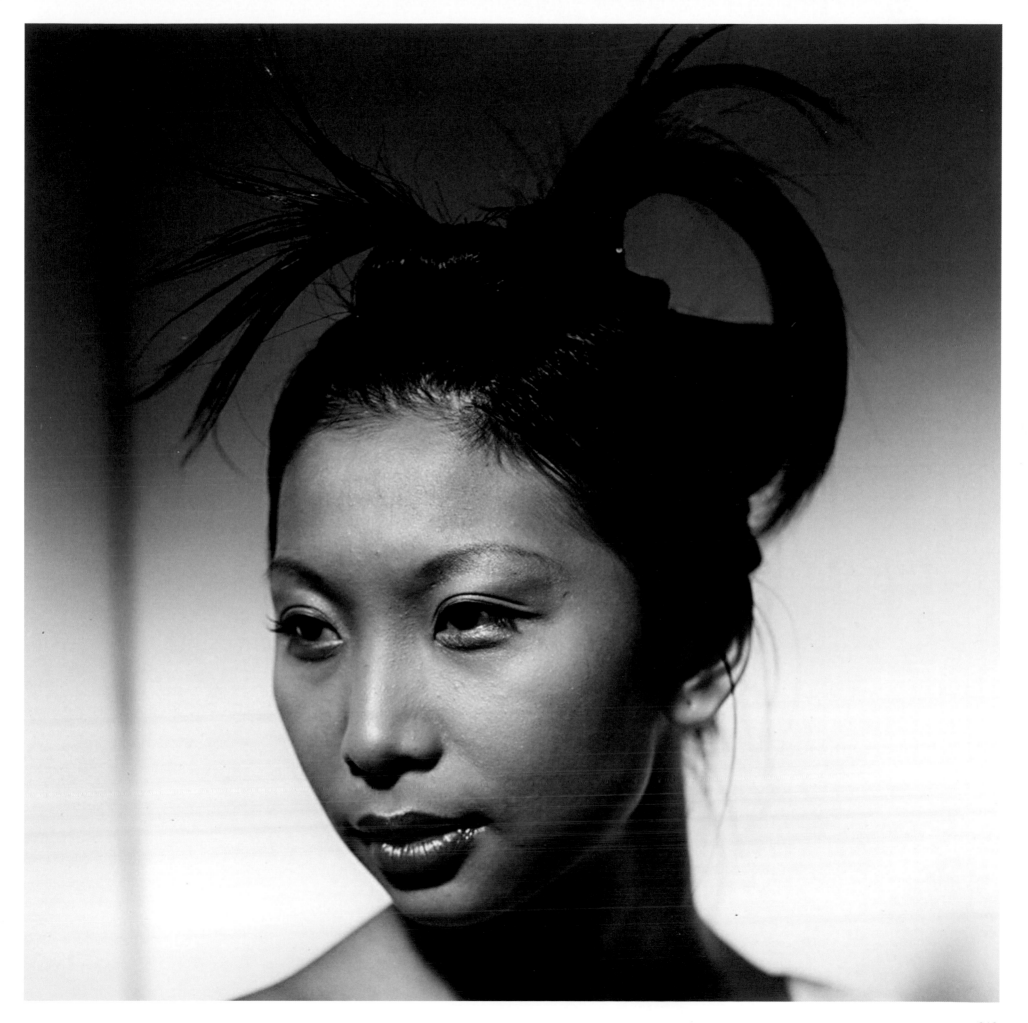

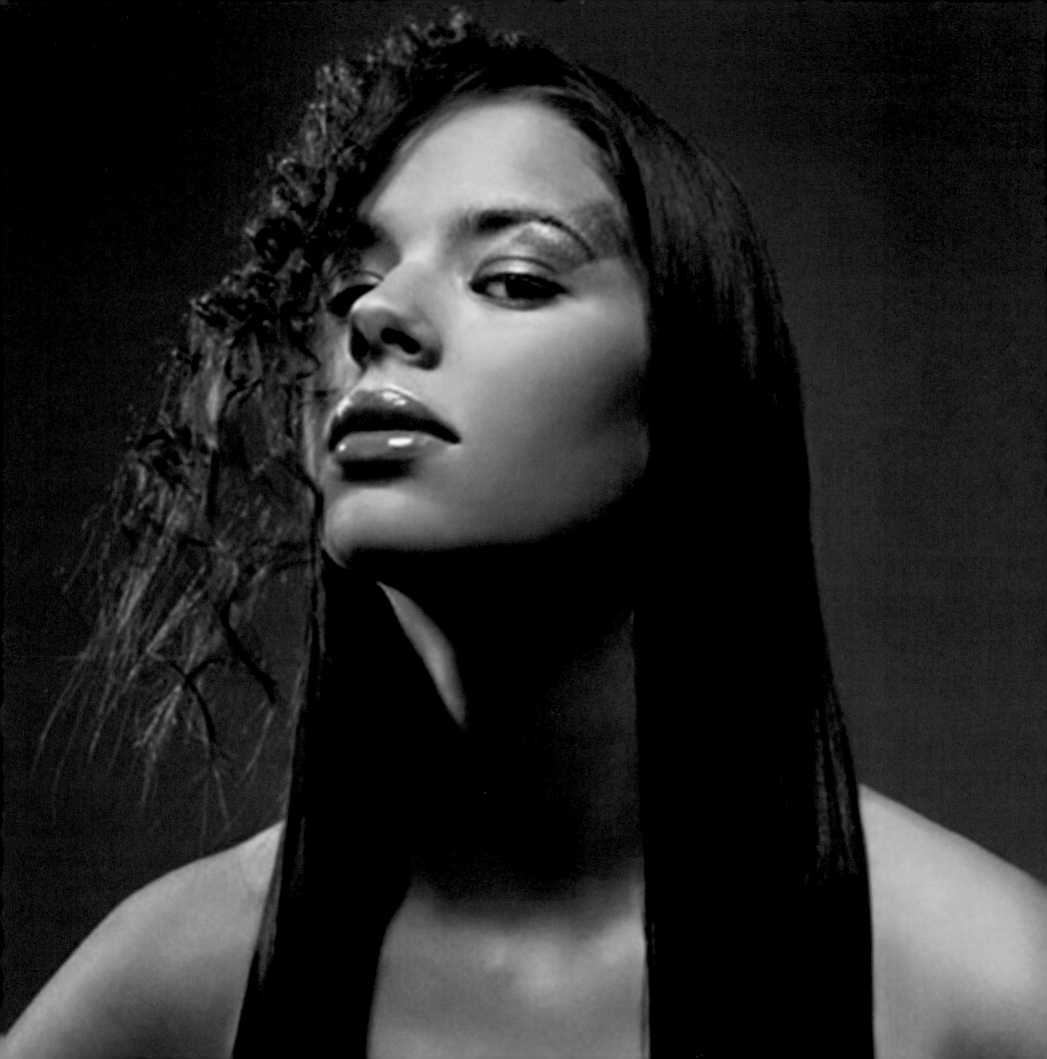

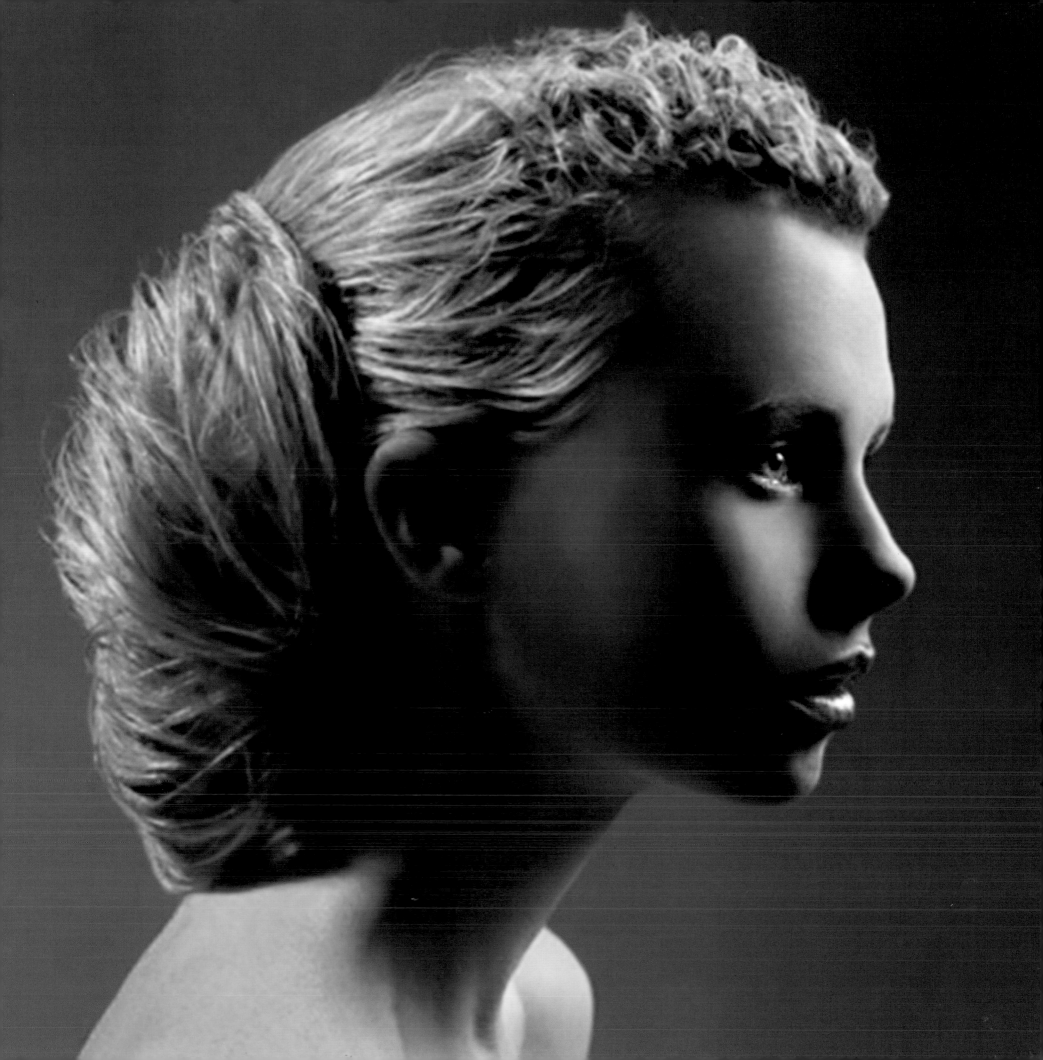

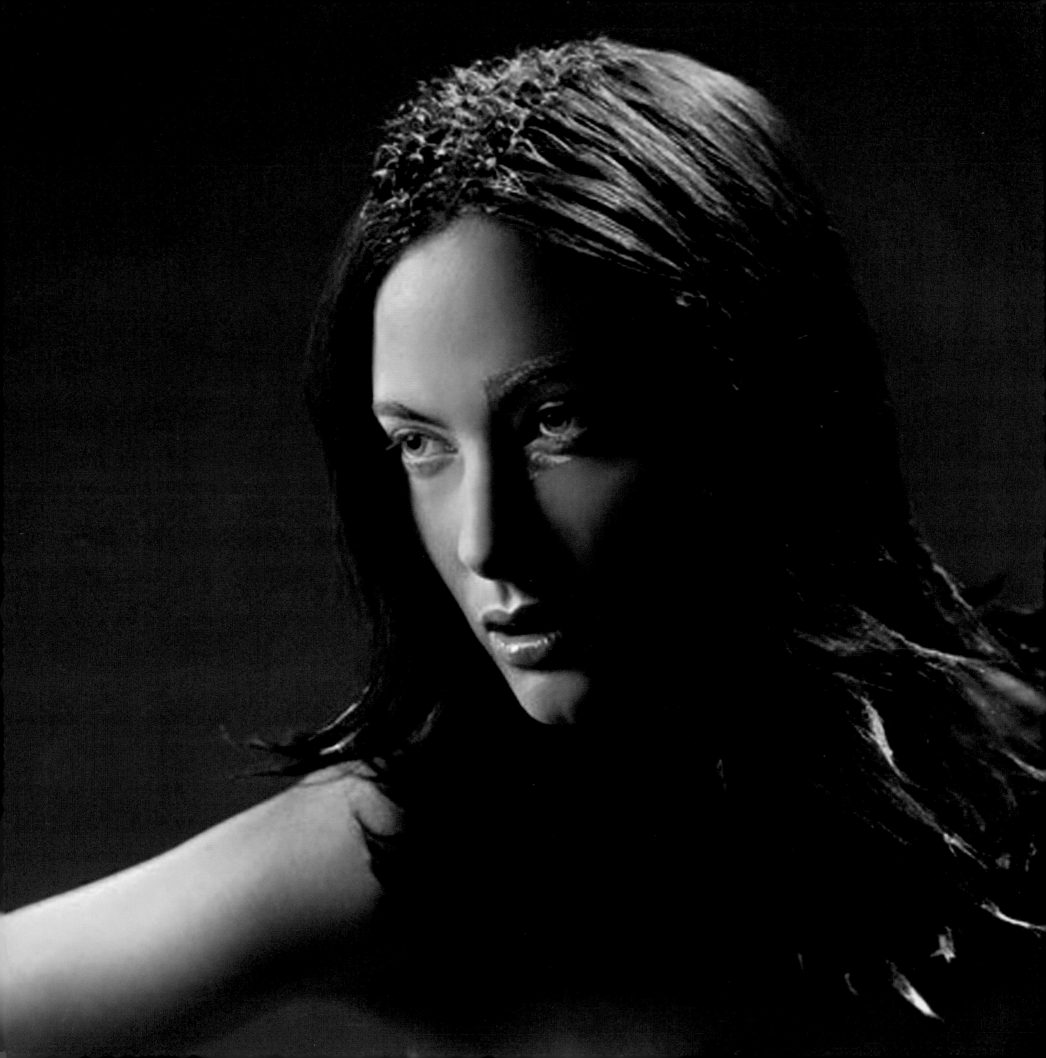

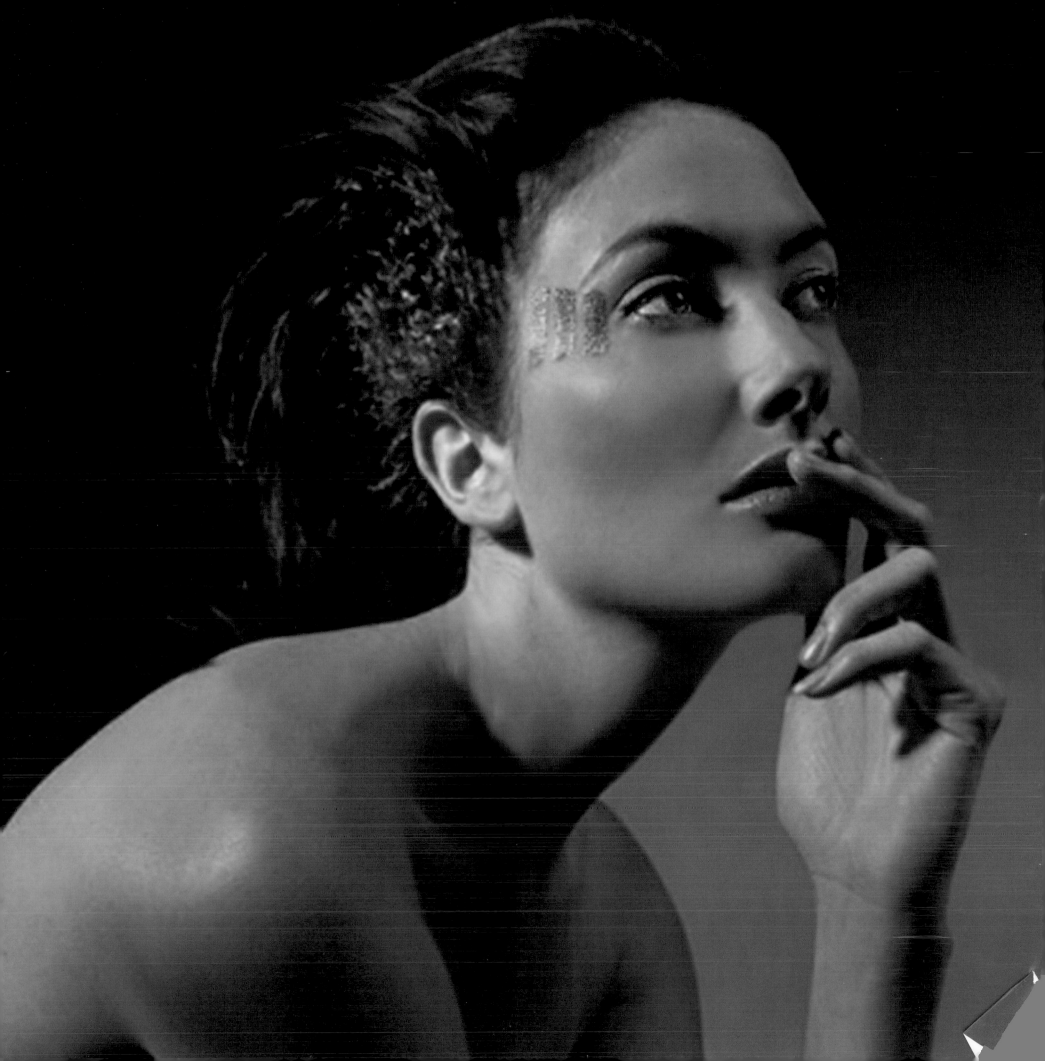

ERROL DOUGLAS pages 224–227

18 Motcomb Street, The Halkins, Knightsbridge, London SW1X 8LB, United Kingdom

Hair: Errol Douglas for Goldwell Professional Haircare
Make-up: Janet Francis
Styling: Jo Barker
Photography: Paul Burley
Products: Goldwell Professional Haircare

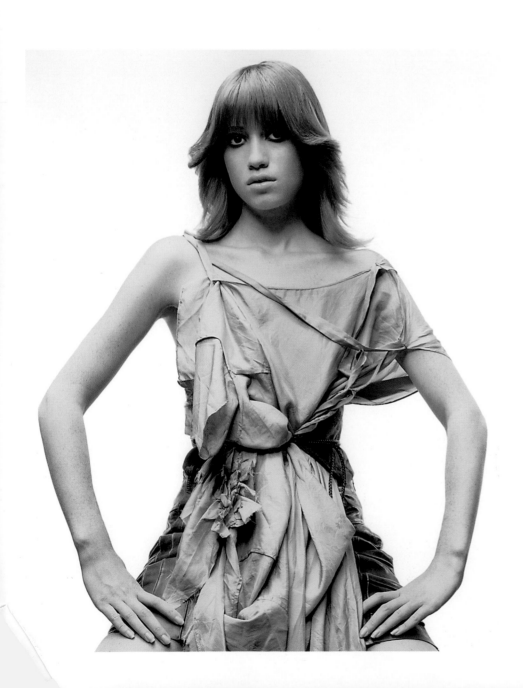

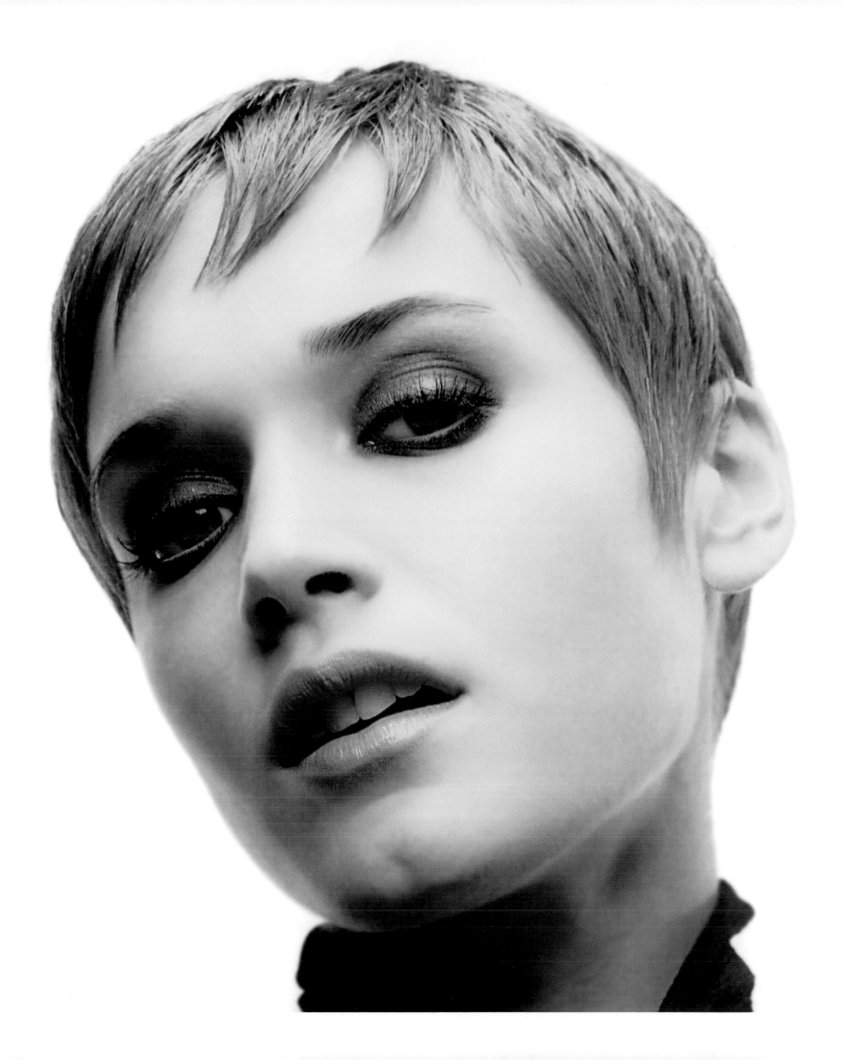

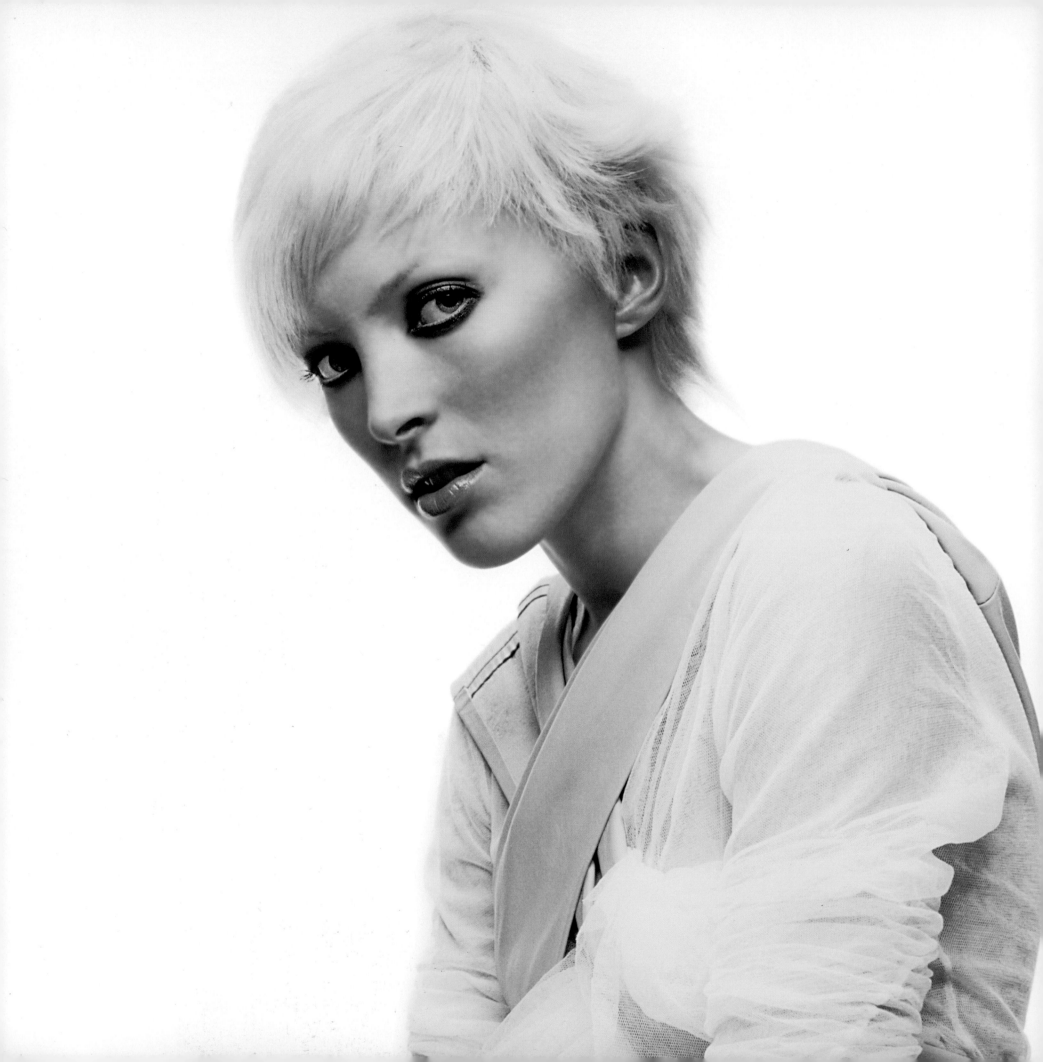

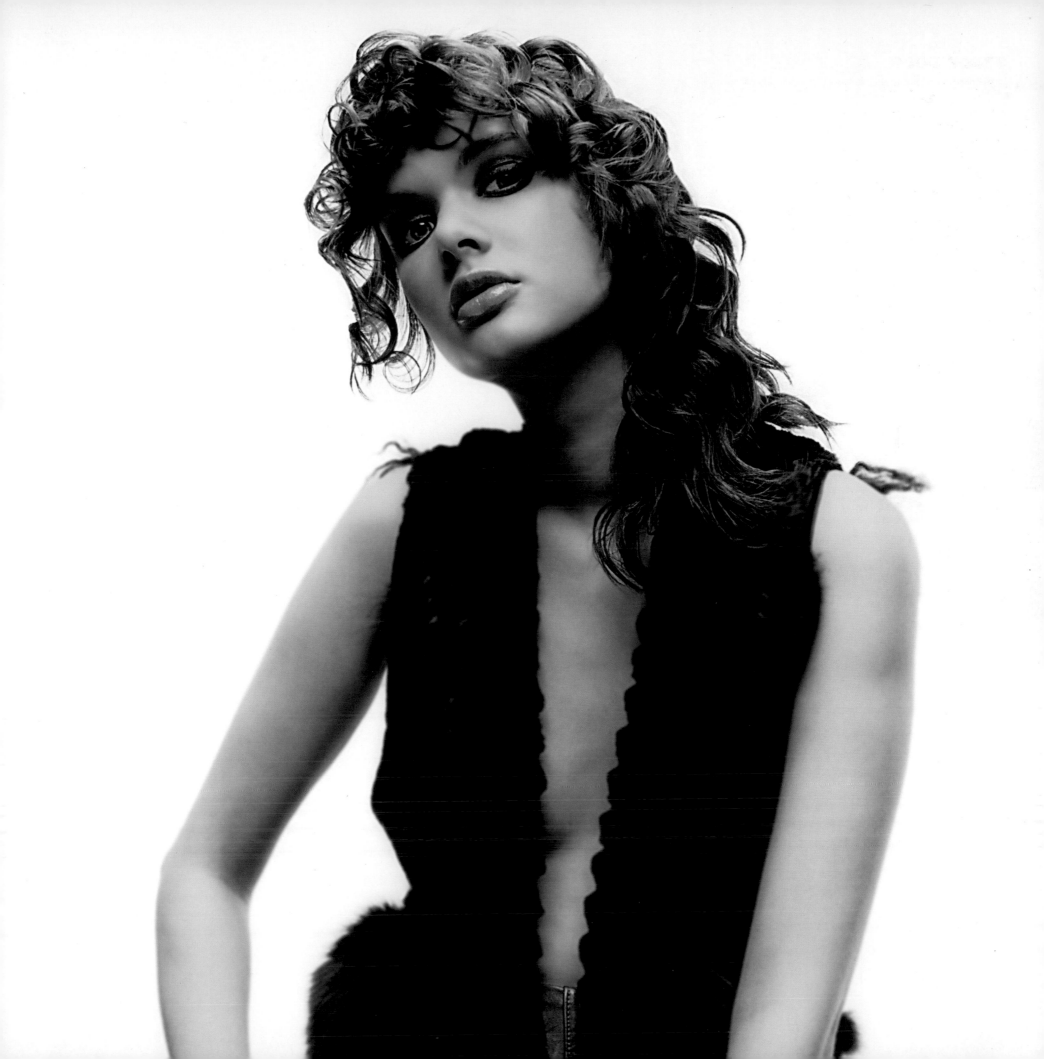

STAGE DOOR pages 228–231

45 Horseferry Road, Westminster, London SW1, United Kingdom, www.stagedoor.co.uk

Hair: Zoe Irwin
Salon: Stage Door
Make-up: Stephanie Picot
Styling: Gayle Rinkoff
Photography: Stuart Weston
Products: L'Oréal Techni.art

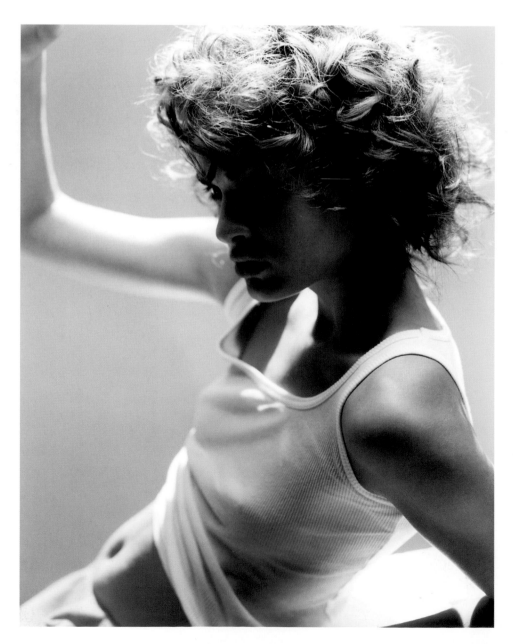

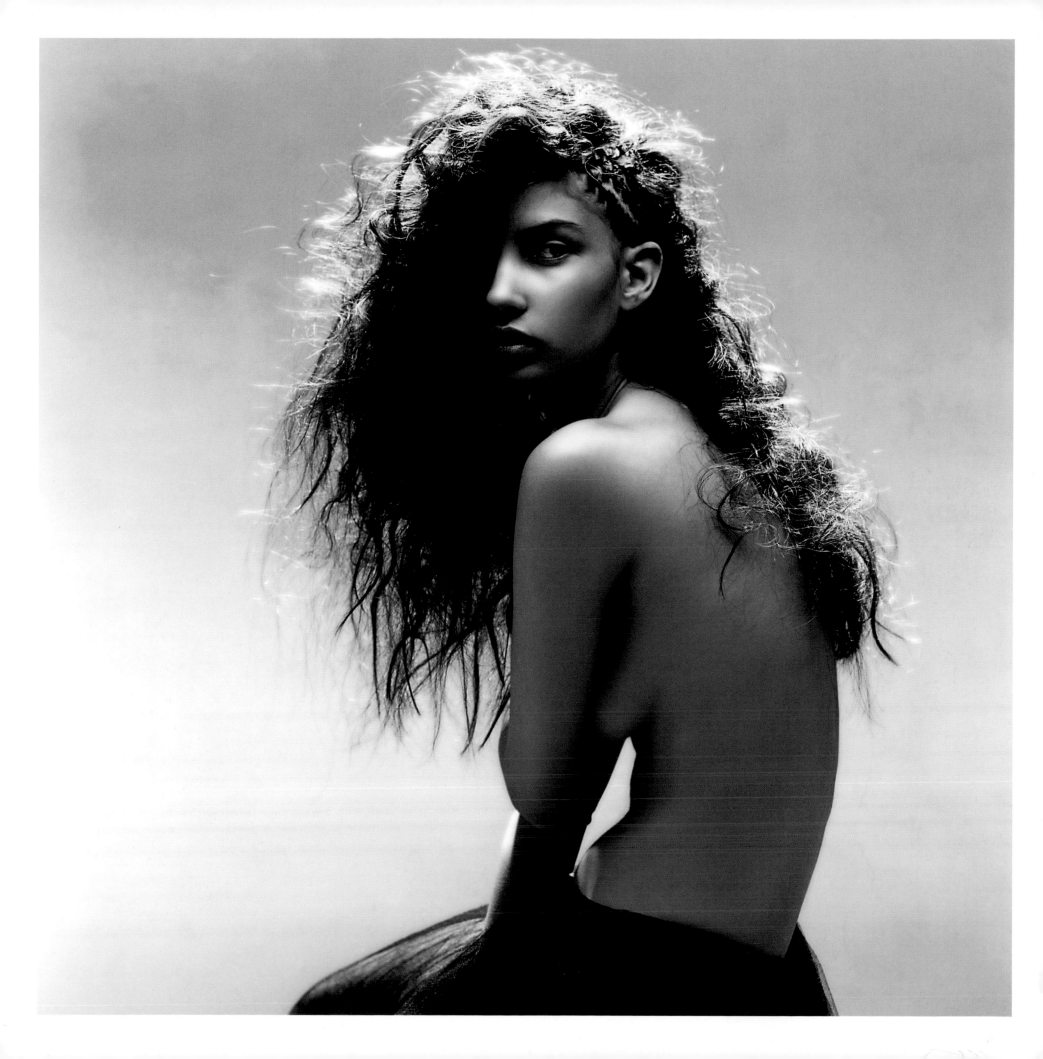

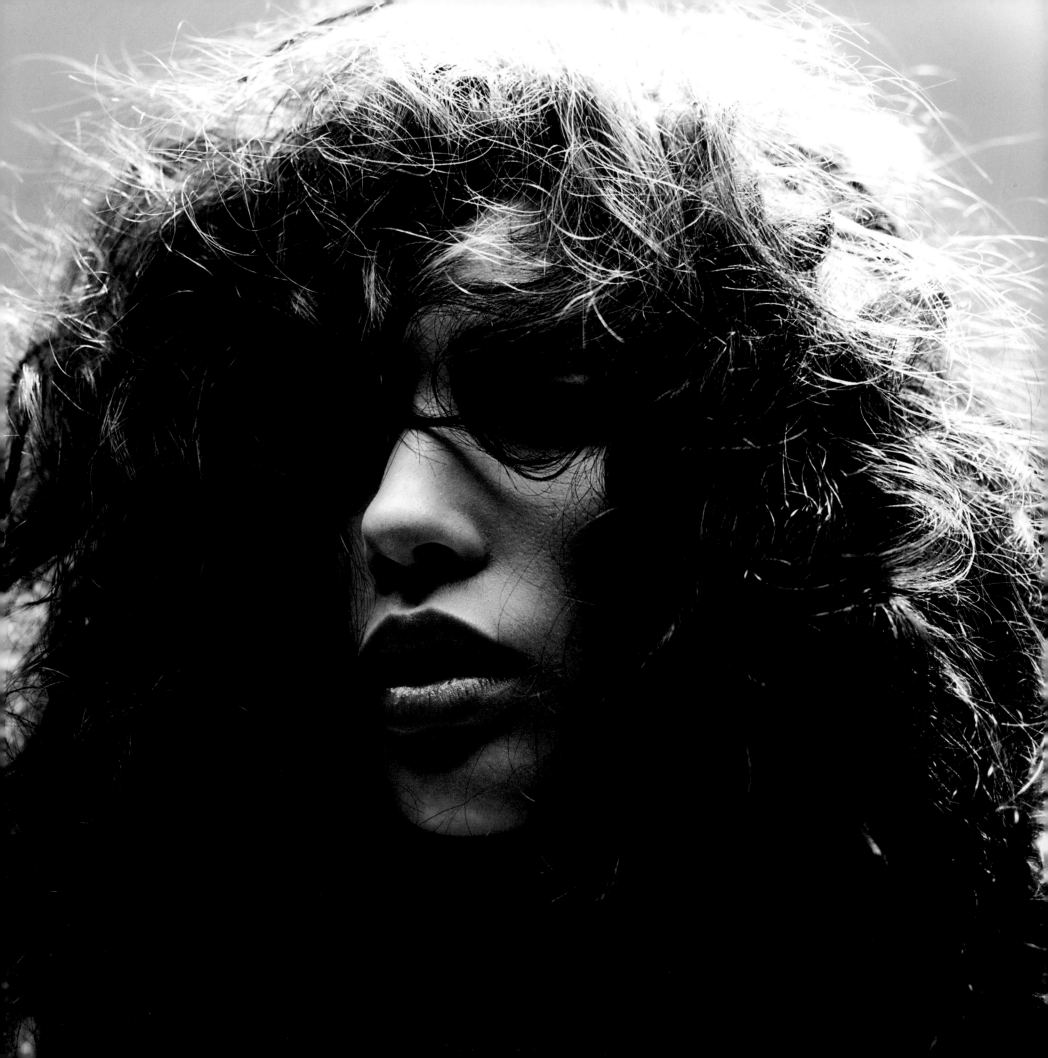

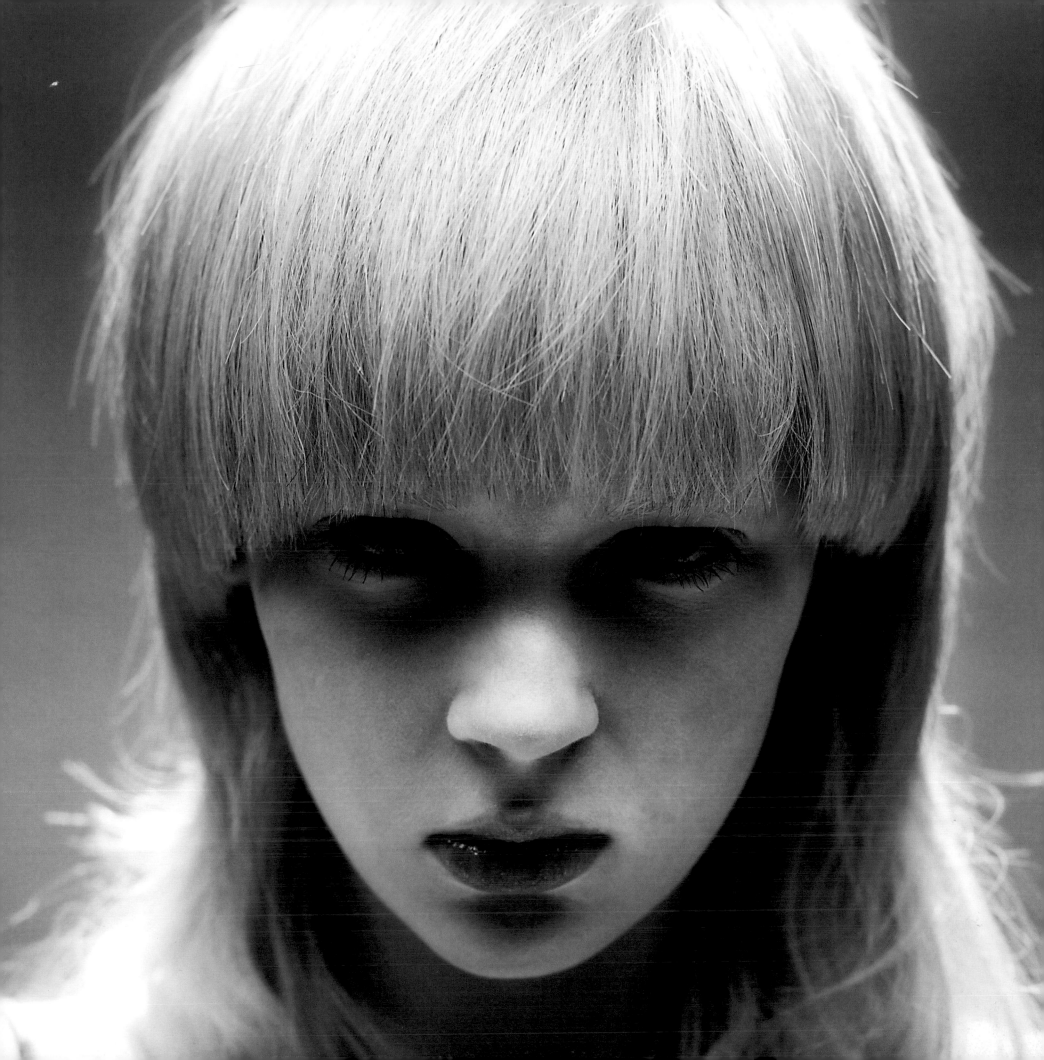

HEADMASTERS pages 232–237

145-155 Ewell Road, Surbiton Surrey KT6 6AW, United Kingdom, www.hmhair.co.uk

Hair: Sharon Landmann, Headmasters, Putney
Salon: Headmasters
Make-up: Melanie Davey
Styling: Annie
Photography: Will Scammell
Products: L'Oréal Professional

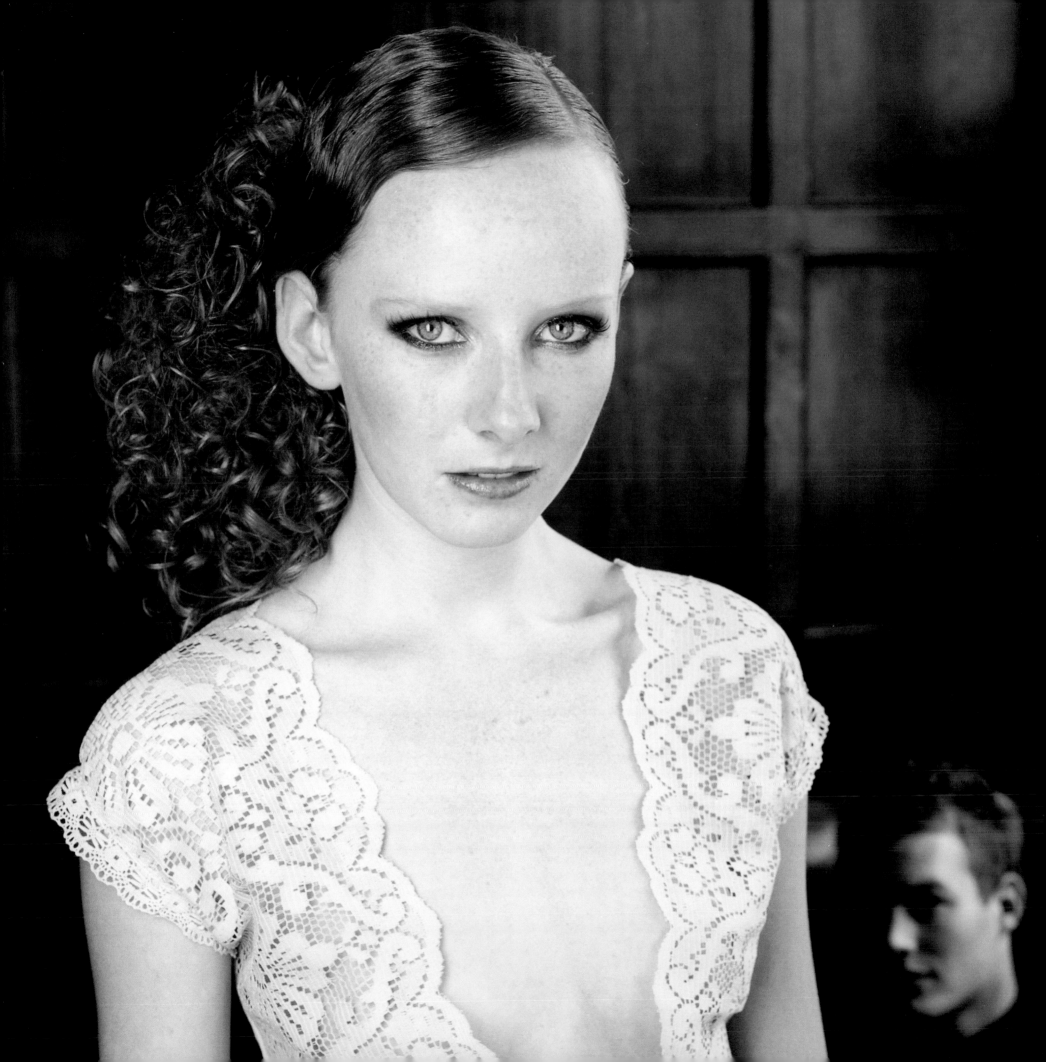

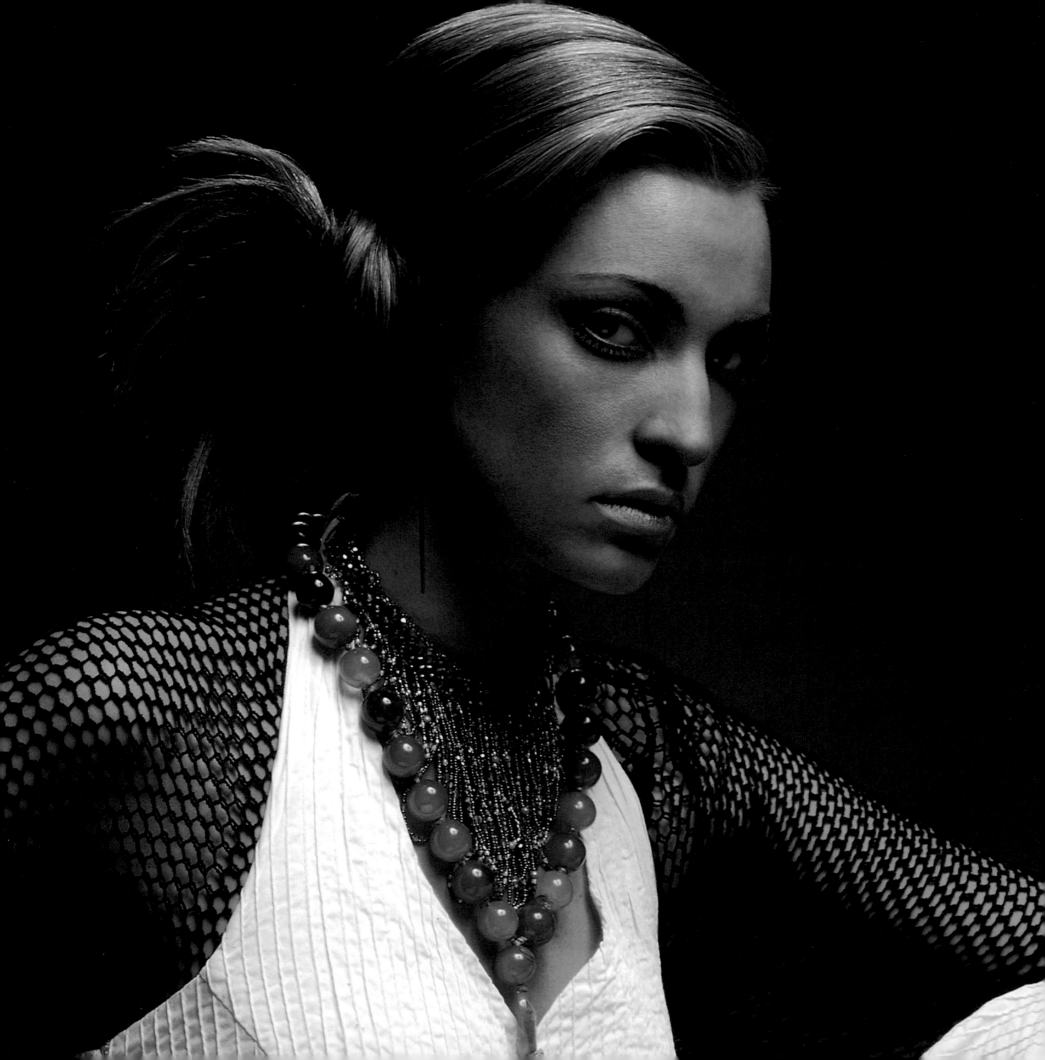

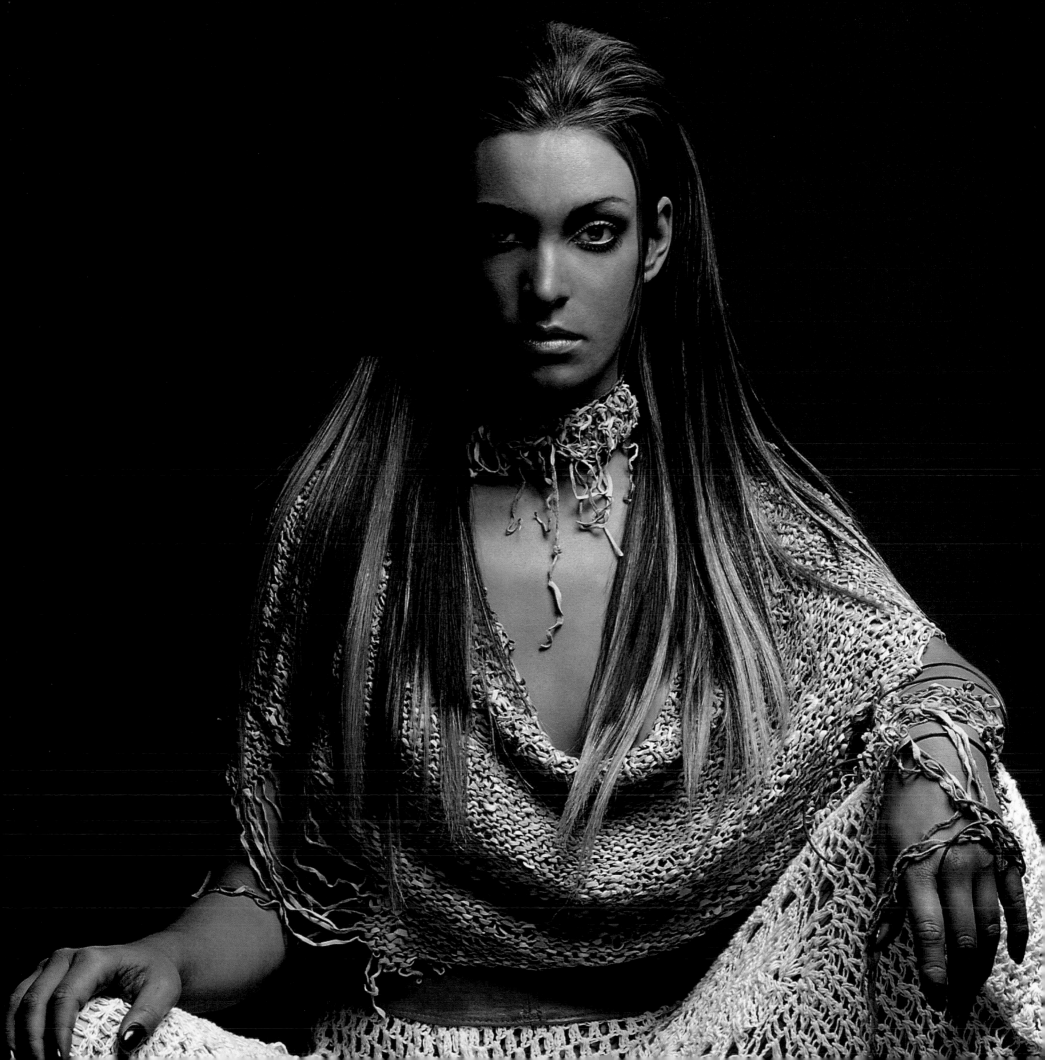

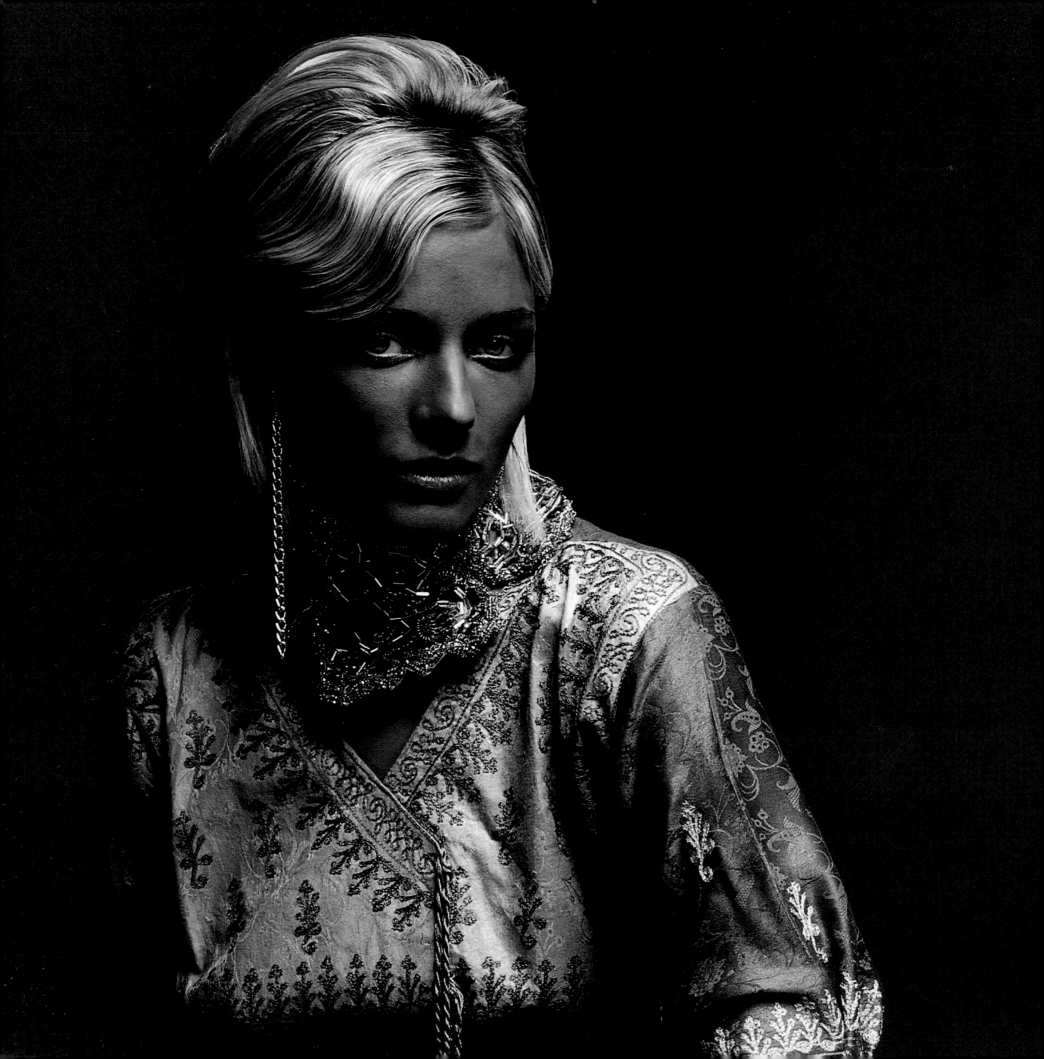

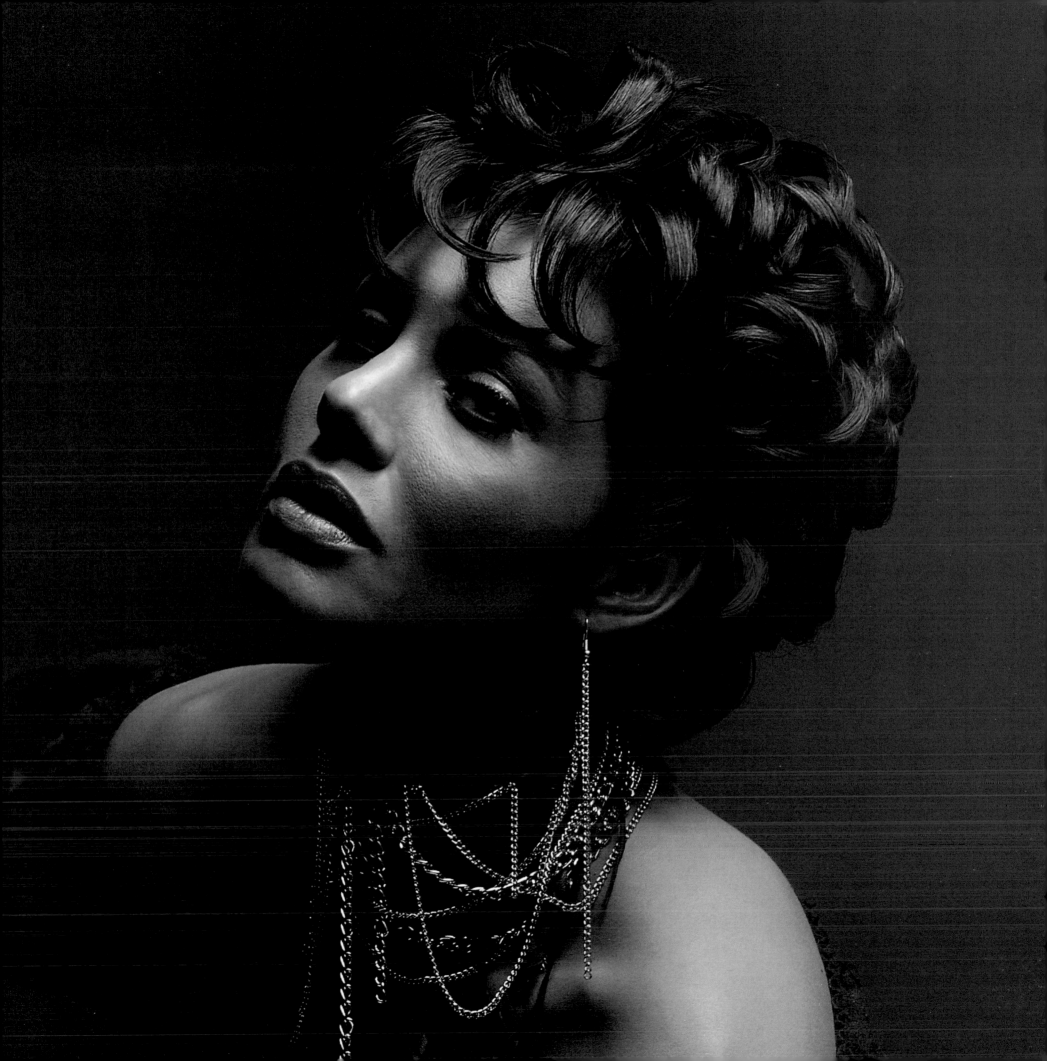

CHARLIE MILLER pages 238–245

13 Stafford Street, Edinburgh EH3 7BR, United Kingdom, www.charliemiller.co.uk

Hair: Jason and India Miller
Salon: Charlie Miller
Make-up: Cheryl Phelps-Gardiner
Styling: Marcella Martinello
Photography: Clive Arrowsmith

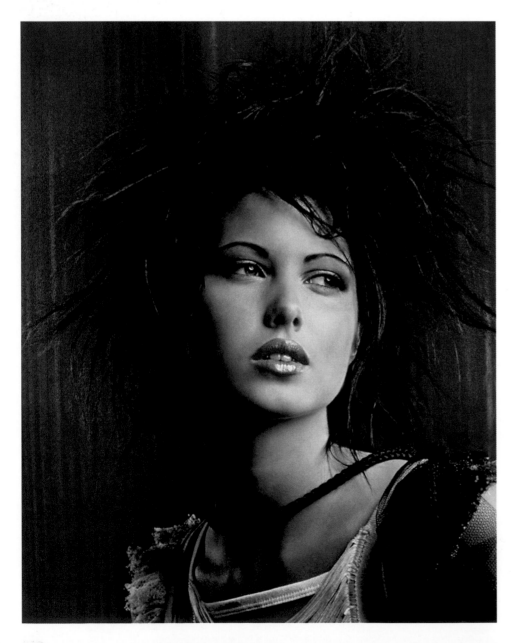

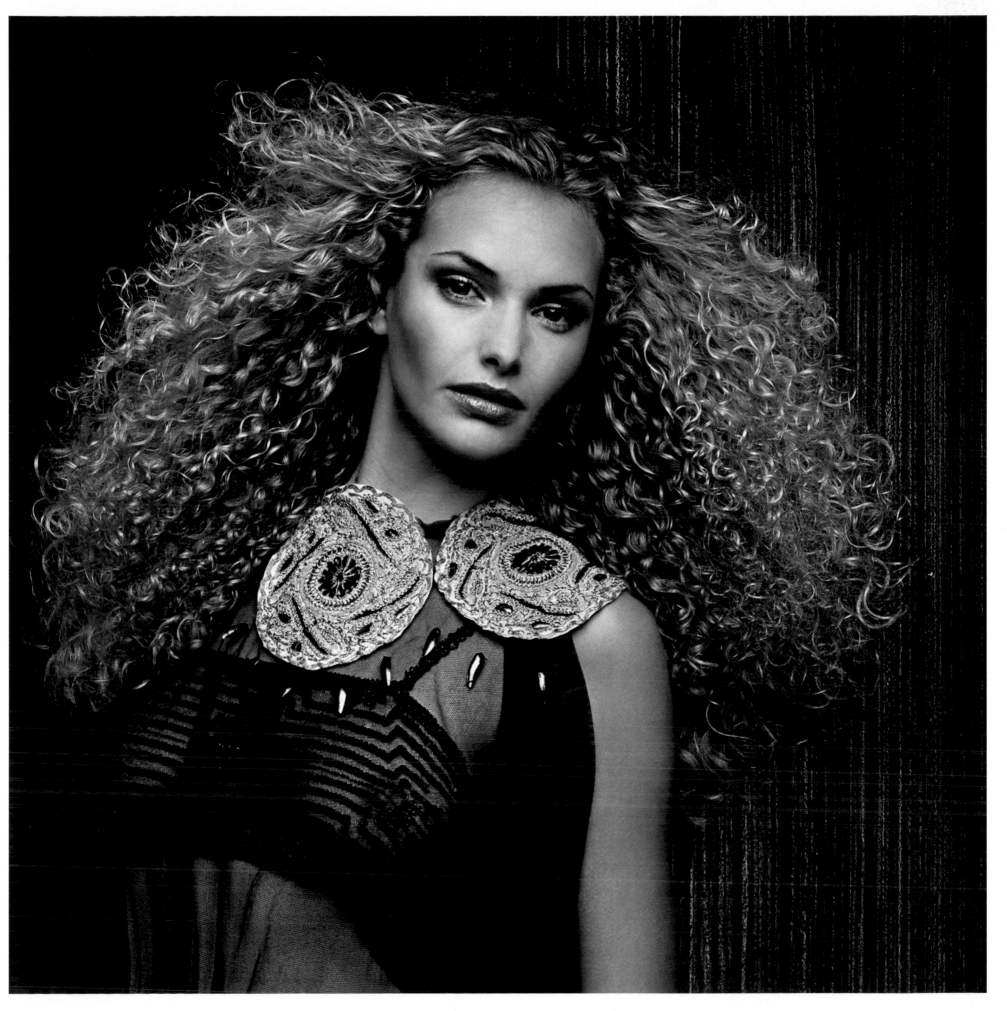

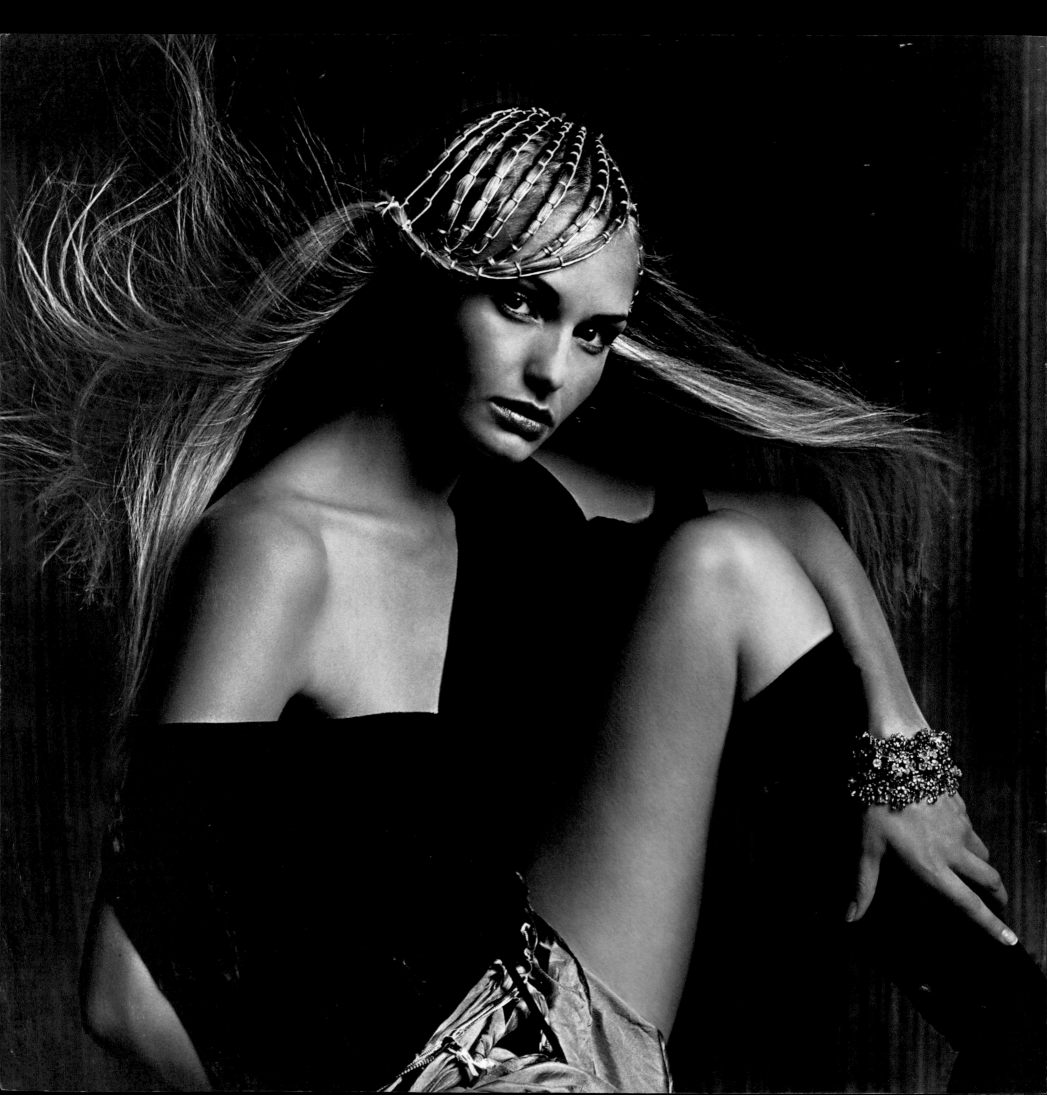

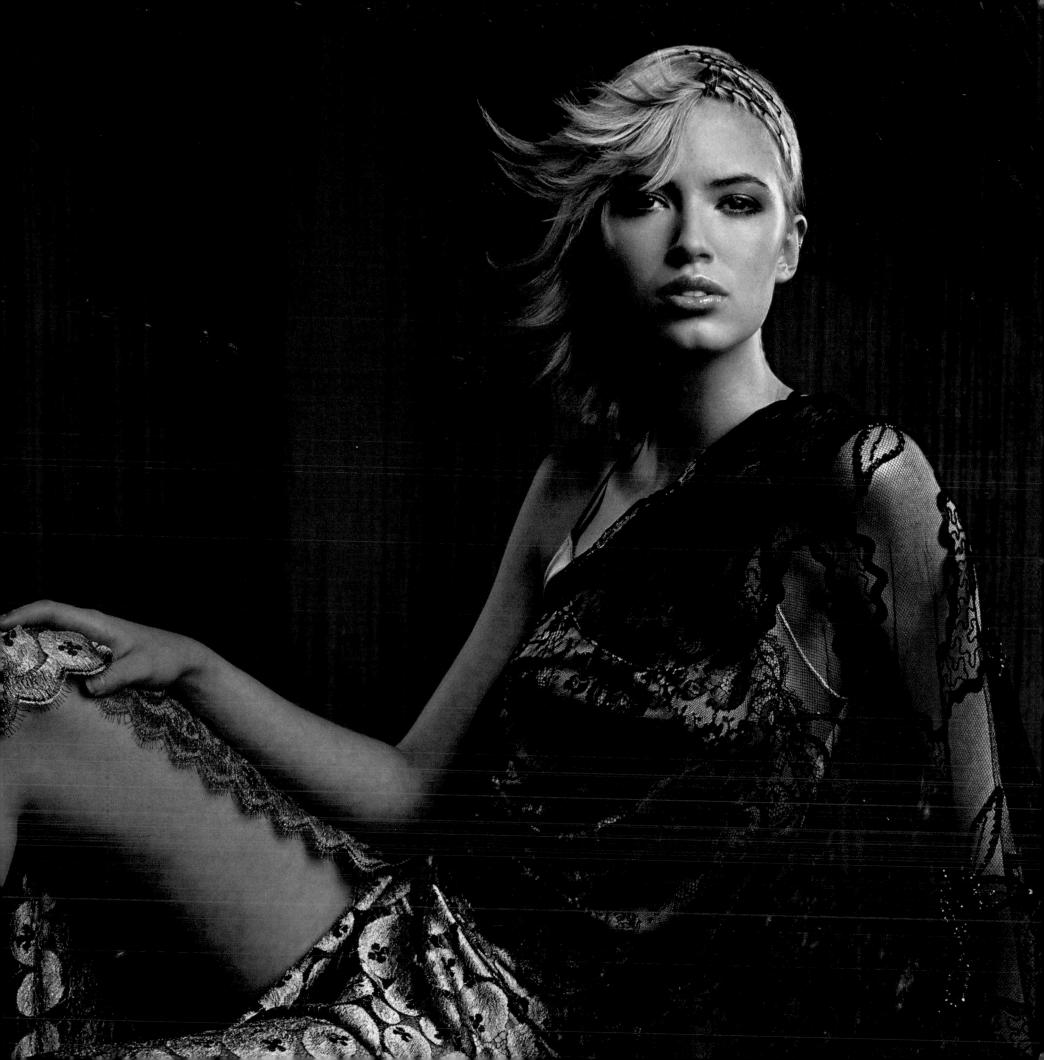

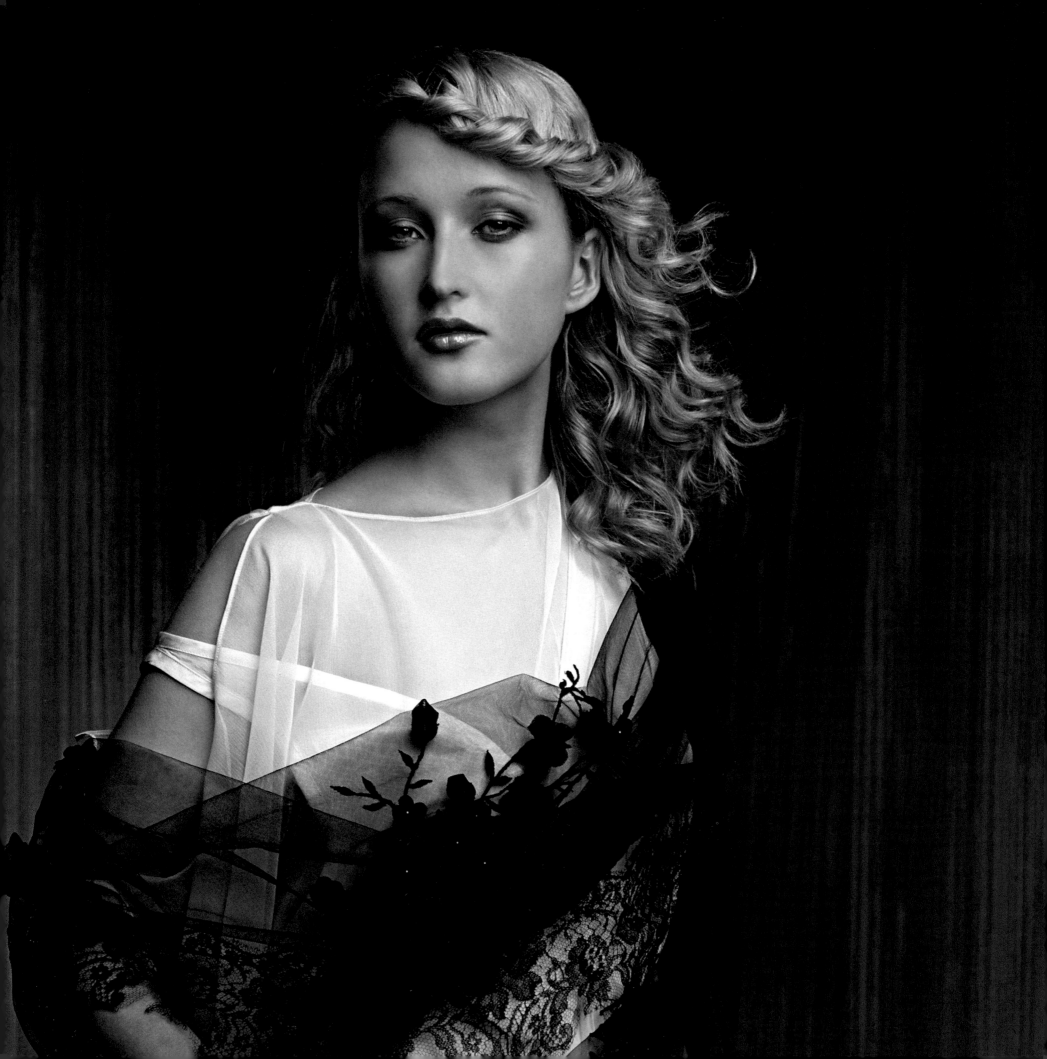

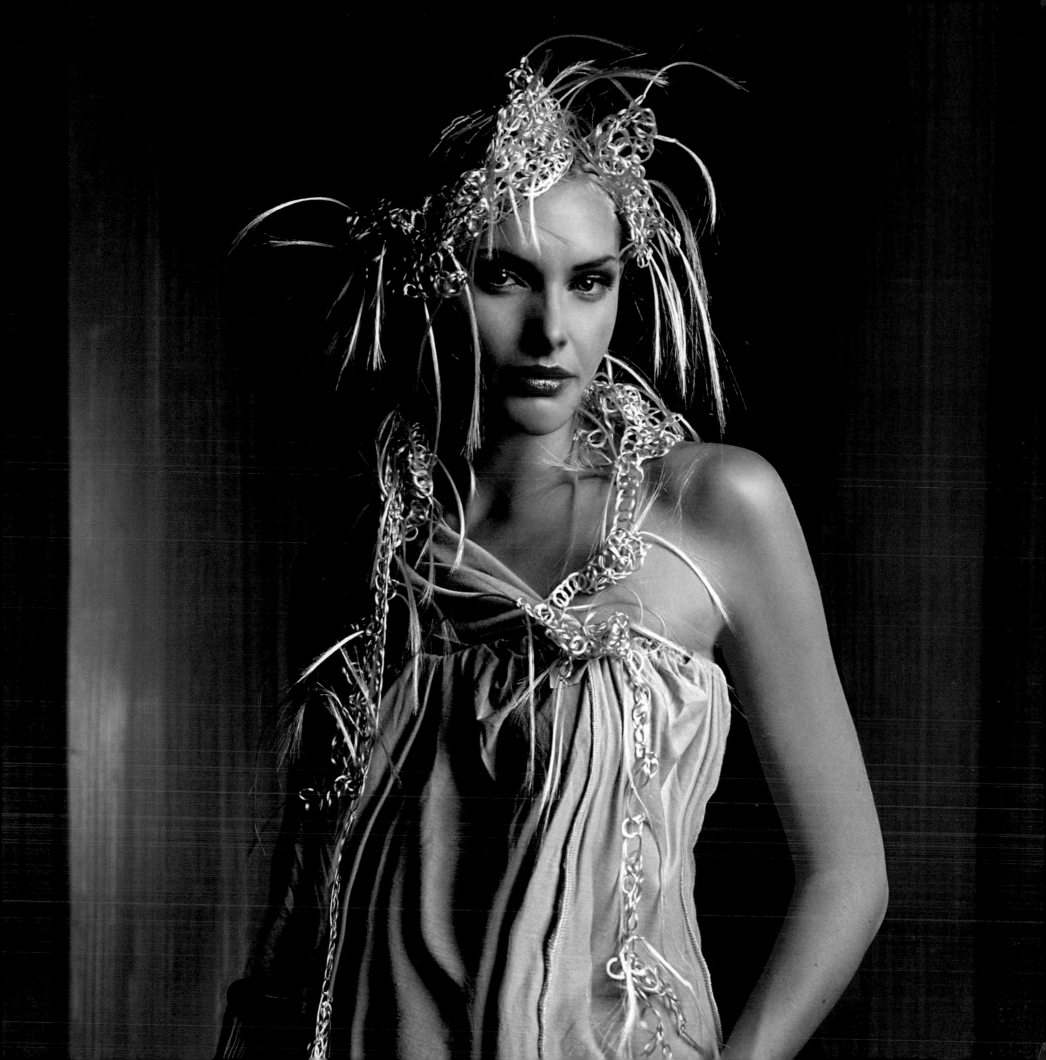

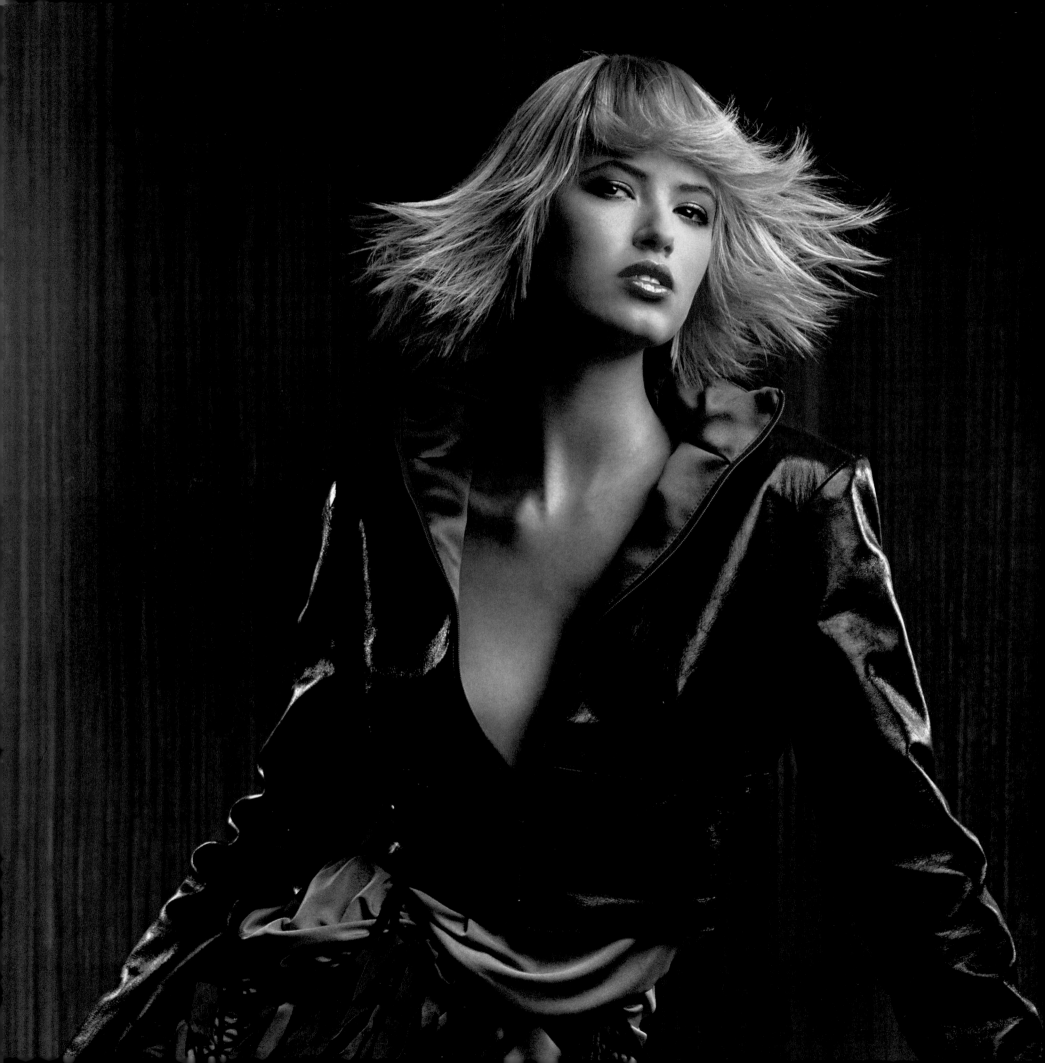

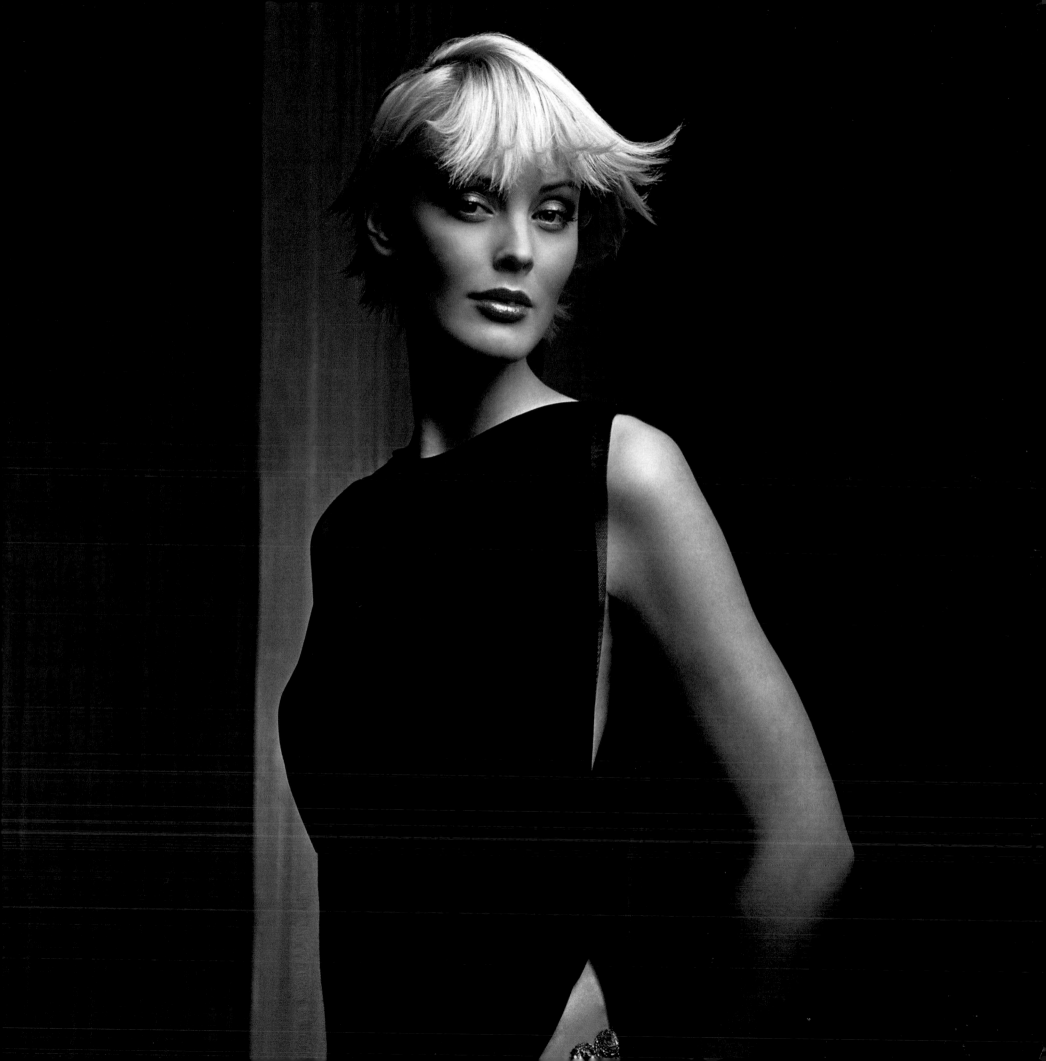

RICHARD WARD pages 246–247

162b Sloane Street, London SW1X 9BS, United Kingdom

Hair: Richard Ward
Salon: Richard Ward Hair & Beauty
Make-up: Melanie Harris, Mark Hayles
Styling: Cannon
Photography: Joseph Oppedisano
Products; L'Oréal Professionnel

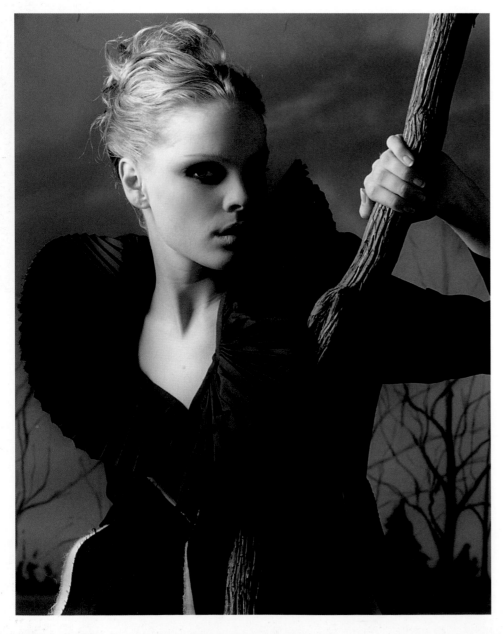

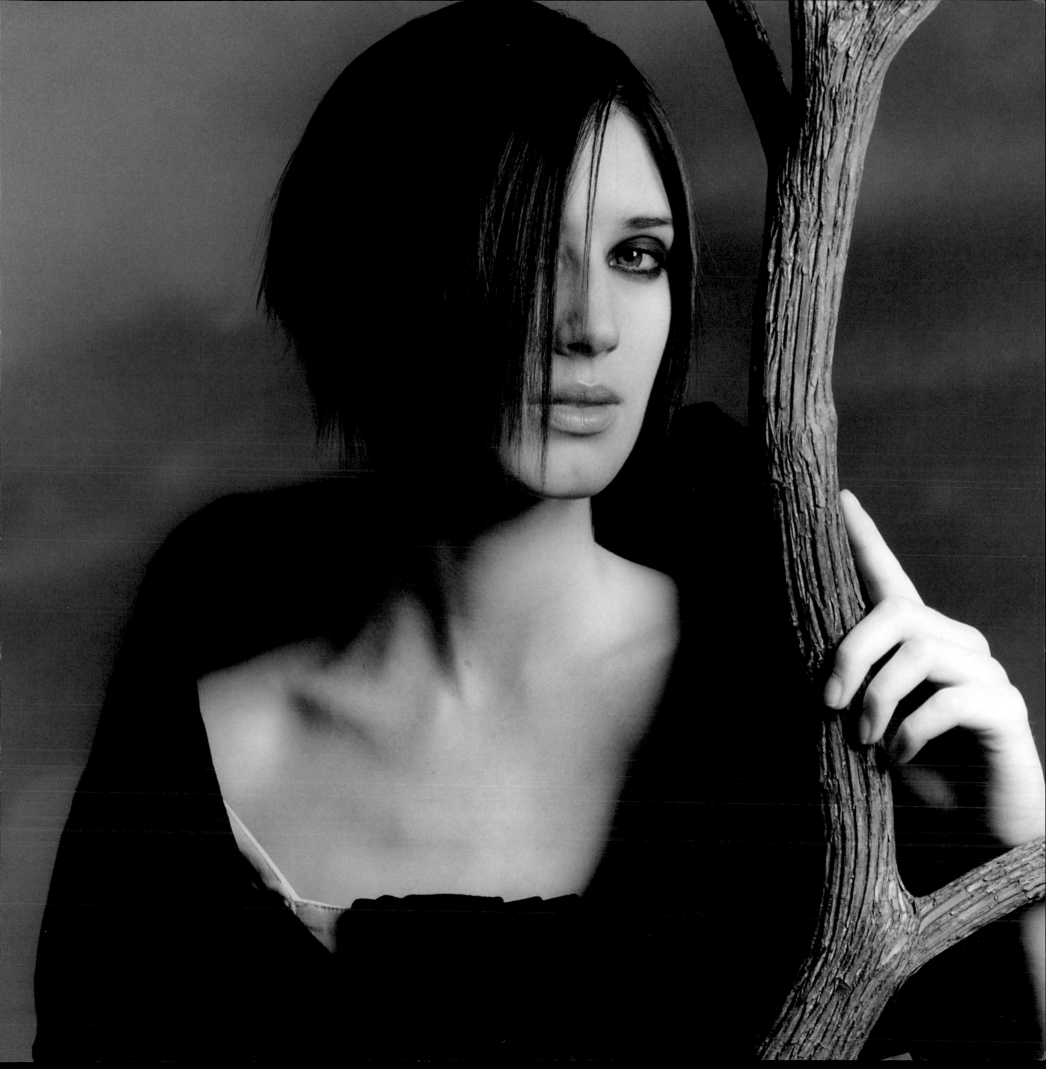

TREVOR SORBIE INTERNATIONAL pages 248–257

27 Floral Street, Covent Garden, London WC2E 9DP, United Kingdom, www.trevorsorbie.com

Hair: Trevor Sorbie (p. 248 - 151) Roberto Perozzi for Trevor Sorbie International (p. 252 - 257)
Salon: Trevor Sorbie International
Make-up: Pat Mascolo (p. 248 - 151) Helen Kalli (p. 252 - 257)
Styling: Wendy Elsmore and Jade Sorbie (p. 248 - 151)
Photography: Anthony Mascolo (p. 248 - 151) Alex Forsey (p. 252 - 257)
Products: Trevor Sorbie Professional

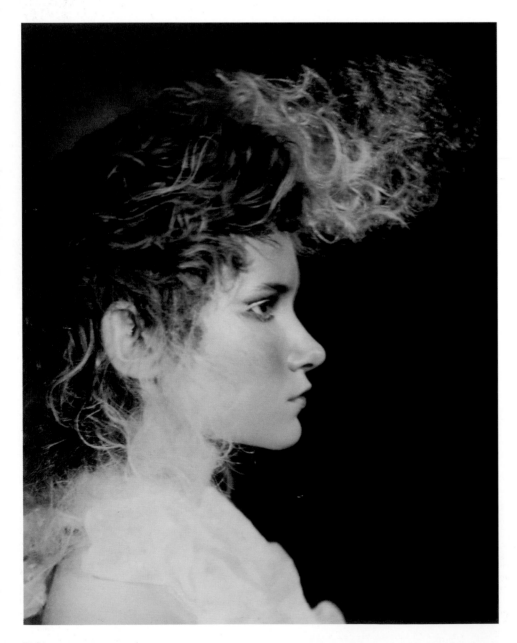

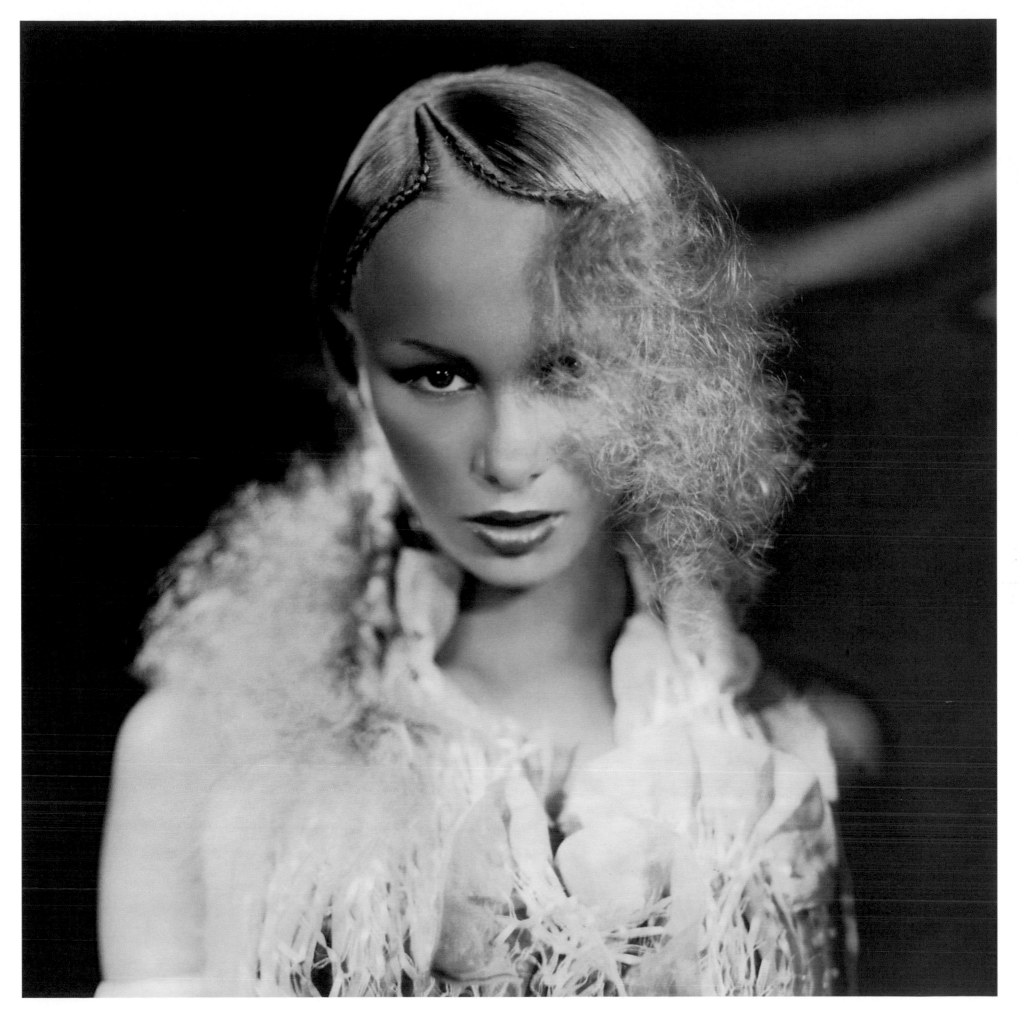

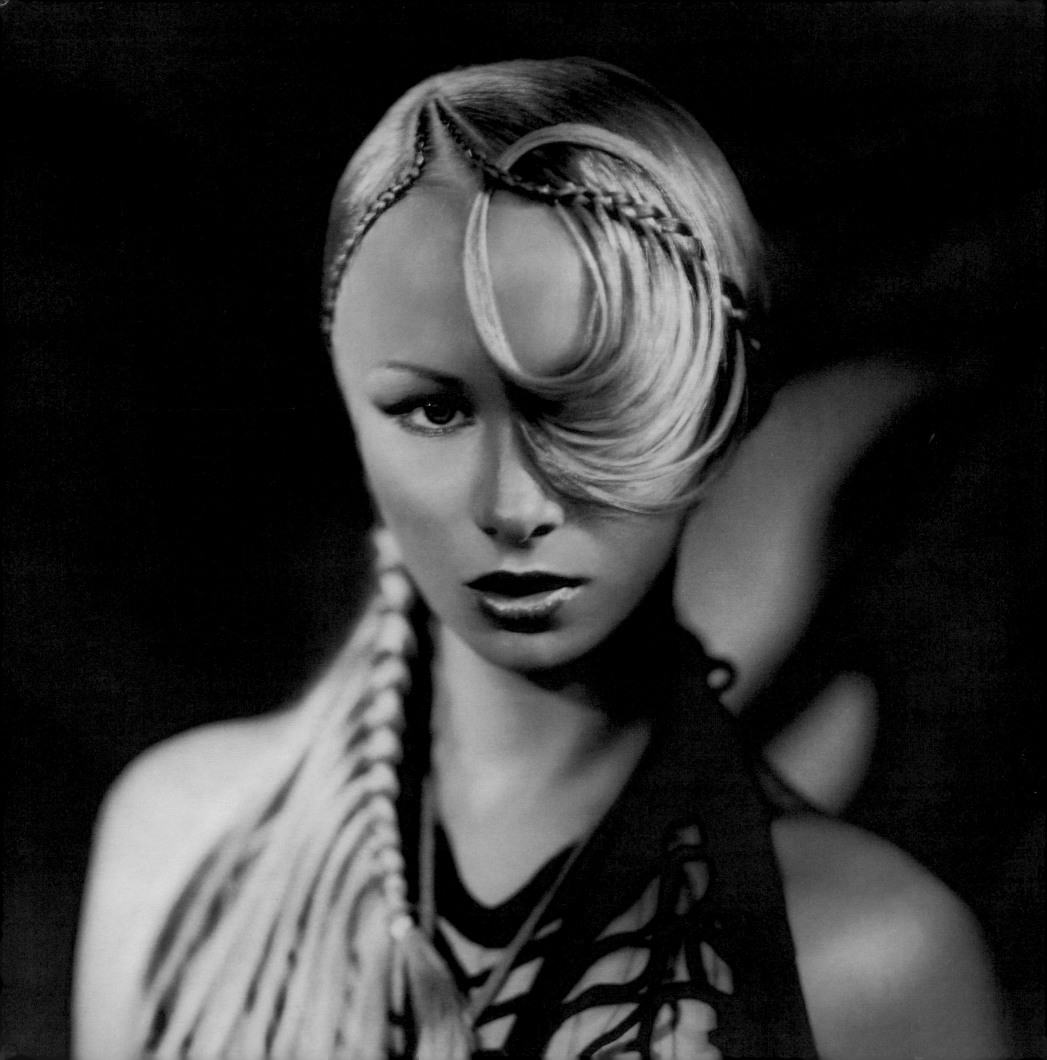

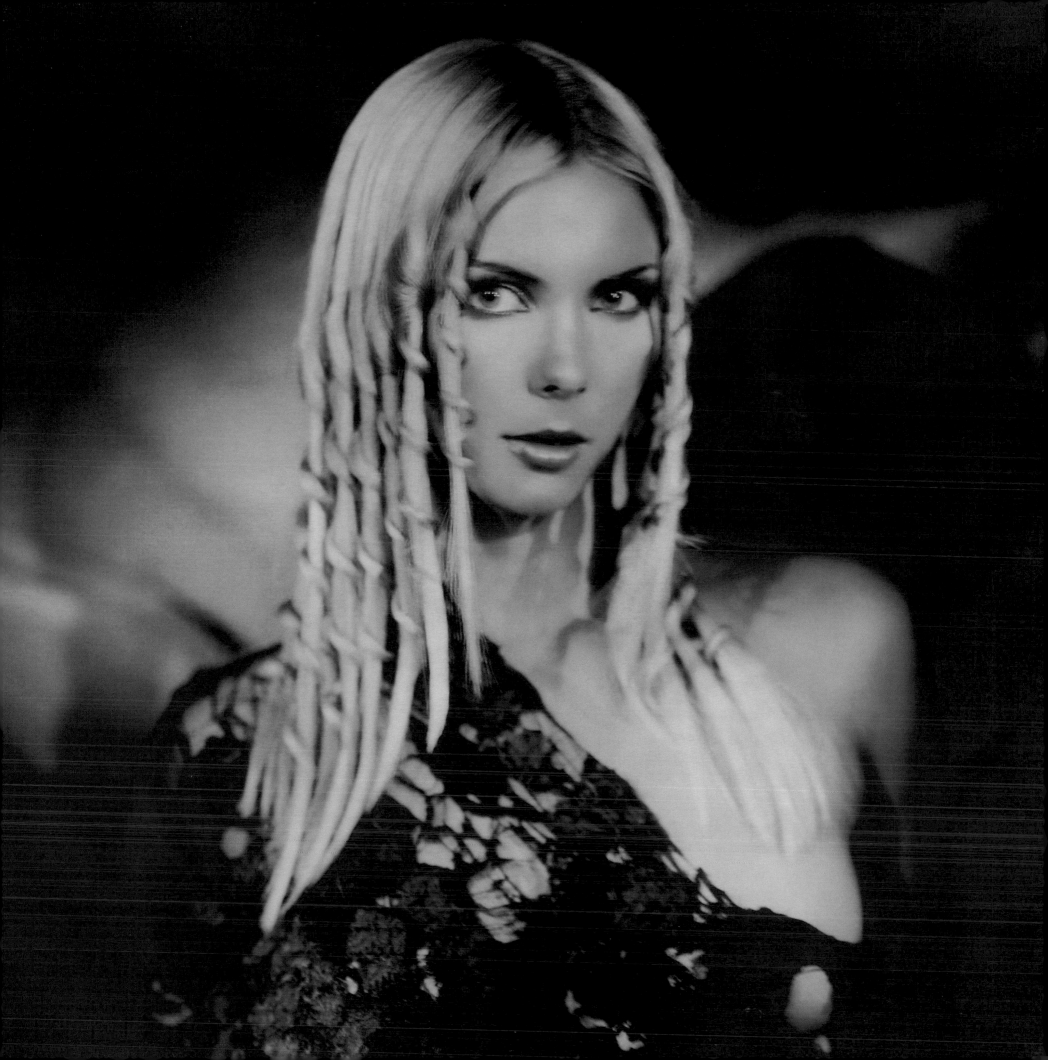

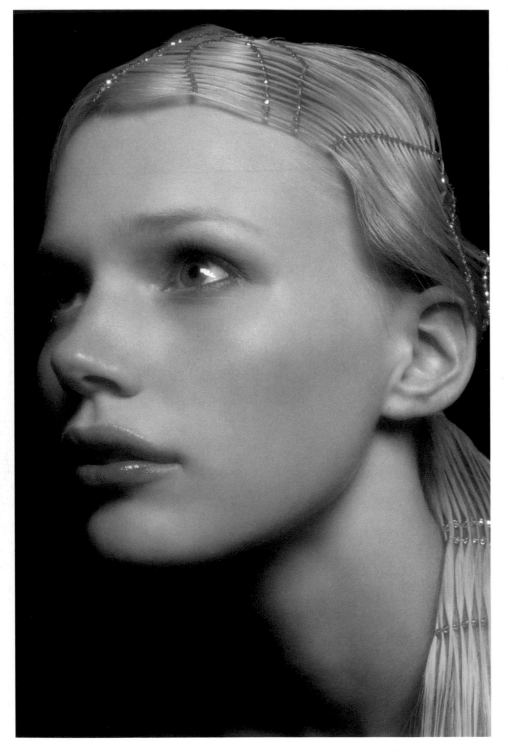
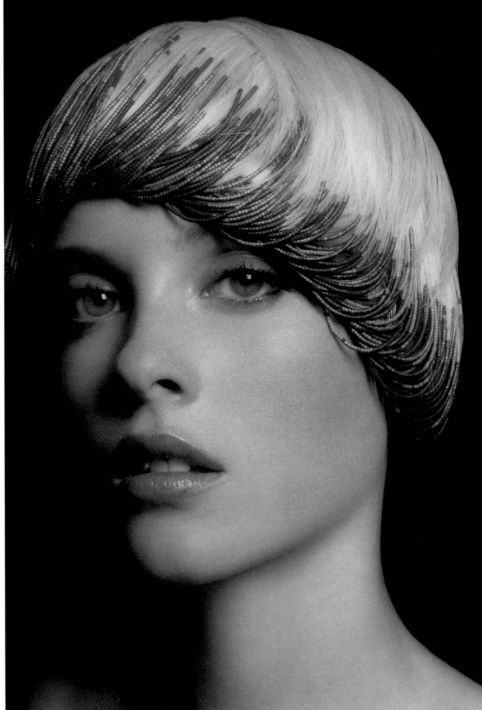

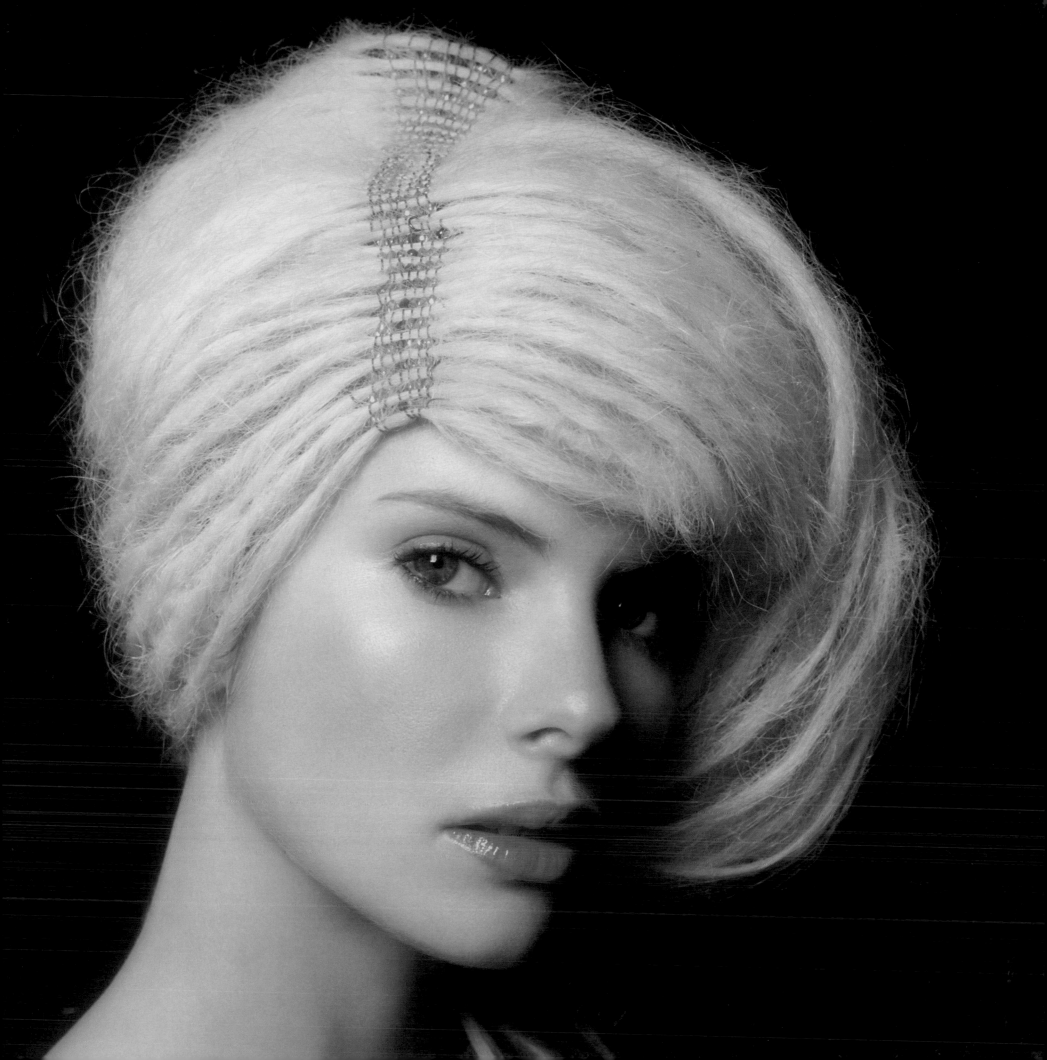

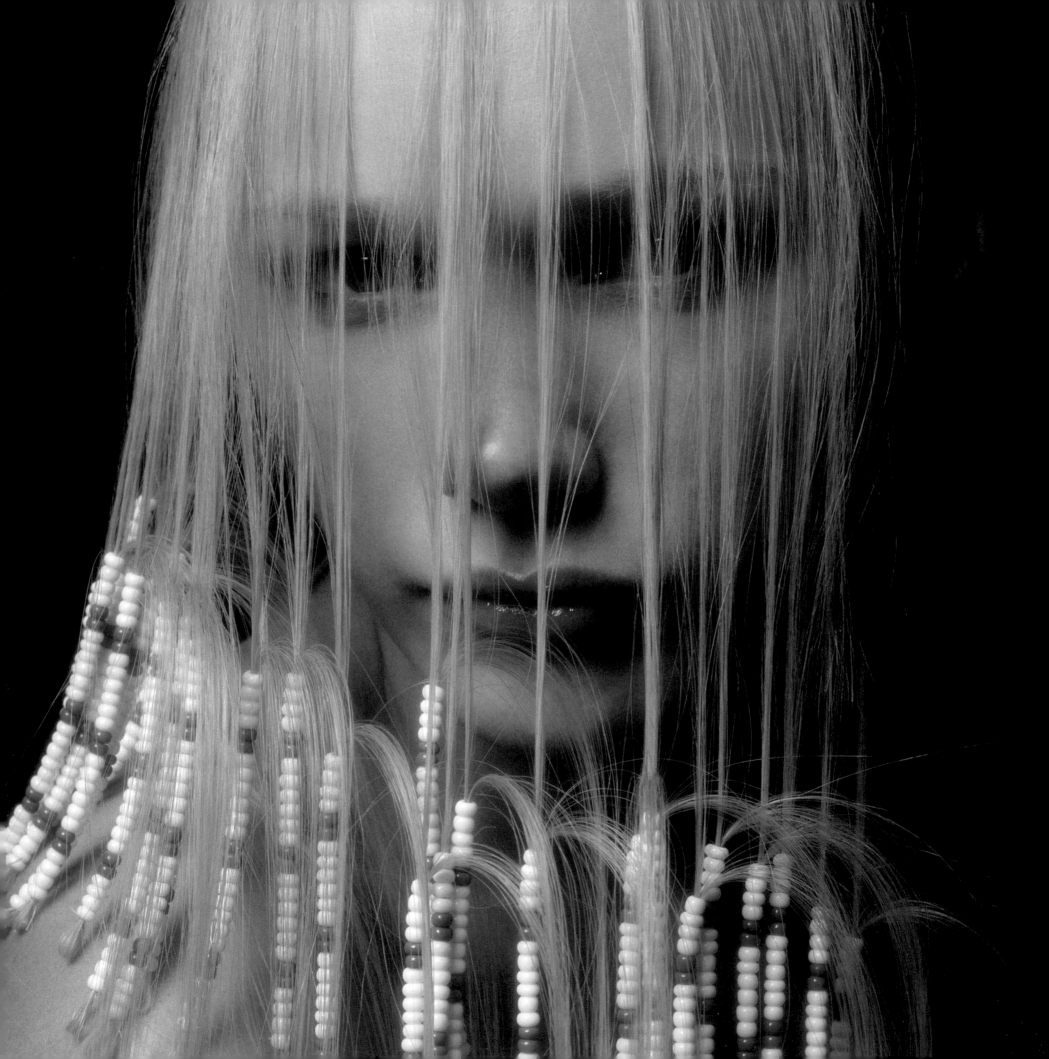

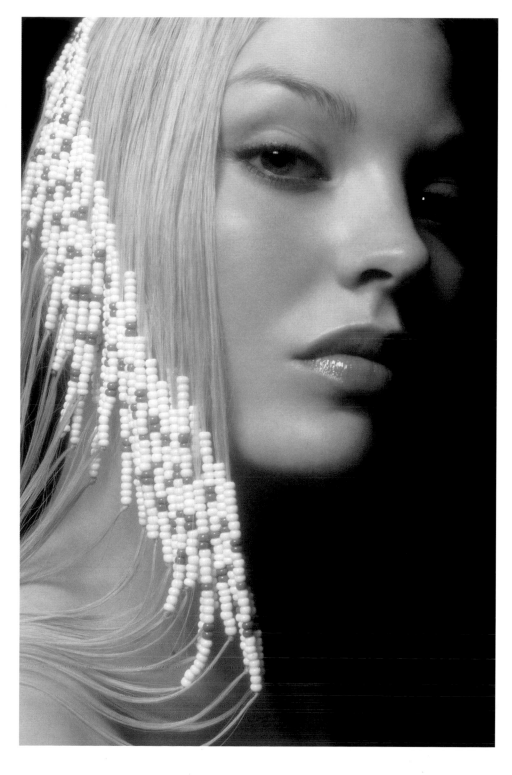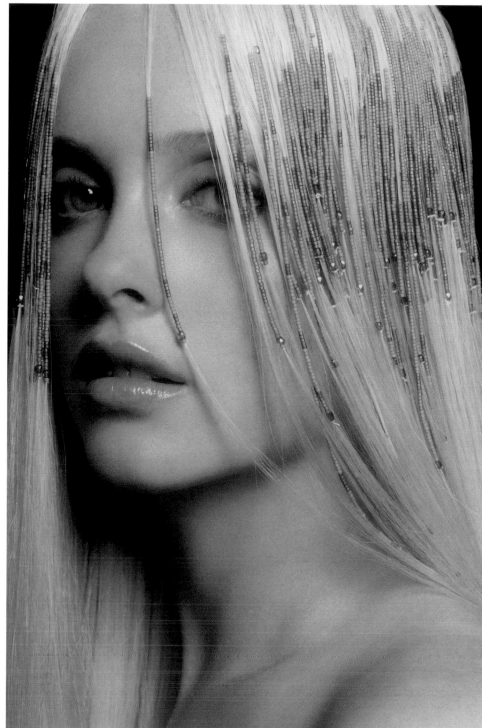

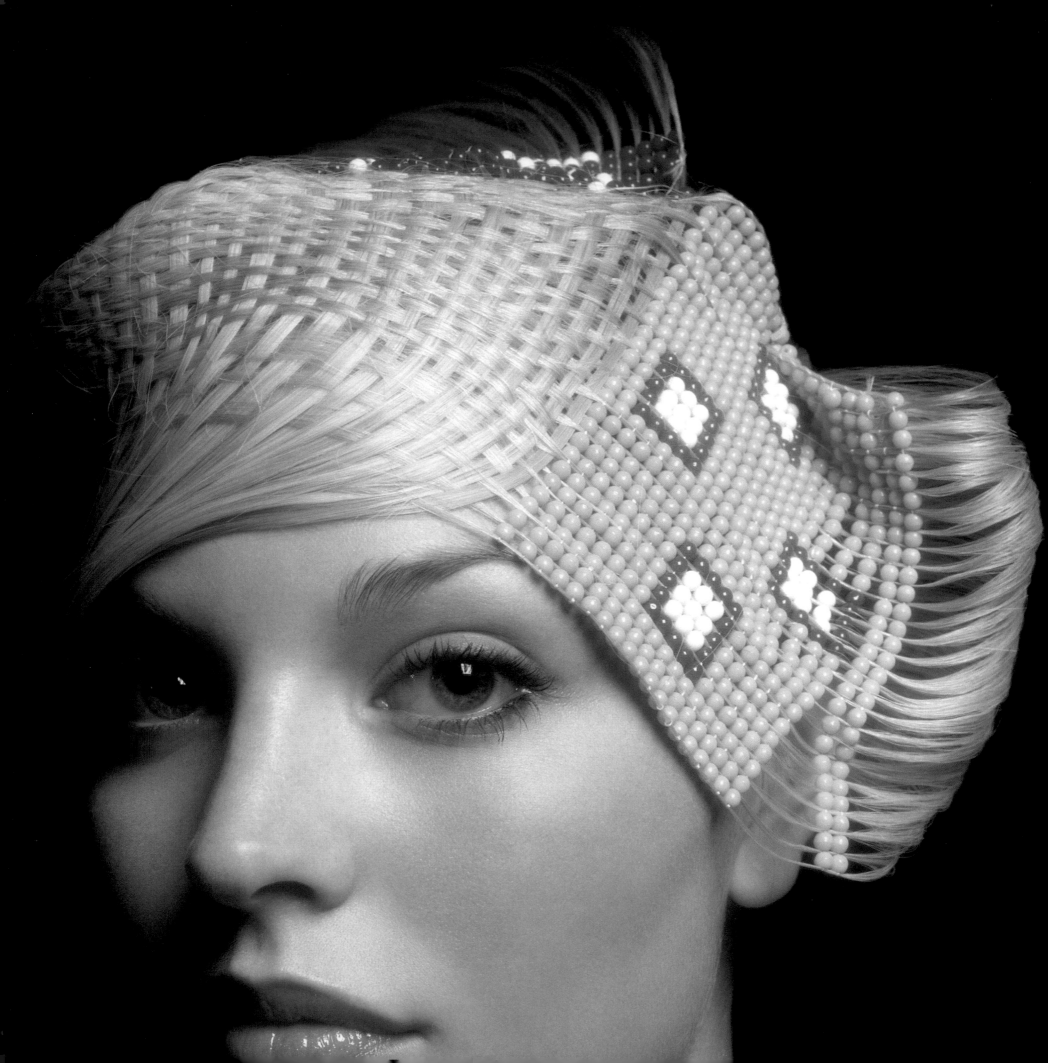

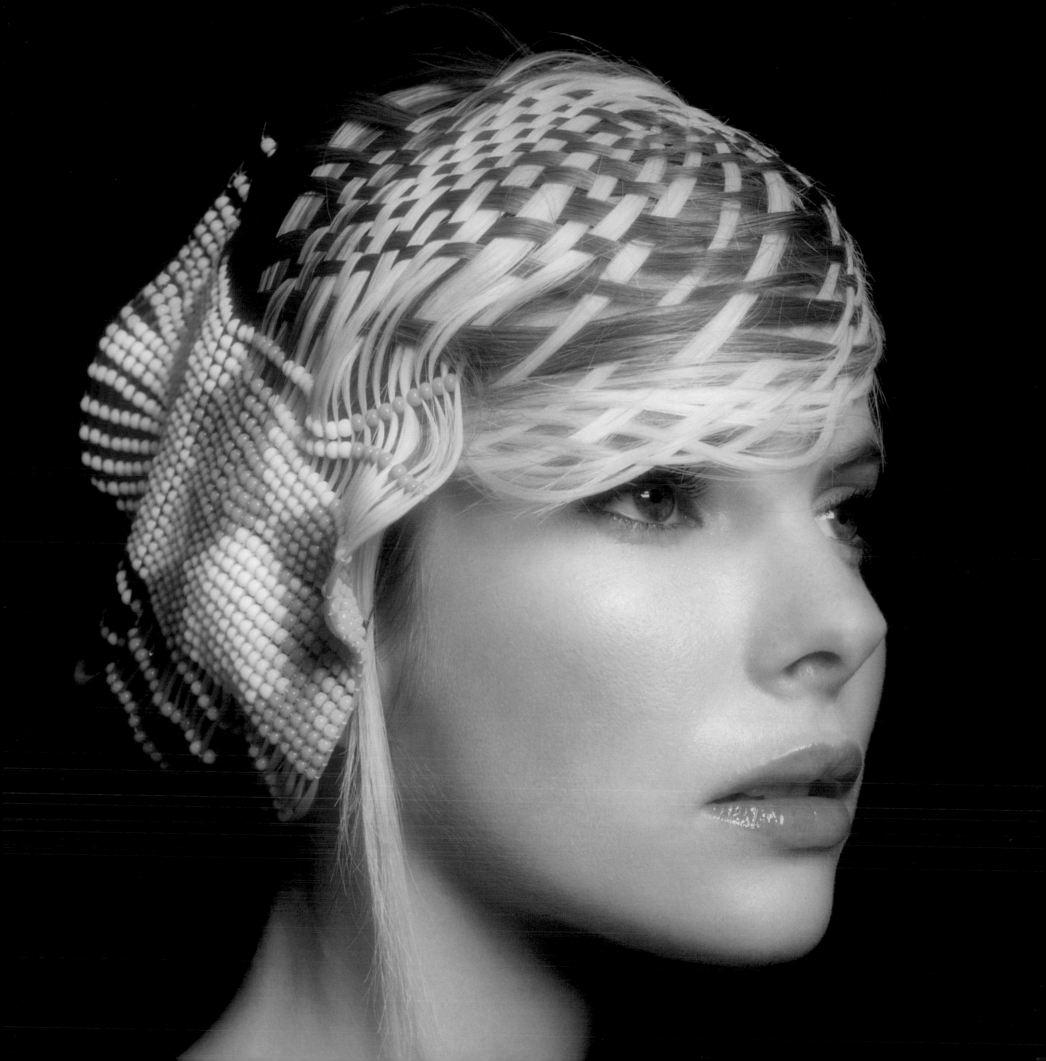

SEAN HANNA pages 258–259

26 The Broadway, Wimbledon, London SW19 1RE, United Kingdom, www.seanhanna.com

Hair: Sean Hanna
Make-up: Joanne Jones
Styling: Yesmin O'Brien
Photography: Dan Connor
Products: L'Oréal Professionnel

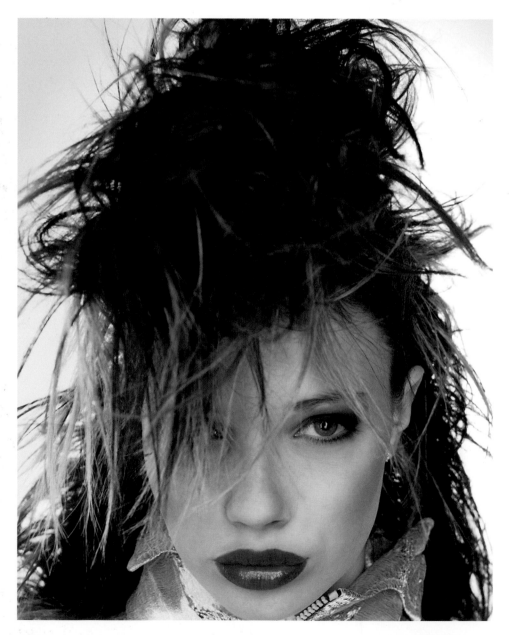

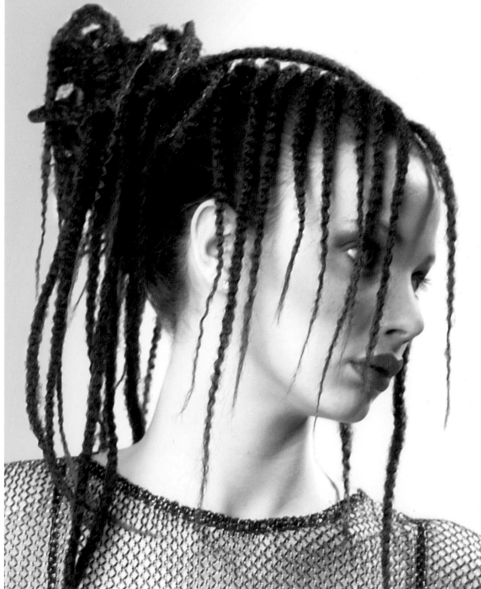

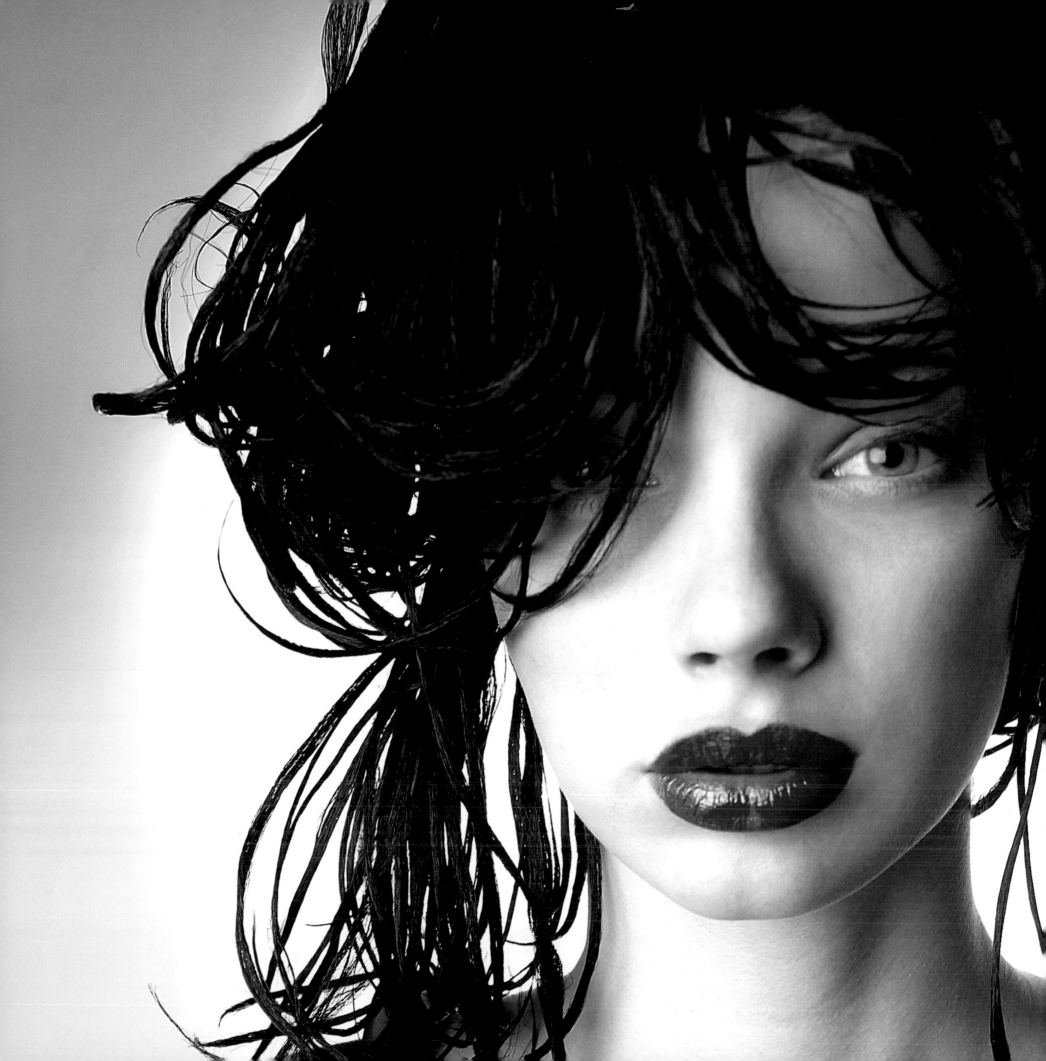

MARK HILL pages 260–261

Mark Hill Salon, Hogg Lane Kirkella, Hull North Humberside HU10 7NU, United Kingdom, www.markhill.co.uk

Hair: Mark Hill Artistic Team
Salon: Mark Hill Salon
Make-up: Cheryl Phelps-Gardiner
Styling: Jonas Halberg
Photography: Malcom Willison
Products: Wella, Schwarzkopf

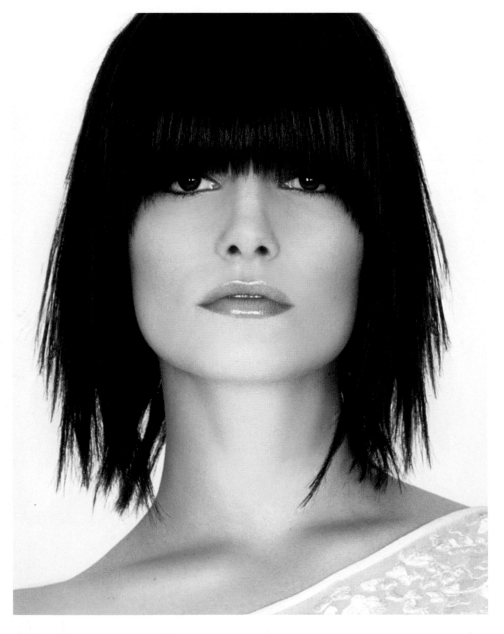

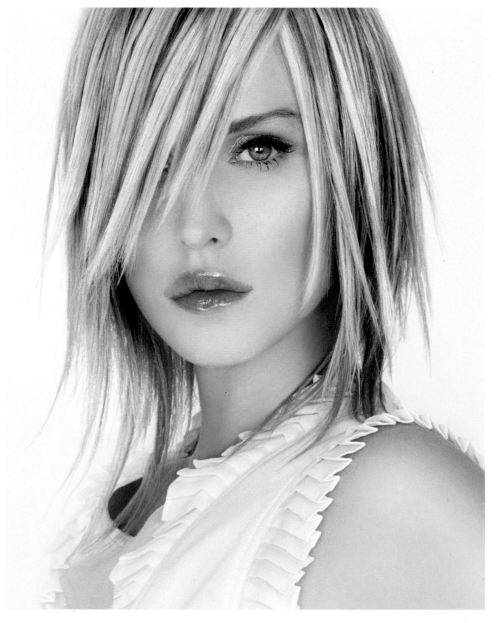

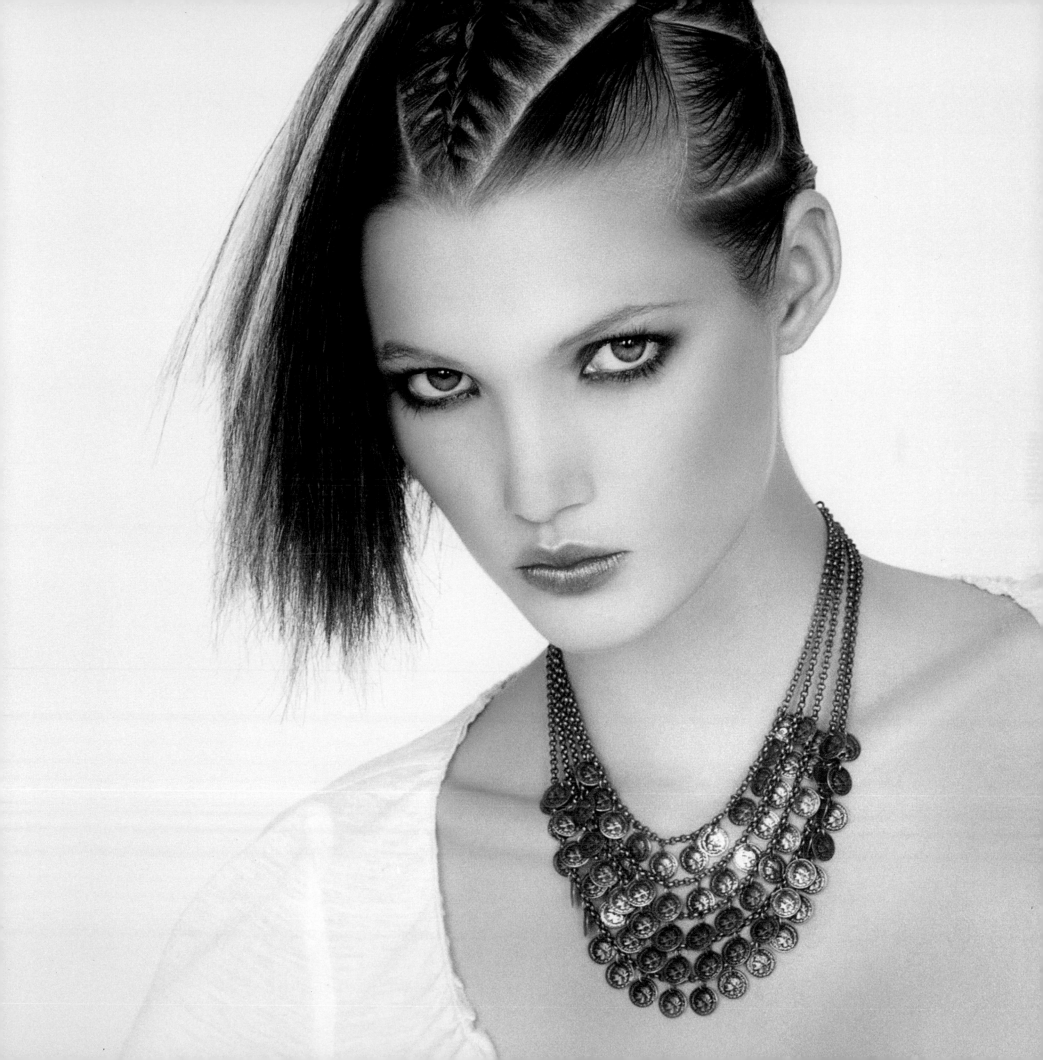

Hair: Jason Atkinson
Colour: Mariesa Ferraro
Make-up: Cathy G.
Photography: Kerry Leonard, BRUIZE

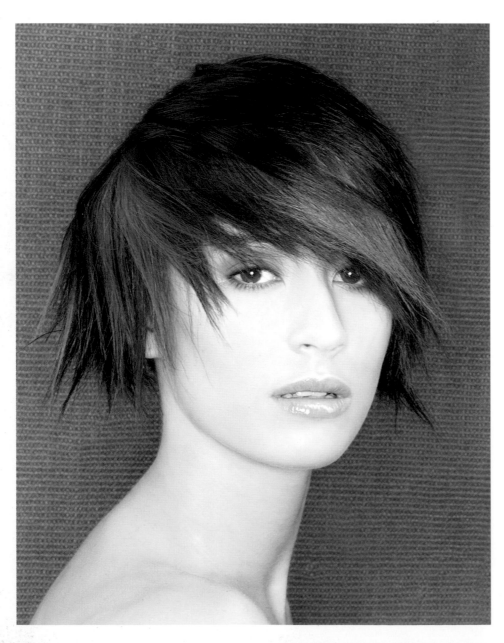

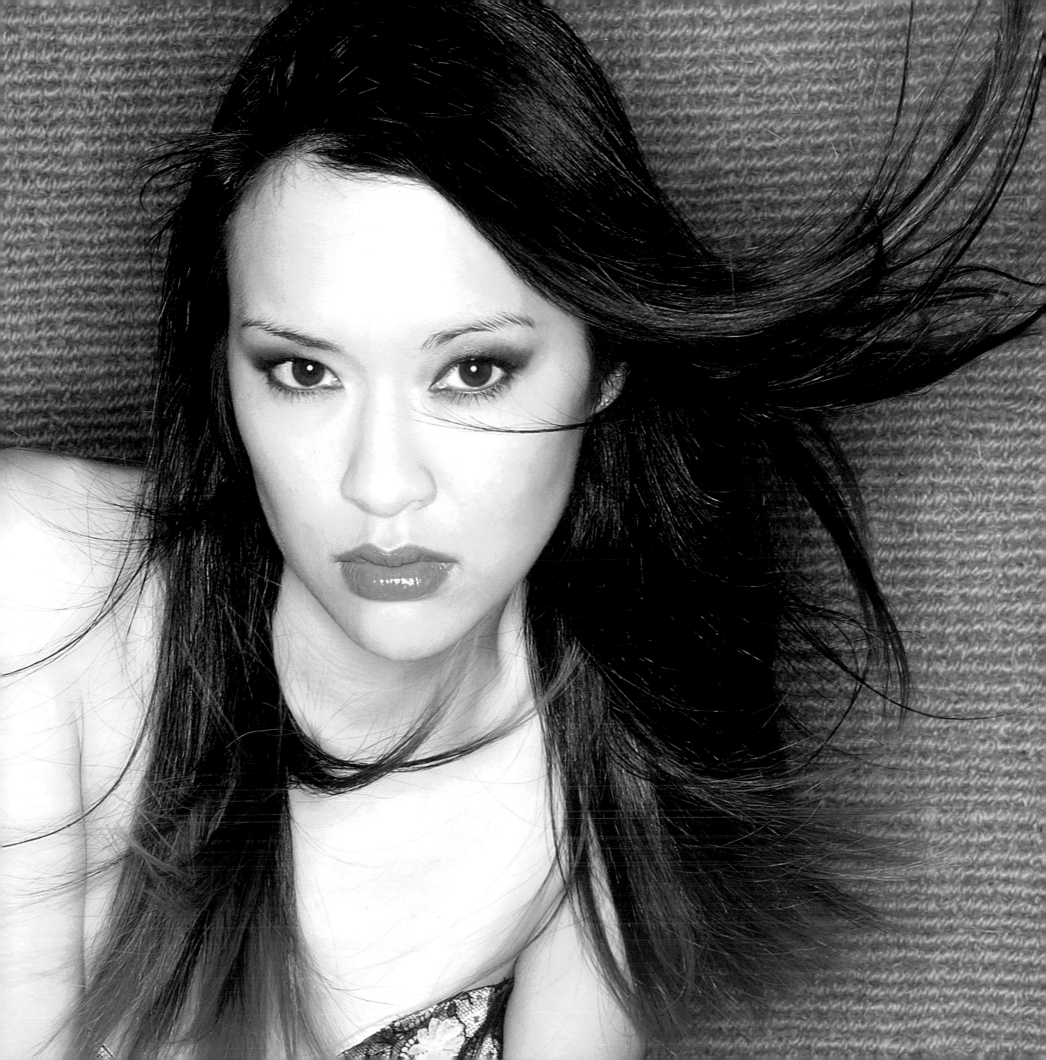

MASSIMO CORSI pages 264–265

Via Roma 123, San Benedetto del Tronto, 63039 AP, Italy, www.massimocorsi.com

Hair: Massimo Corsi
Make-up: Guillermina Carinelli for Massimo Corsi
Styling: Antonella Maroni
Photography: Massimo Corsi
Products: Paul Mitchell

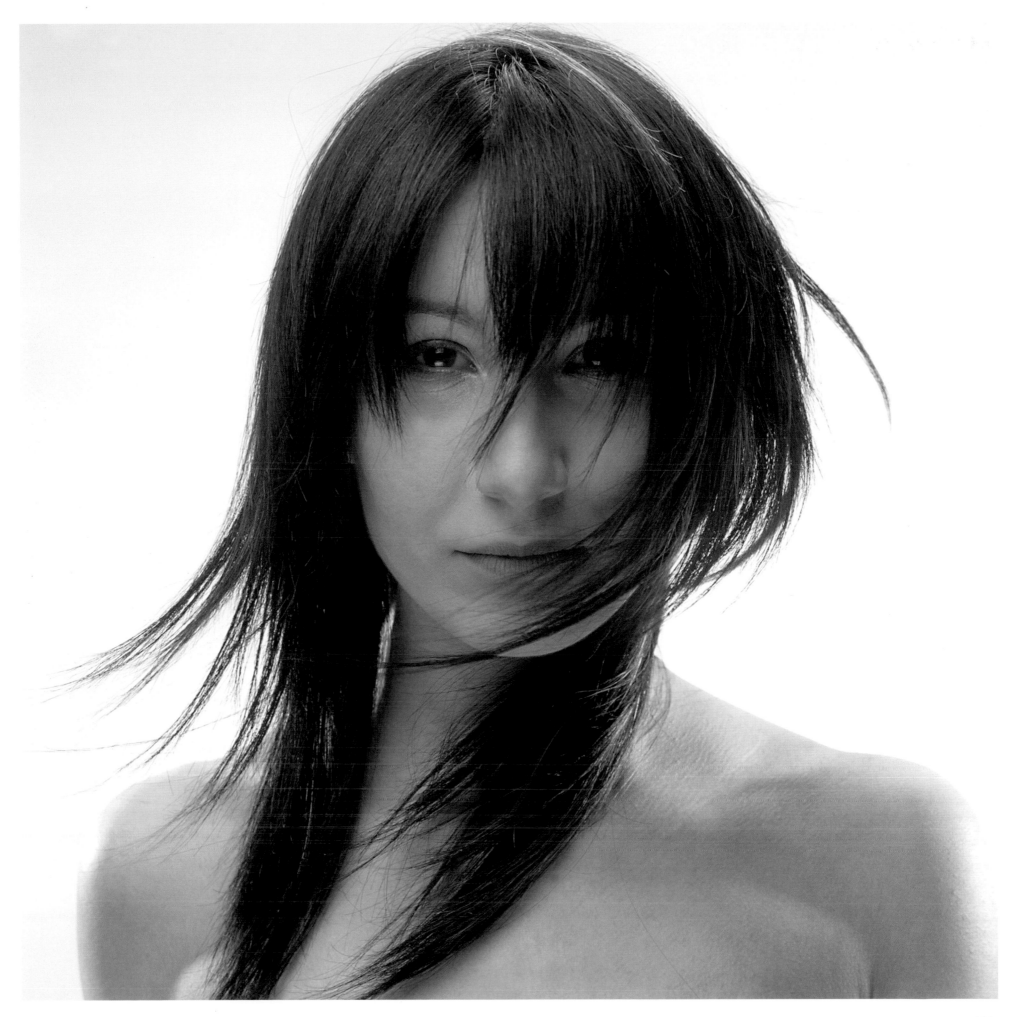

TERY DOUGHERTY pages 266–267

1227 Muirkirk Court, Folsom California 95630, USA, www.teridougherty.com

Hair: Tery Dougherty
Styling: Bill Conti
Photography: Valtz Kleins Latvia
Models: Usta (p. 266) Evita (p. 266) Inessa (p. 267)

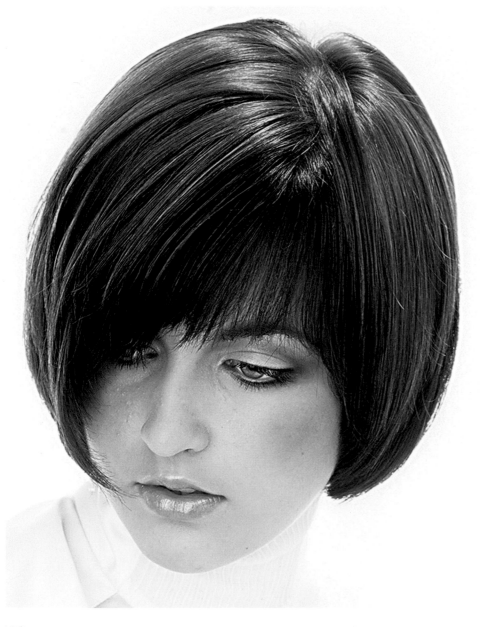

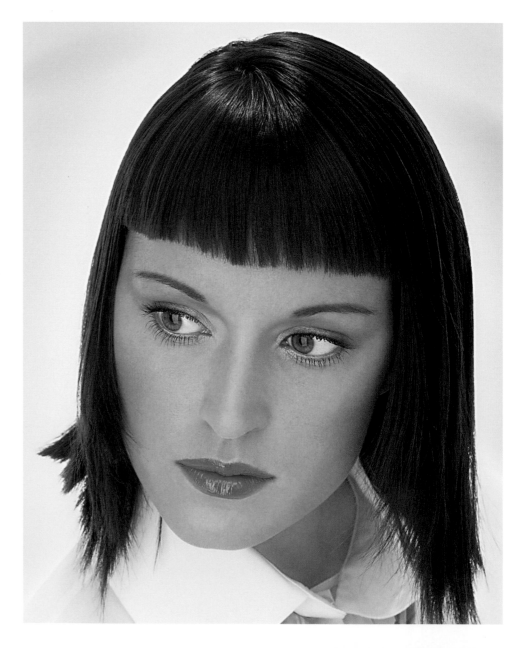

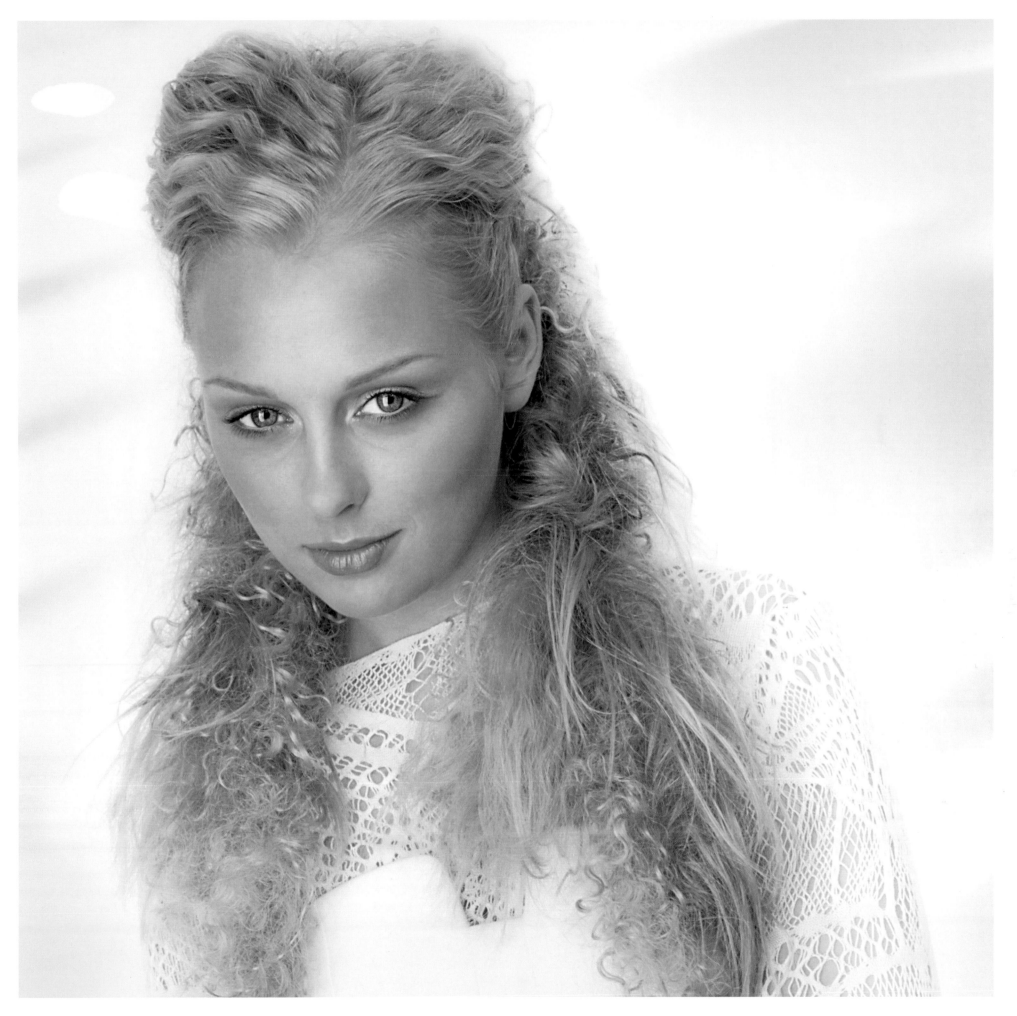

TSIKNARIS HAIR pages 268–269

169-171 Elizabeth Street, Brisbane QLD 4000, Australia, www.tsiknarishair.com

Hair: Bill Tsiknaris
Salon: Tsiknaris Hair
Make-up: Sarah Laidlaw
Styling: Mary Tsiknaris

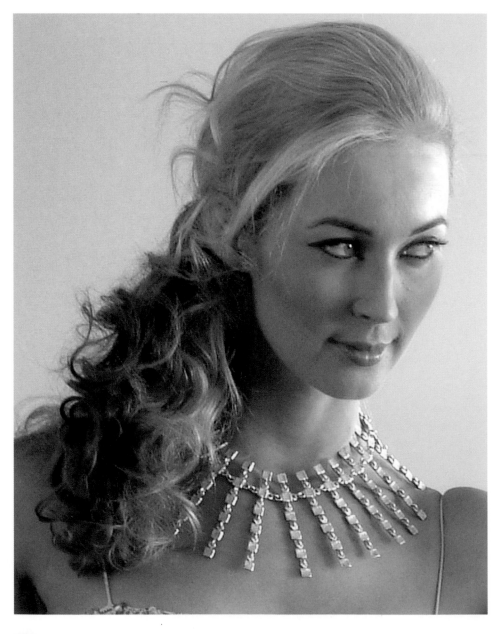
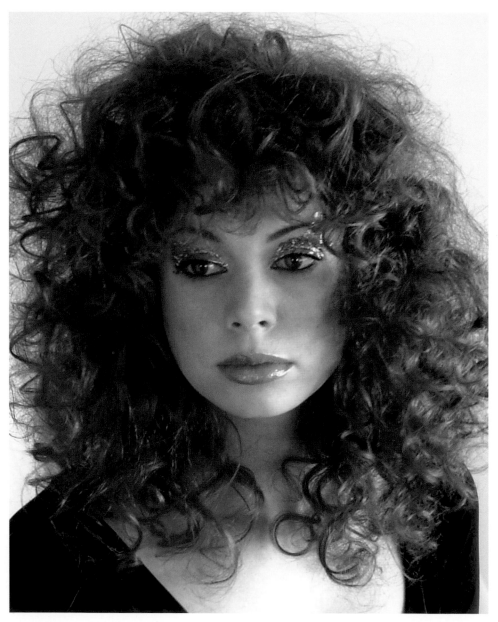

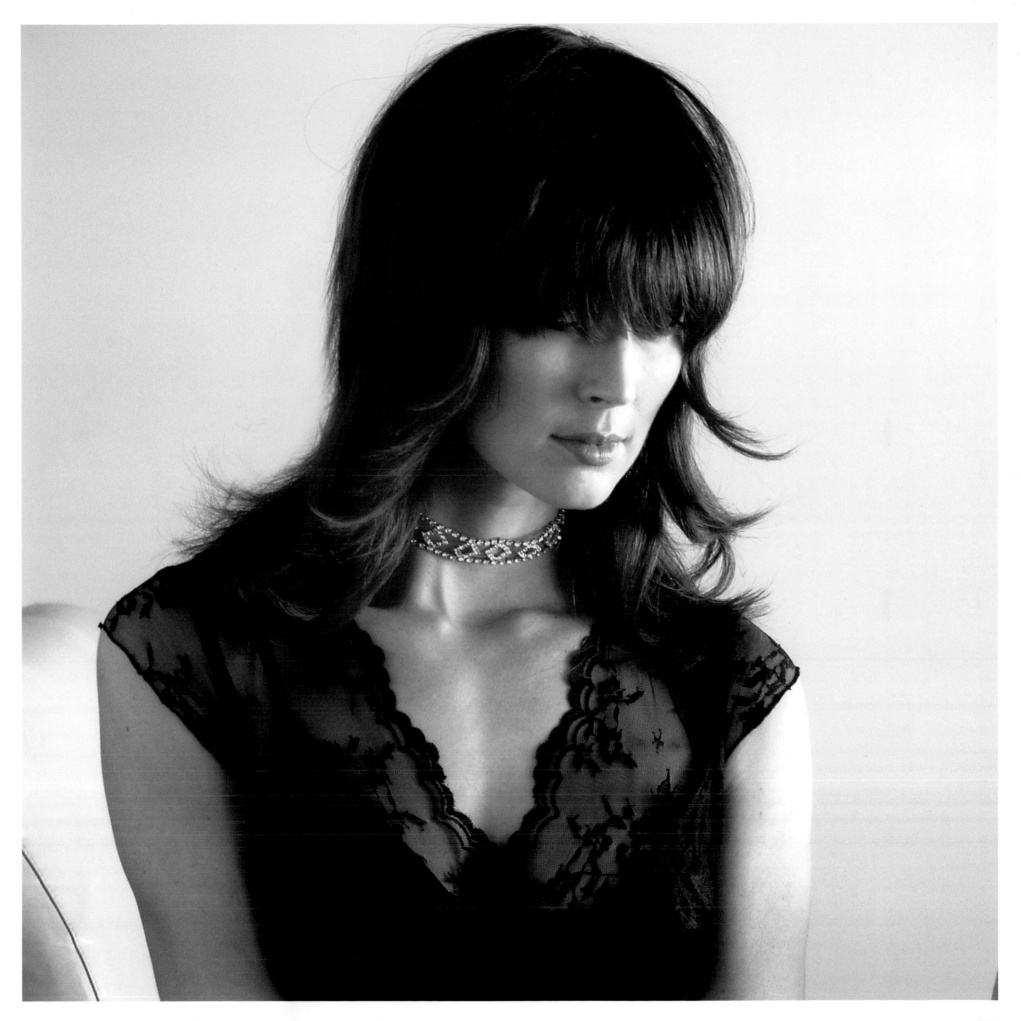

ANTOINETTE BEENDERS pages 270–271

The Urban Retreat, 174 High Holborn, London WC1 7AA, United Kingdom

Hair: Antoinette Beenders for Aveda
Colour: Ana Karzis for Aveda
Make-up: Sinden
Styling: Damian Foxe
Photography: Chris Dunlop

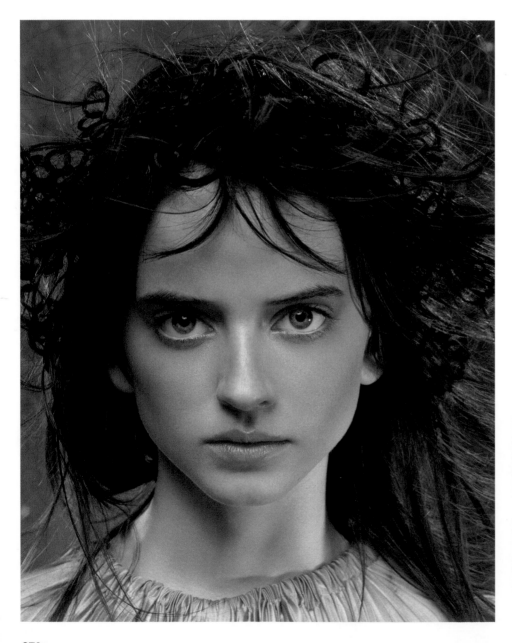

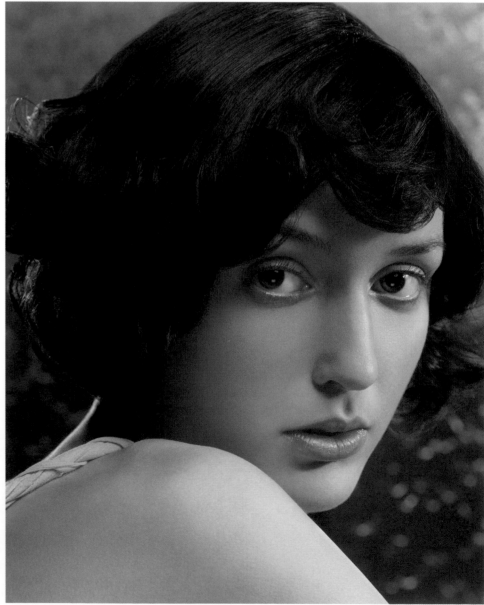

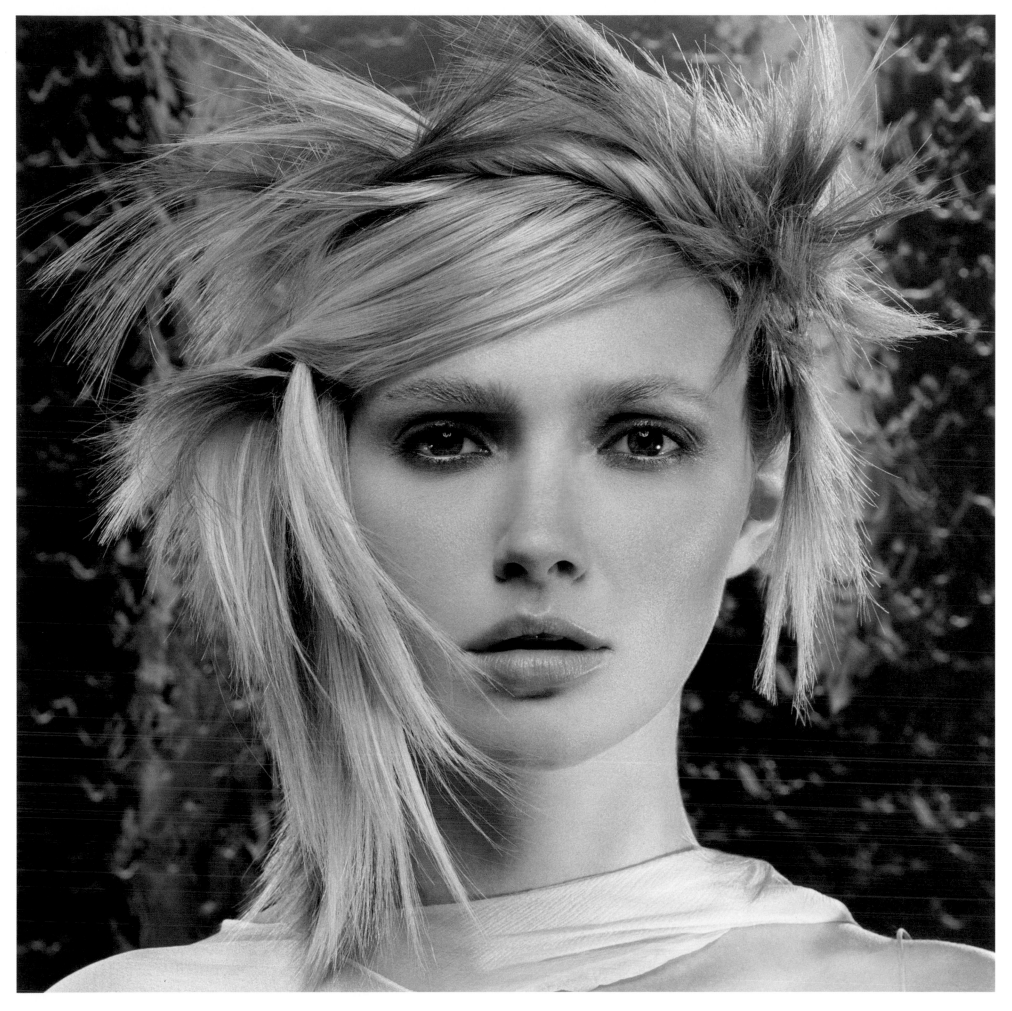

JEAN VALLON pages 272–273

Centre Perform, 28 Blvd. Jeu de Paume, 34000 Montpellier, France, www.jeanvallon.com

Hair: Jean Vallon
Make-up: Coco
Styling: Christian for Mea Culpa
Photography: JP Duretz

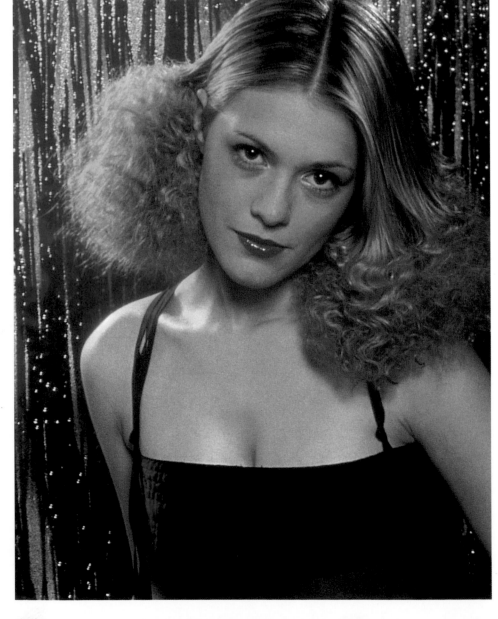

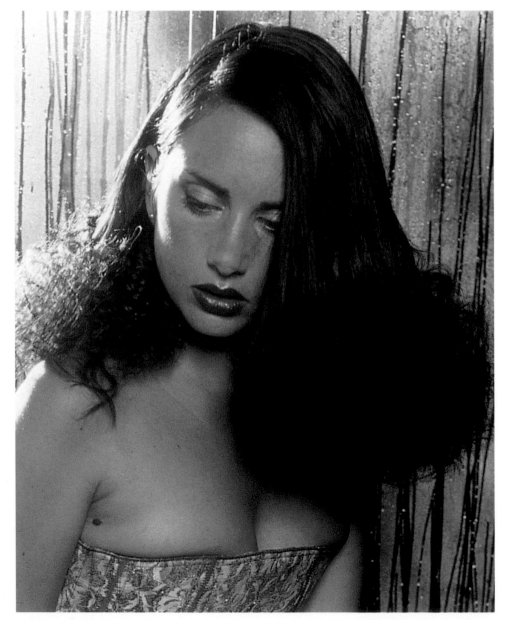

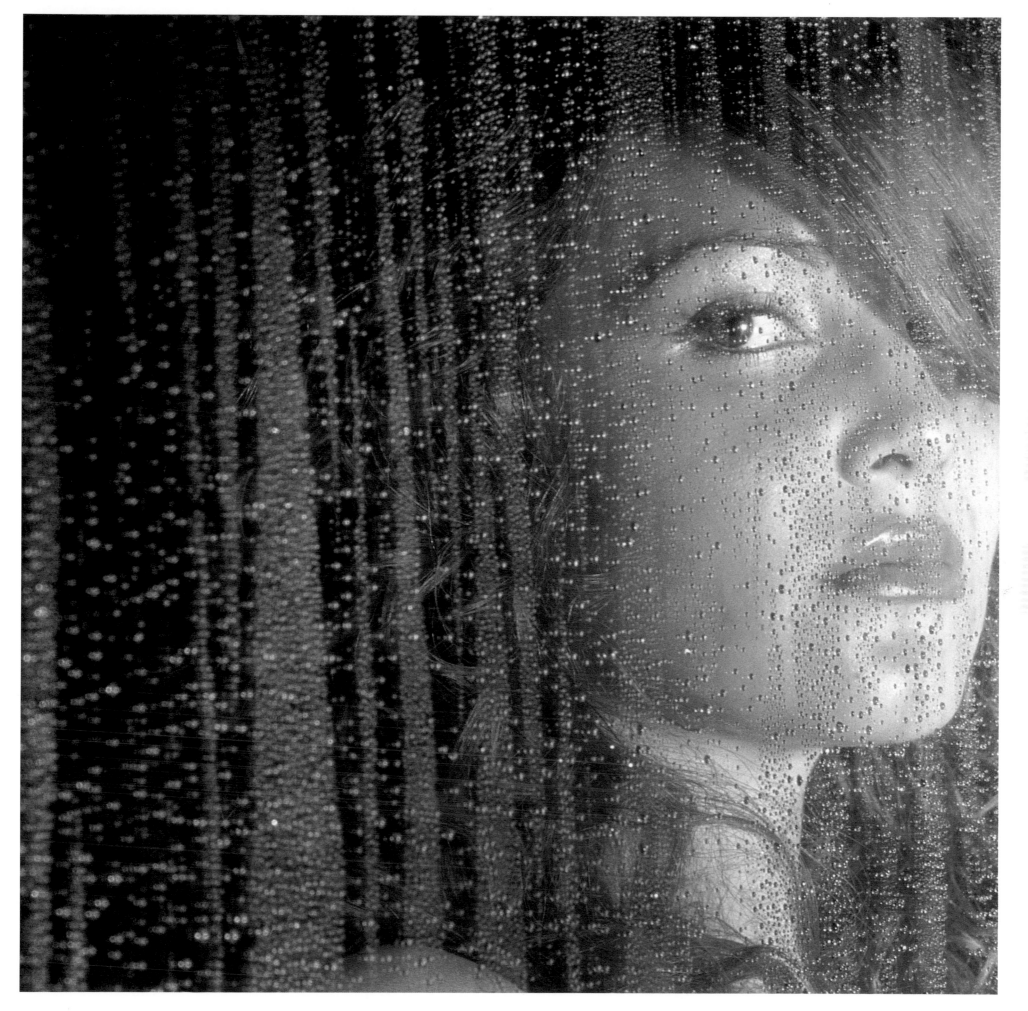

BY BEYER THE HAIR pages 274–275

Beyer Friseur GmbH, Friedrich-Ebert-Straße 66, 45468 Mülheim am Ruhr, Germany, www.bybeyer.de

Hair: Gaby Beyer, Martin Borger
Make-up: Renata Steffens, Palma de Mallorca
Styling: Claudia Joest, Palma de Mallorca
Photography: Silvia Klebon, Palma de Mallorca
Models: Philip and Kelly
Products: L'Oréal

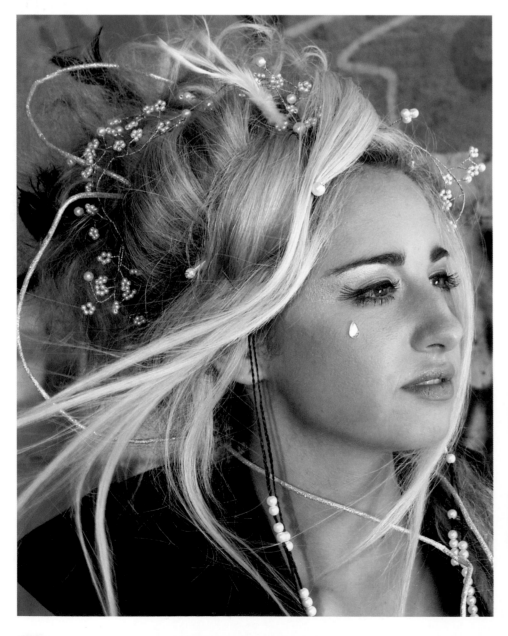
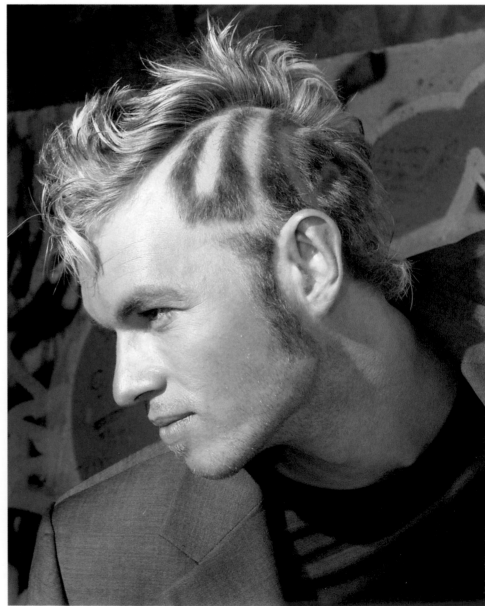

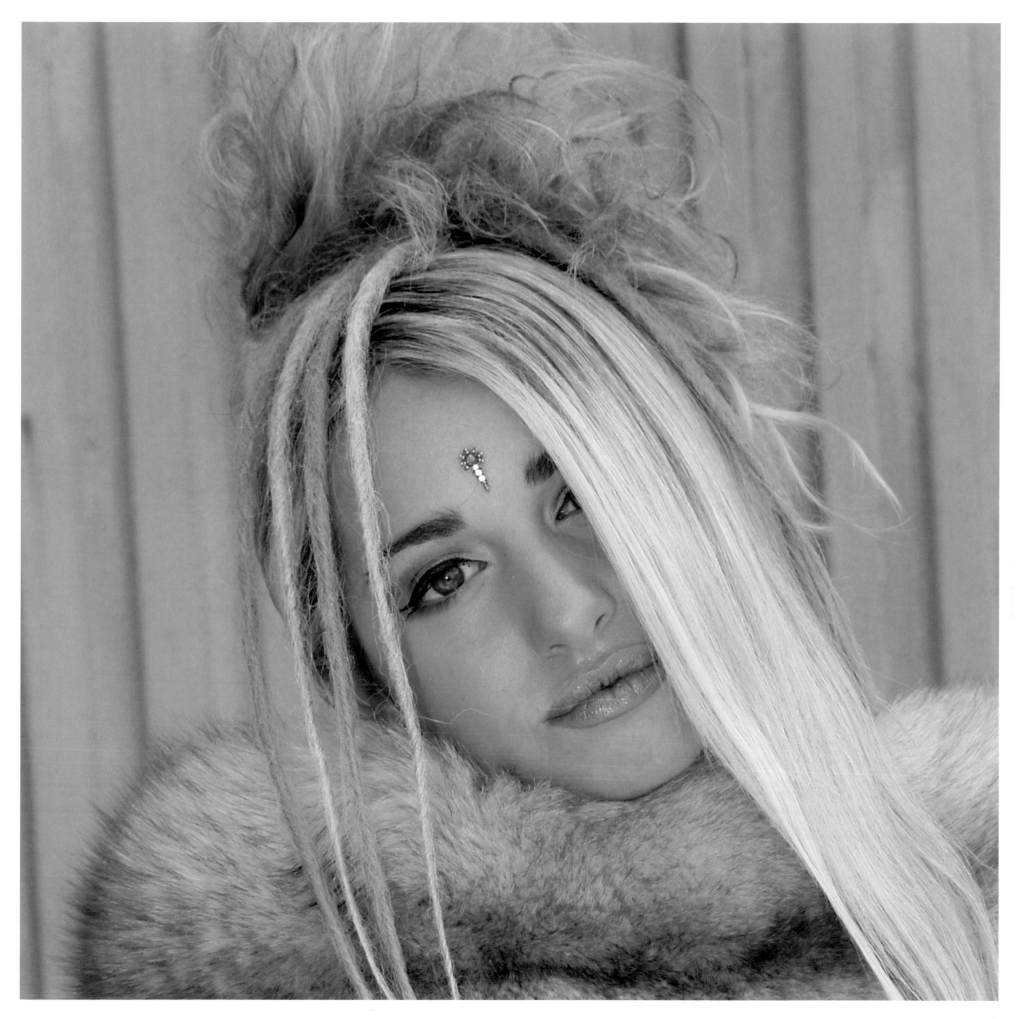

MCINTYRE HAIRDRESSING pages 276–279

50 Union Street, Dundee DD1 4BE, United Kingdom, www.mcintyres.co.uk

Hair: Kay McIntyre
Salon: McIntyre Hairdressing
Make-up: Cheryl Phelps-Gardiner
Styling: Viviana Rullo
Photography: Trevor Leighton

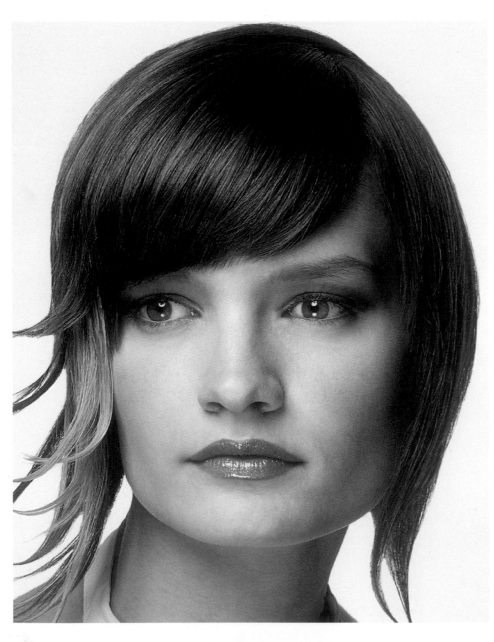

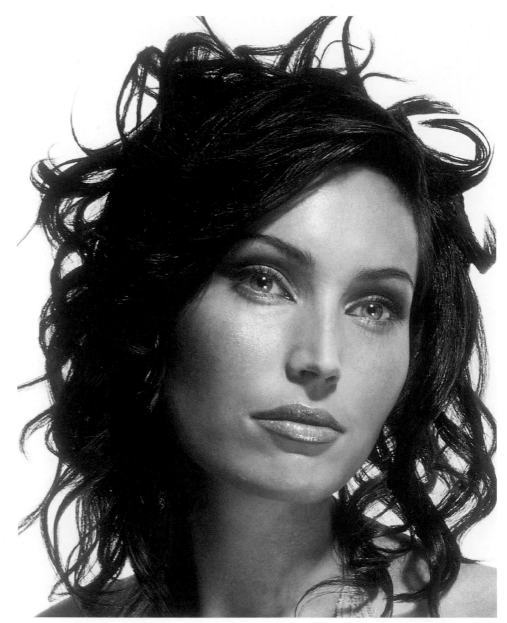

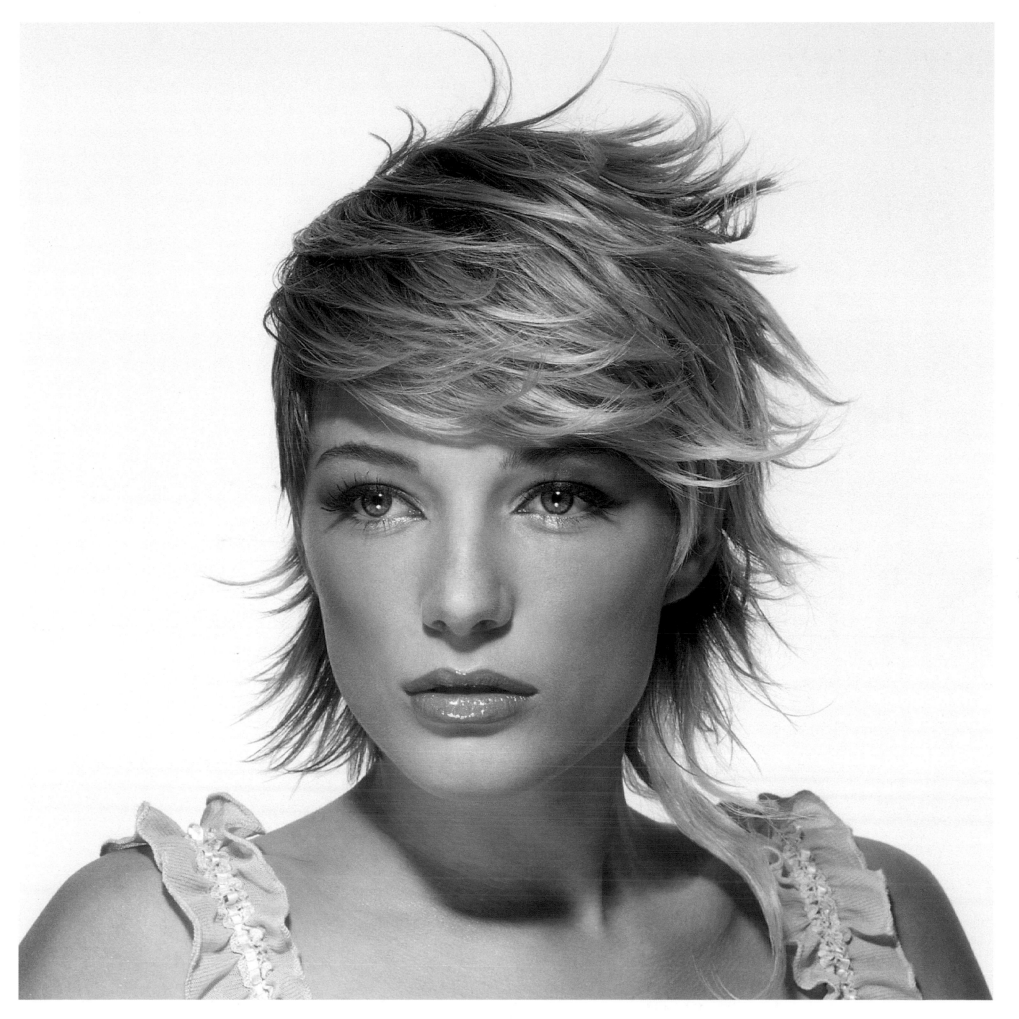

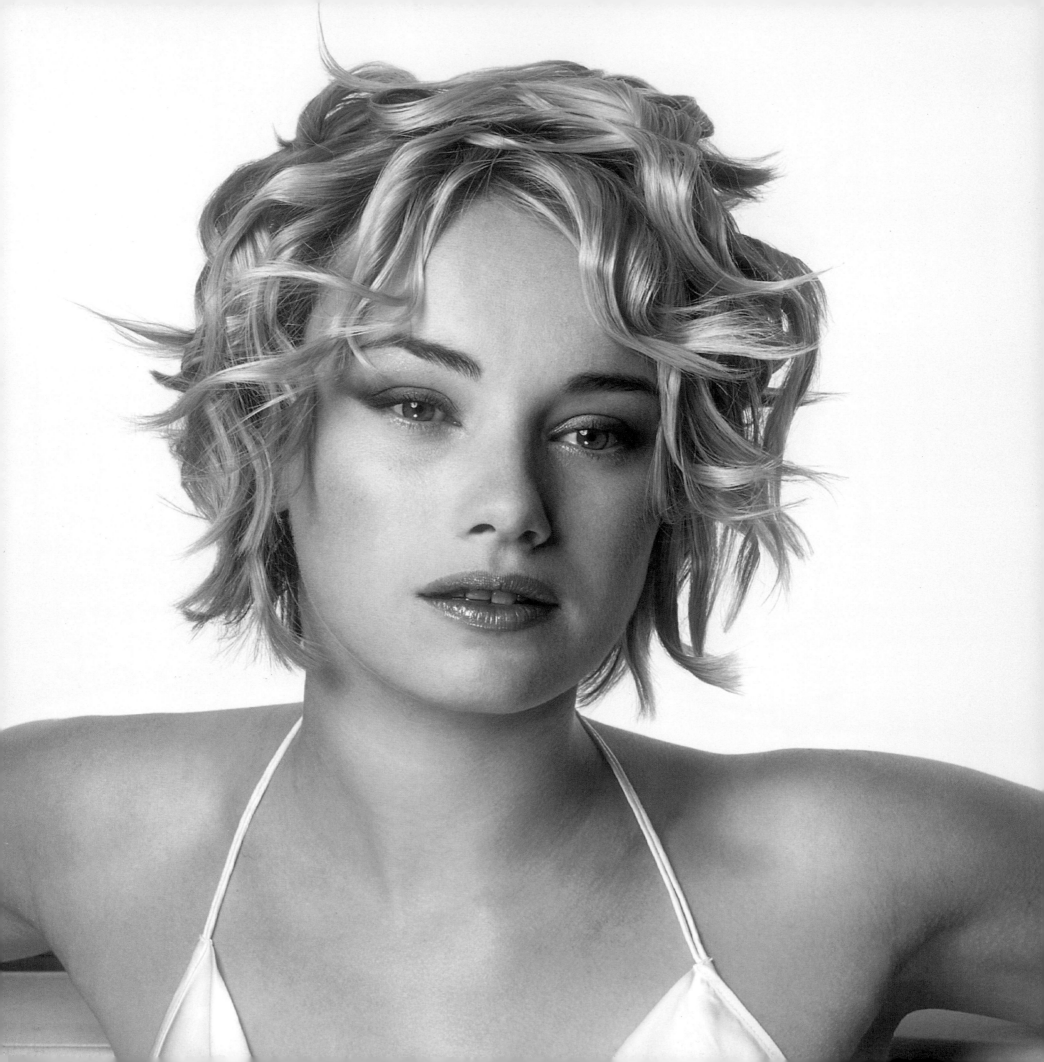

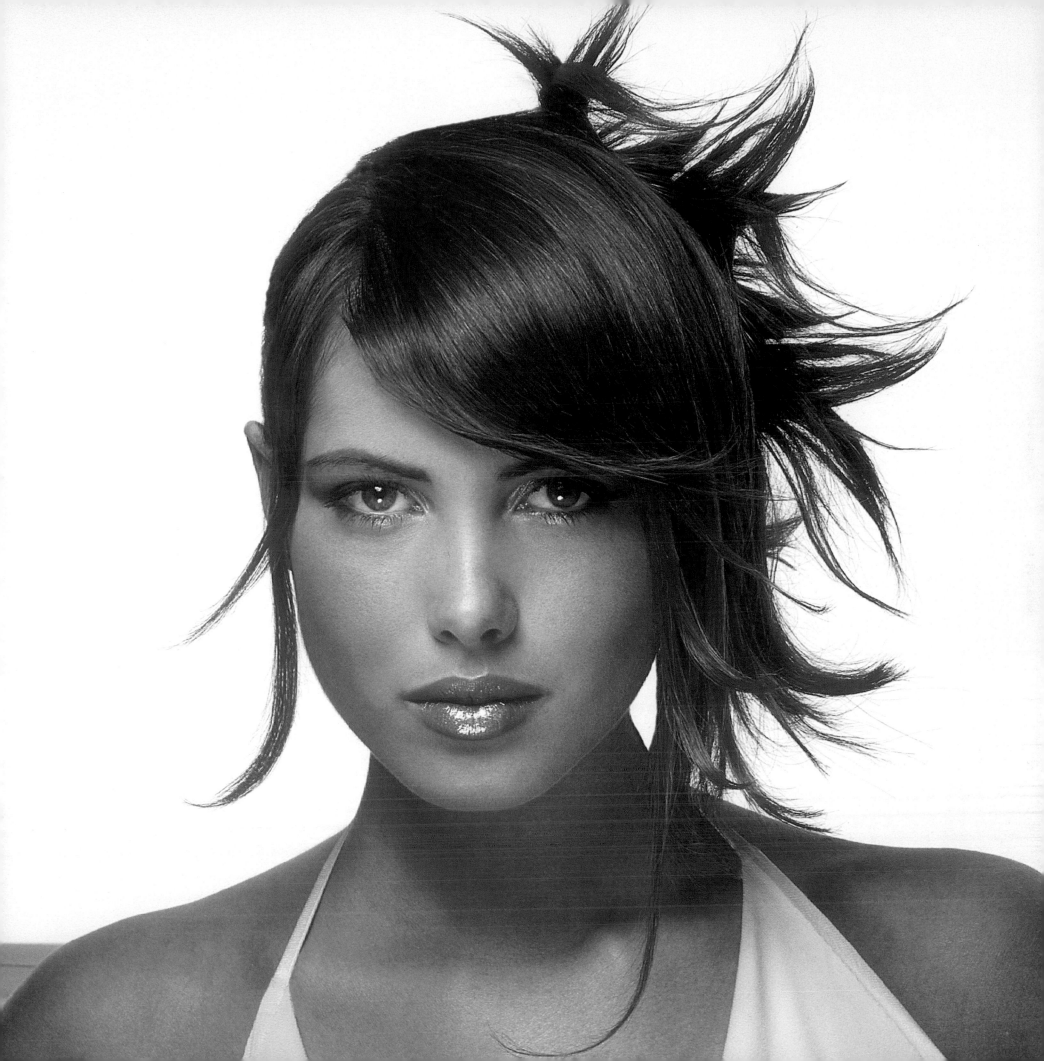

UMBERTO GIANNINI pages 280–281

Warick House, 159 Lower High Street, Stourbridge DY8 1TT, United Kingdom, www.umbertogiannini.co.uk

Hair: Umberto Giannini
Photography: Andrew O'Toole

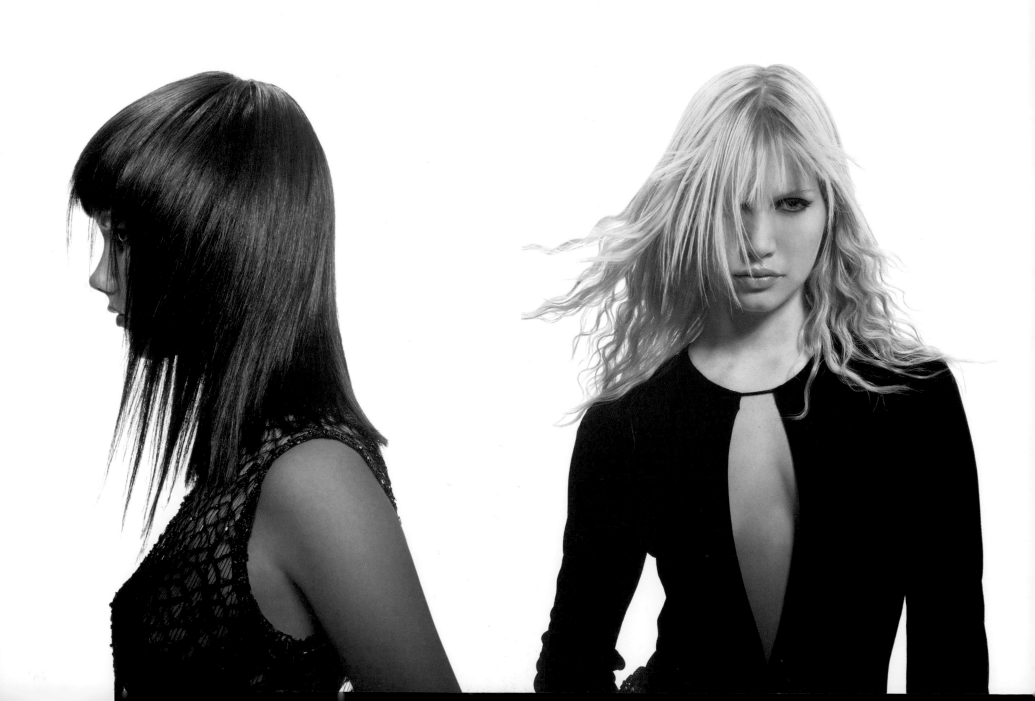

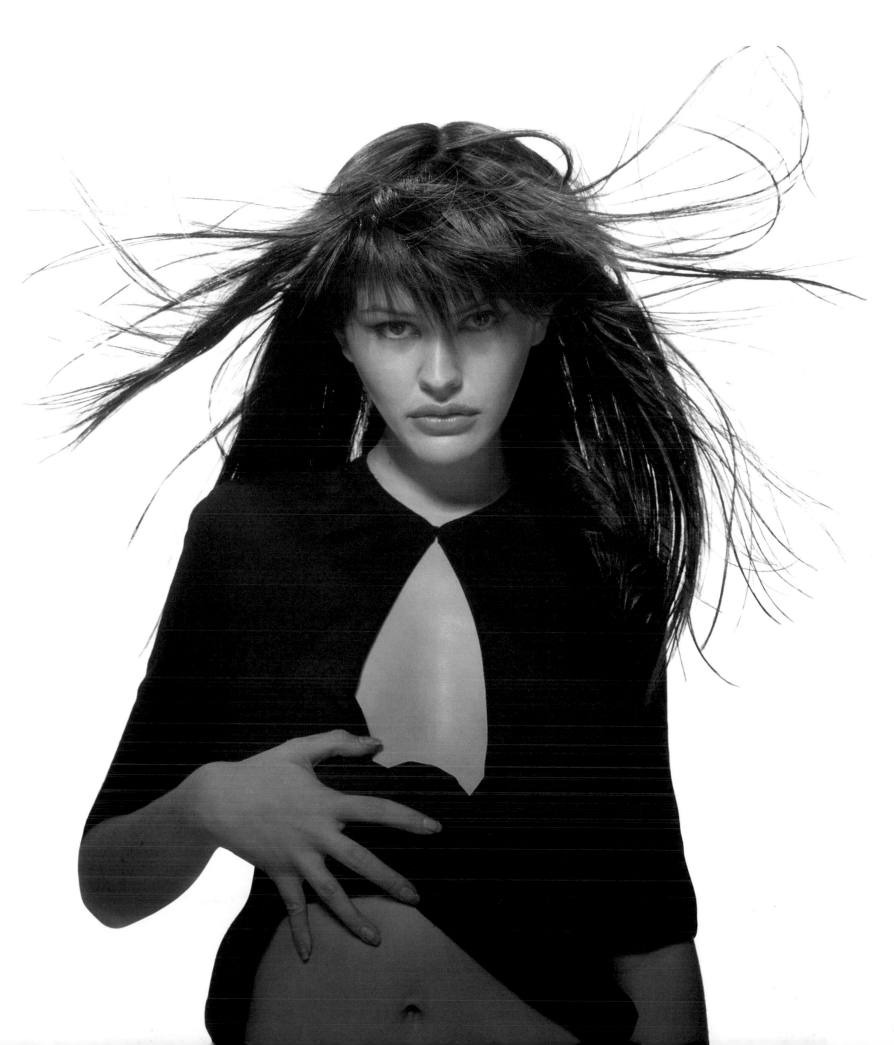

HARINGTONS pages 282–283

Haringtons Hairdressing, 31 Green Lane, Northwood Middlesex HA6 2PX, United Kingdom, www.haringtons.com

Hair: Esti Carton, Louise Maxwell
Make-up: Emily Newsome
Styling: Wendy Dina
Photography: Jason Eggby
Products: L'Oréal Professionel

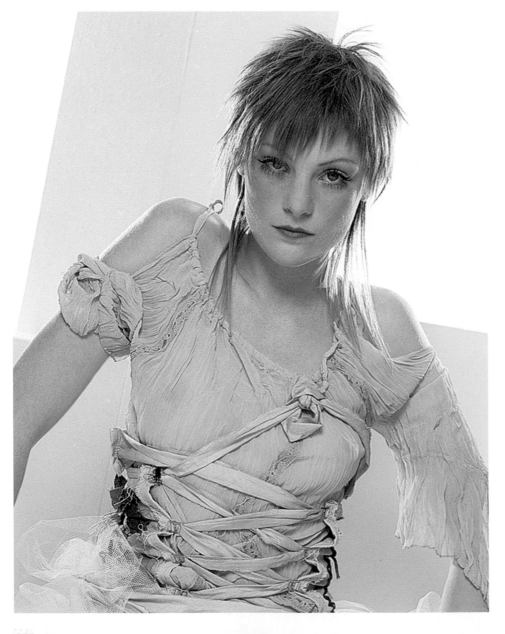

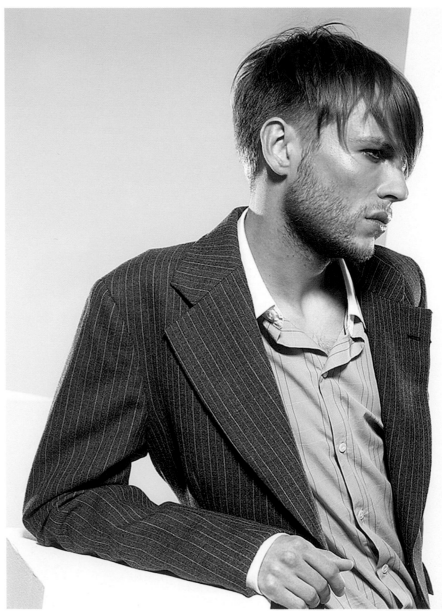

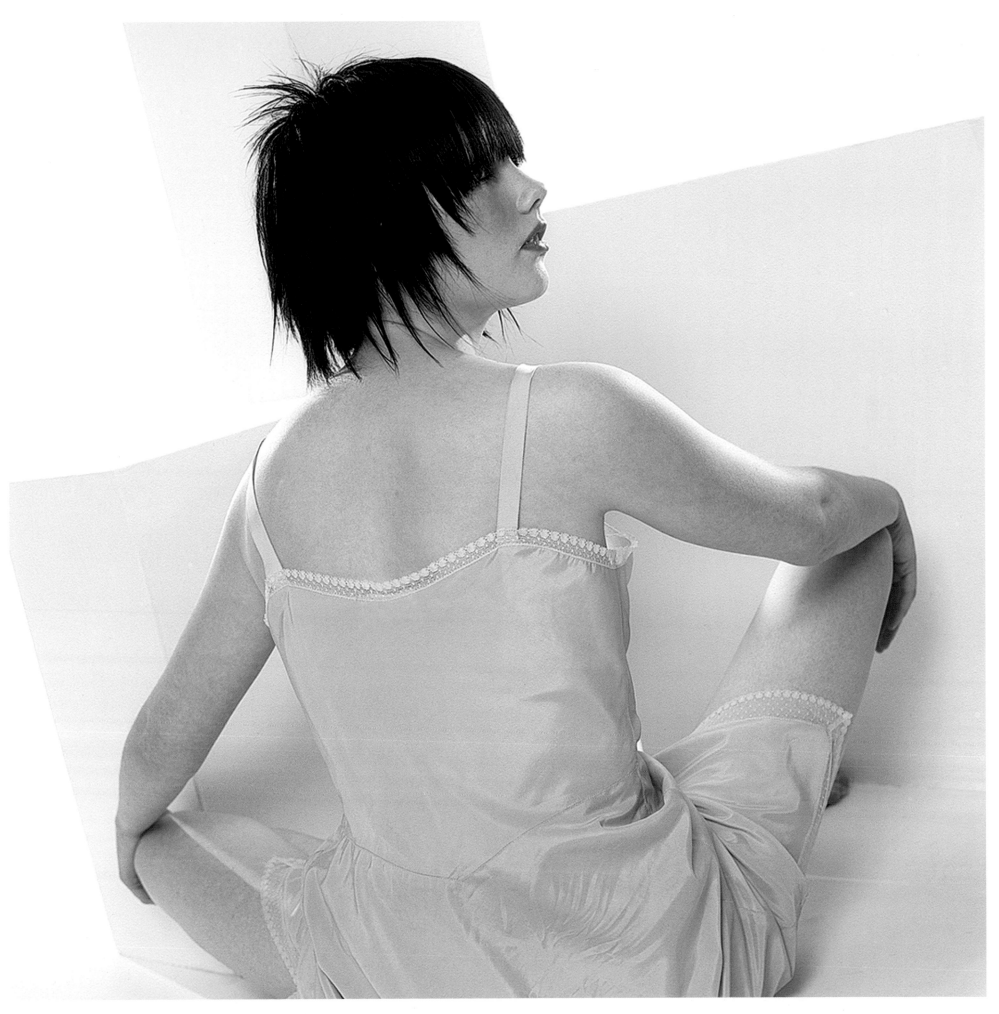

KELLER THE SCHOOL pages 284–285

Sindelfinger Straße 28, 71032 Böblingen, Germany, www.keller-company.de

Hair: Keller The School
Academy: Keller The School
Make-up: Stefan Armbruster and Melanie Mornhinweg (p. 284) Paddy Nitschke (p. 284, 285)
Styling: Frank Oberberger
Photography: Vlado Golub

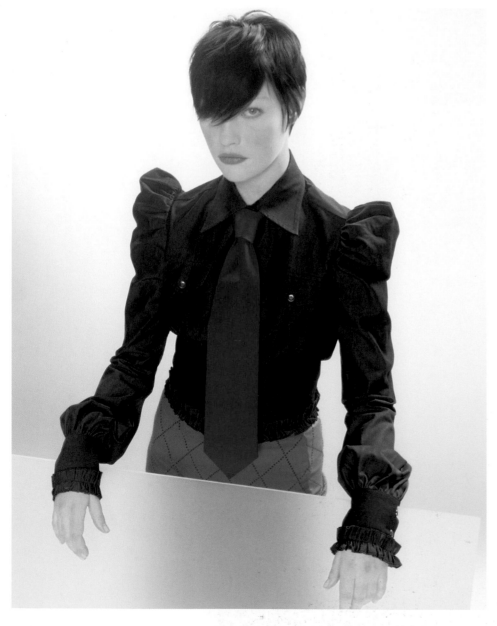

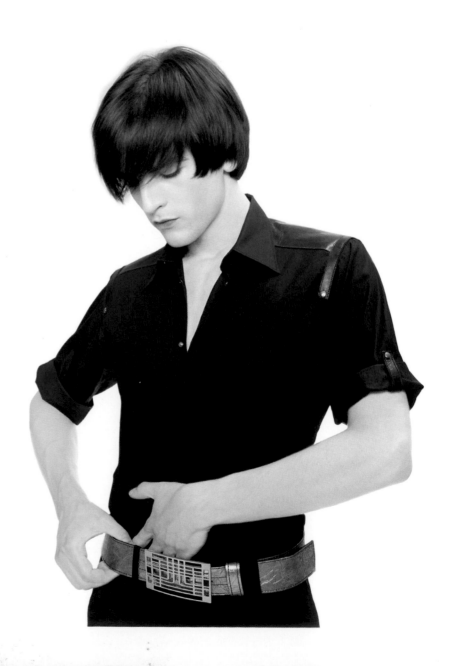

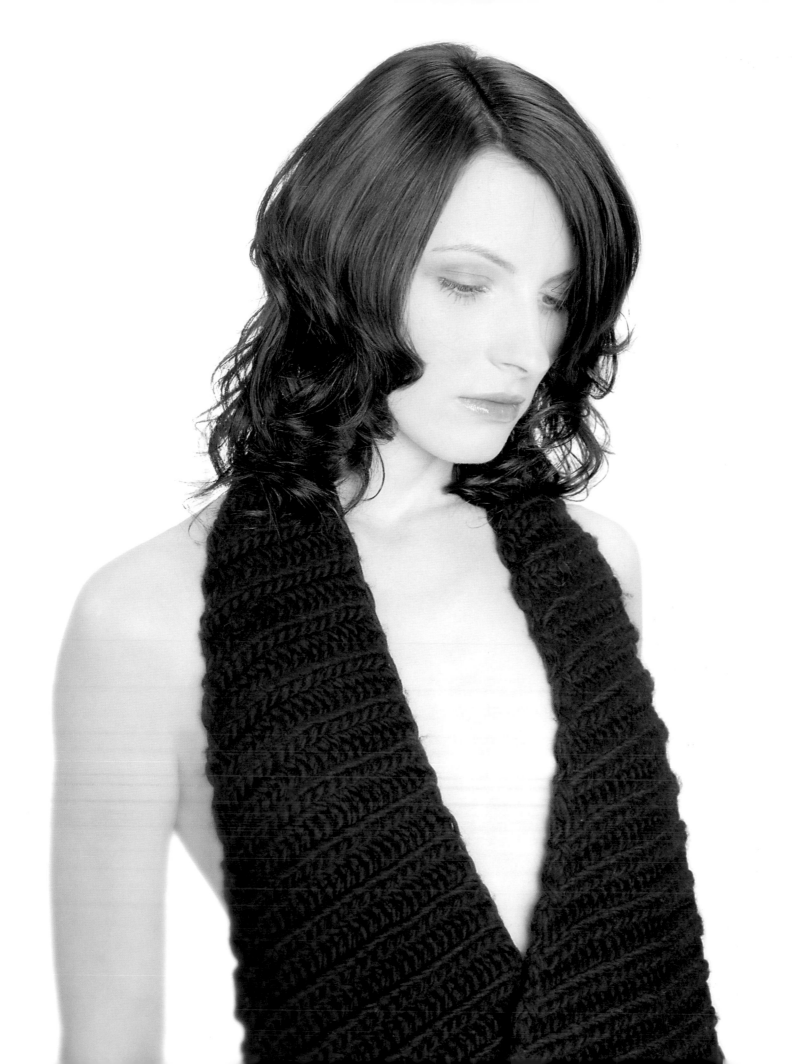

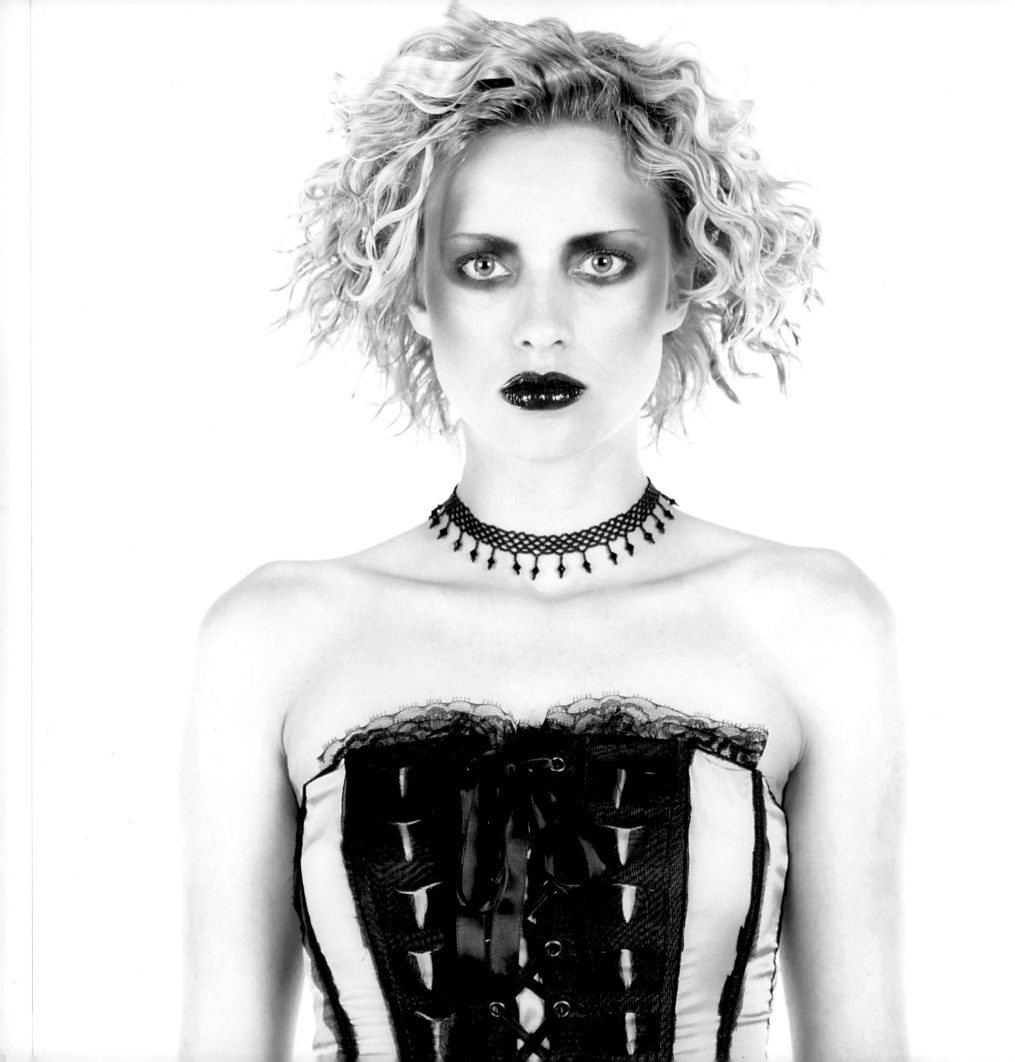

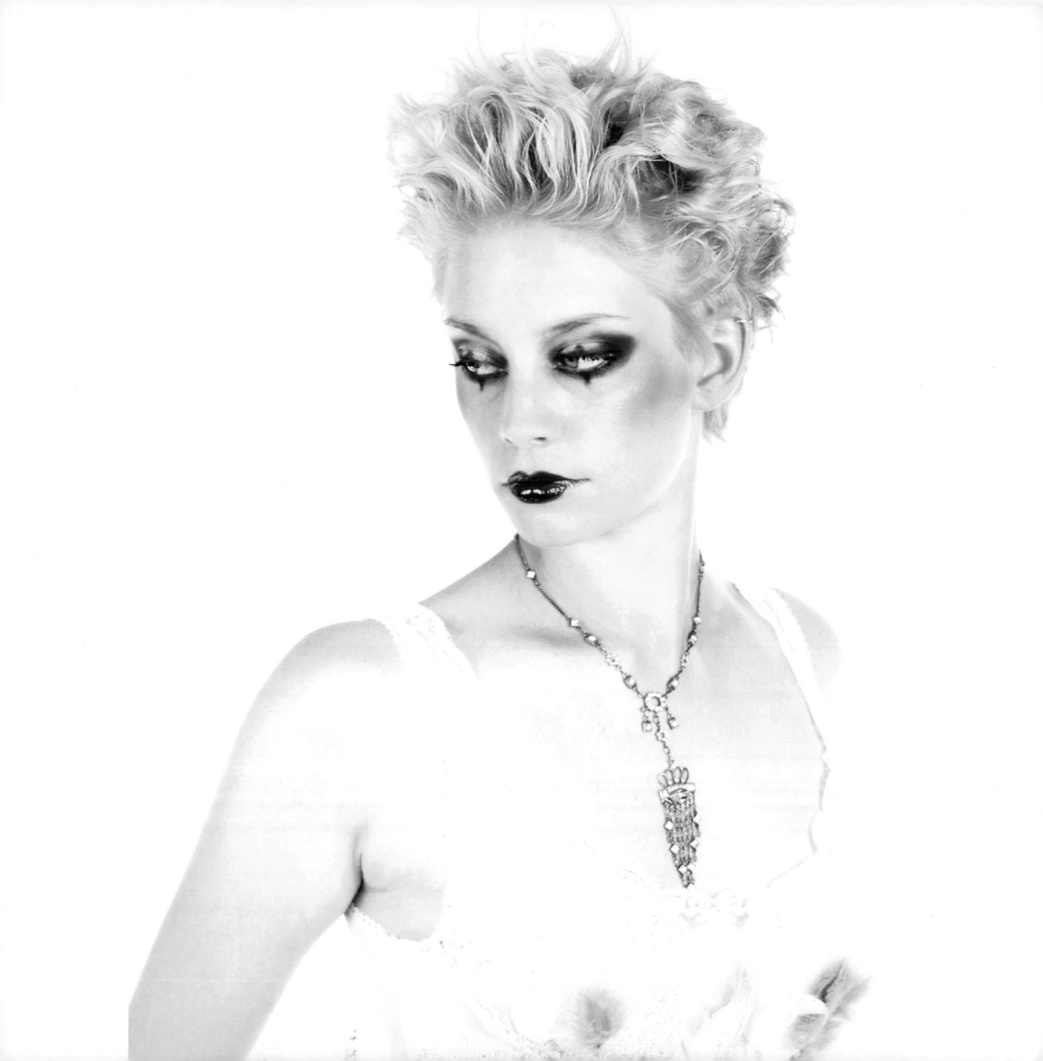

CLIPSO pages 290–295

57 Queens Road, Watford, Herts WD17 2QN, United Kingdom, www.clipso.demon.co.uk

Hair: Jane Collins for Clipso (p. 290 - 293) Clipso Art team (p. 294 - 295)
Salon: Clipso, Hemel Hempstead
Make-up: Janet Francis (p. 290 - 293) Astrid at Carol Hayes (p. 294 - 295)
Styling: Angela Barnard (p. 290 - 293) Mellana at Carol Hayes (p. 294 - 295)
Photography: Martin Evening
Products: L'Oréal Professionnel

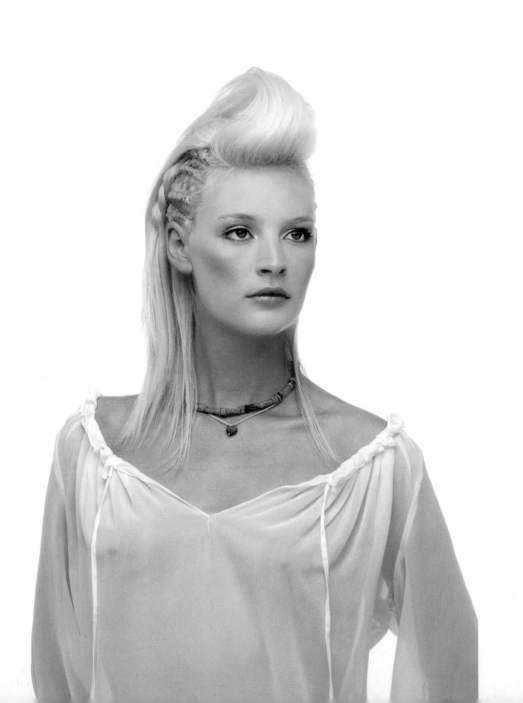

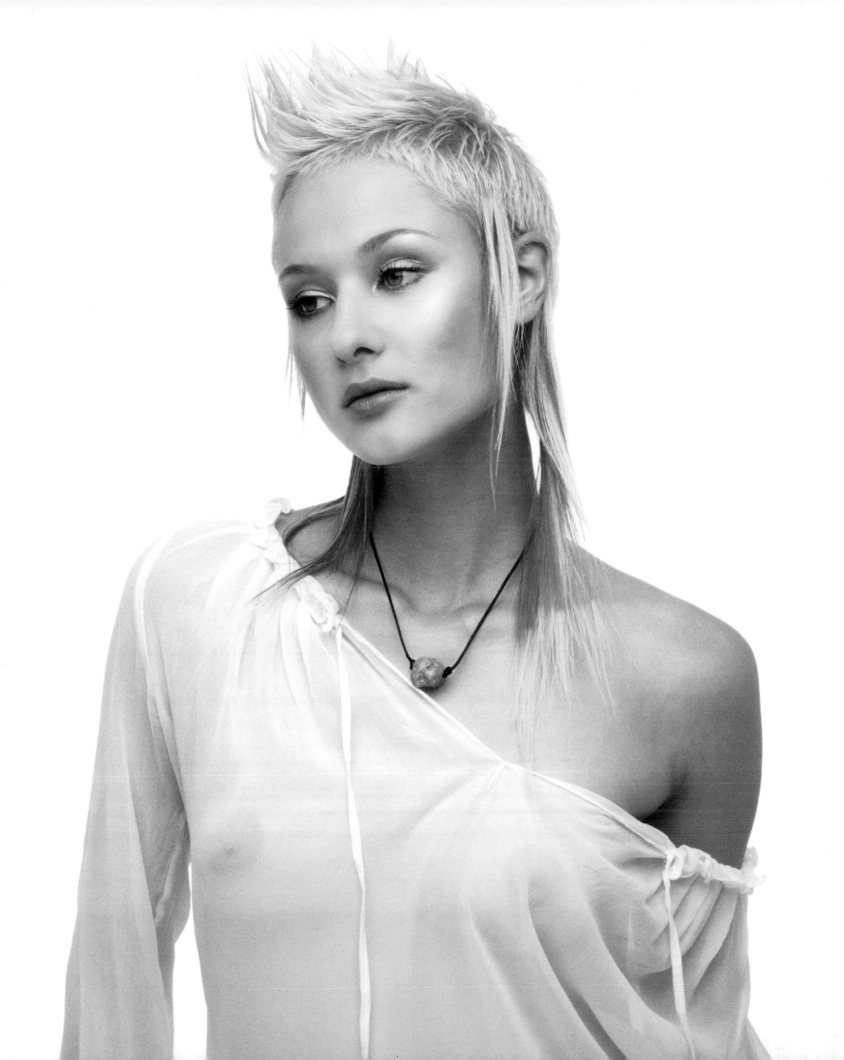

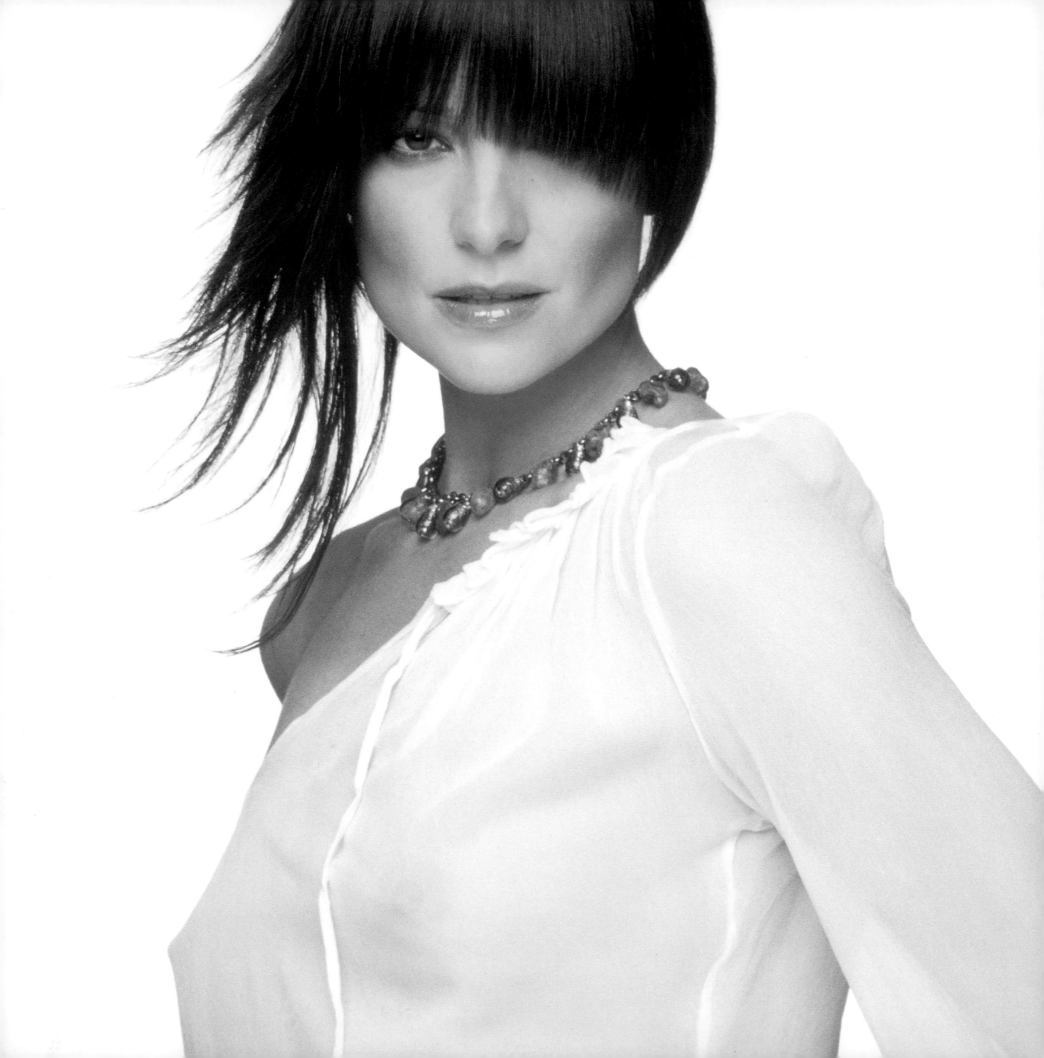

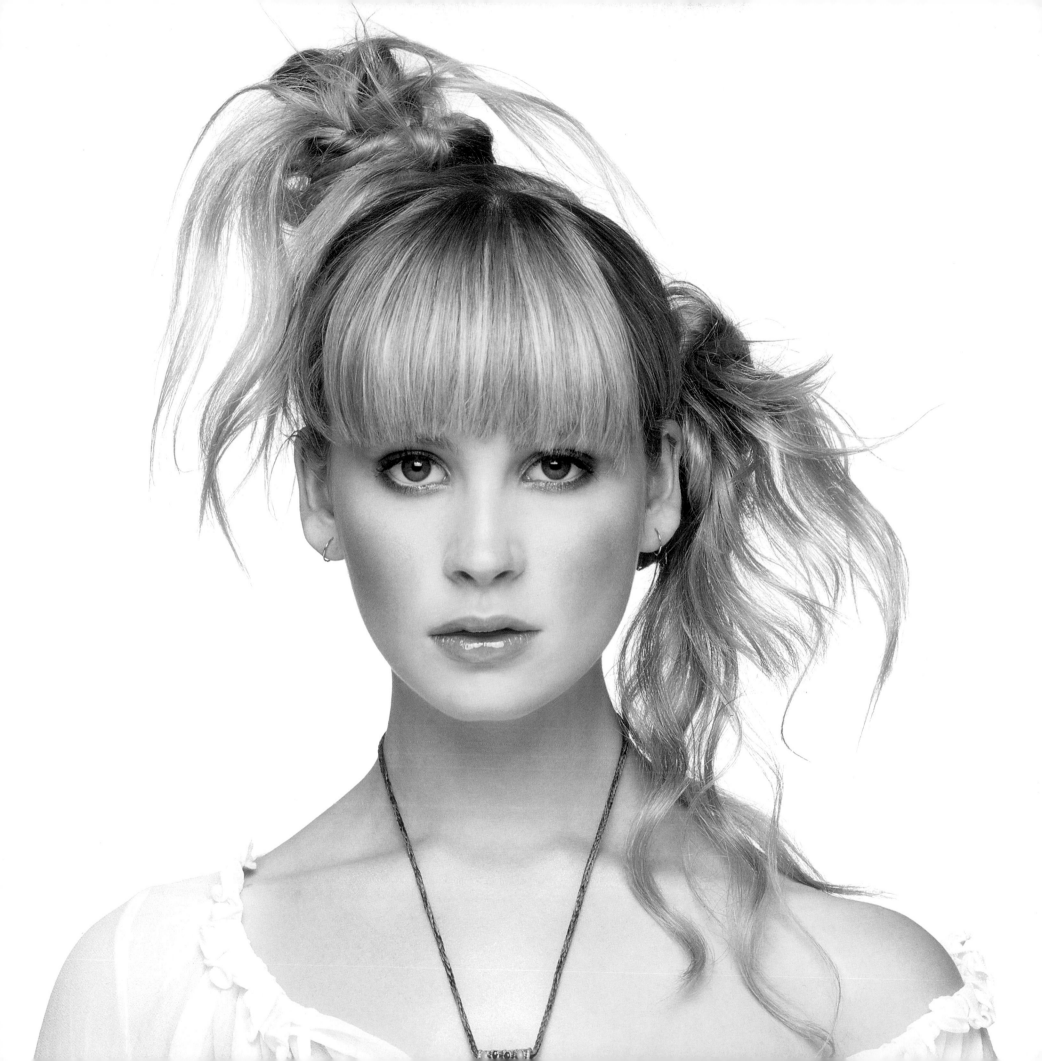

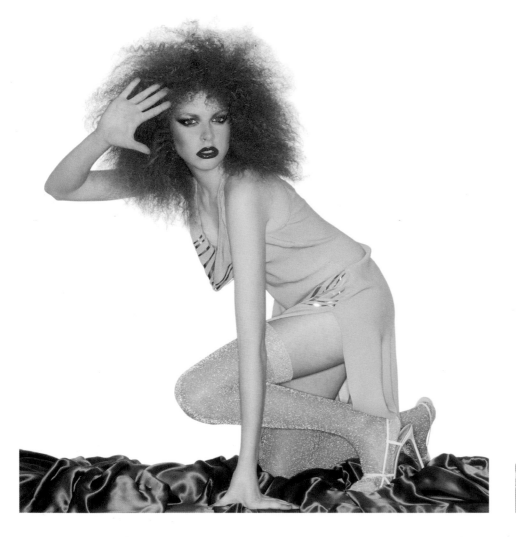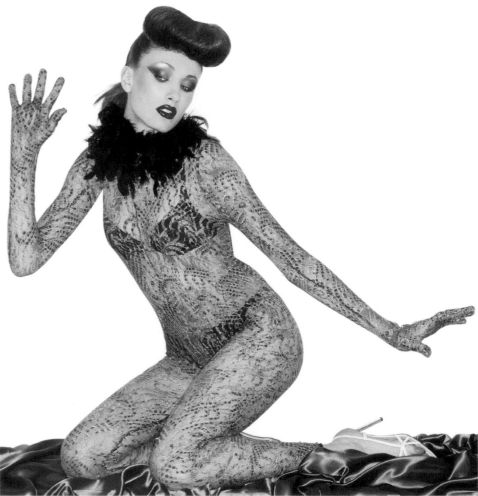

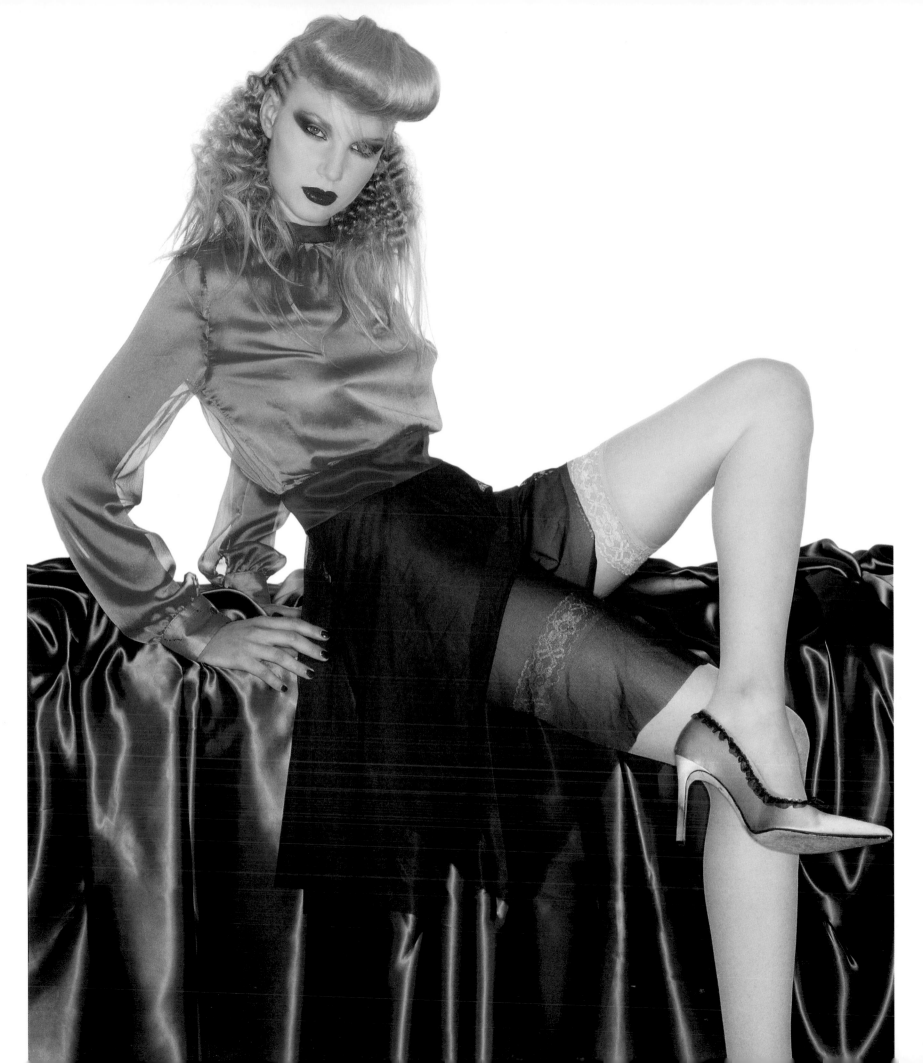

SEBASTIÁN FERRER pages 296–297

Av. Vitacura 5656, Vitacura, Santiago,Chile, www.sebastianferrer.cl

Hair: Sebastián Ferrer
Salon: Sebastián Ferrer Peluquerias
Make-up: Poli Picó
Photography: Mr. Julio Donoso
Production: Verónica Padilla
Products: L'Oréal Professionnel

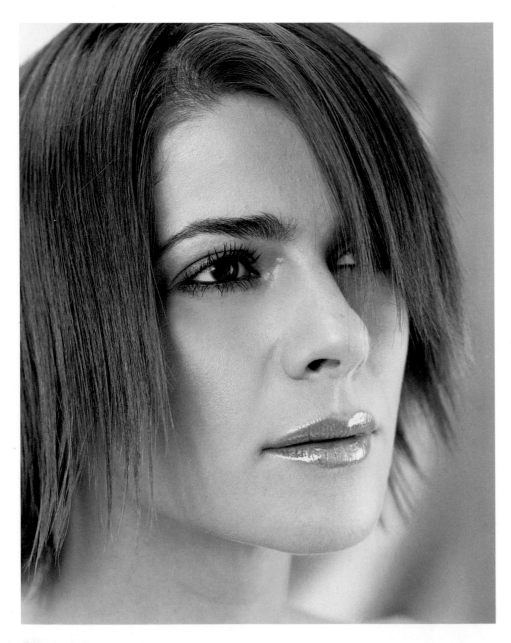

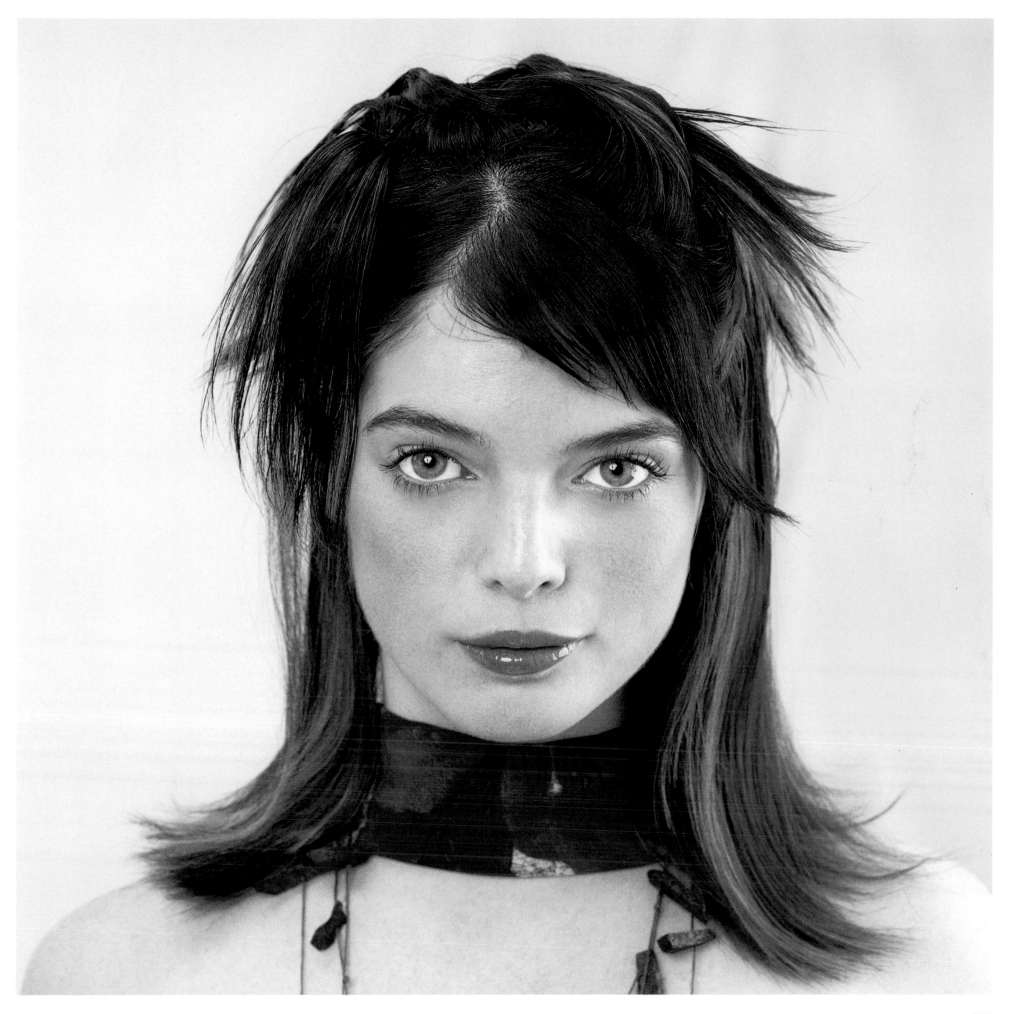

Hair: Heading Out
Make-up: Bernadette Fisher
Styling: Mark Wasiak
Photography: Gerard O'Connor
Products: L'Oréal

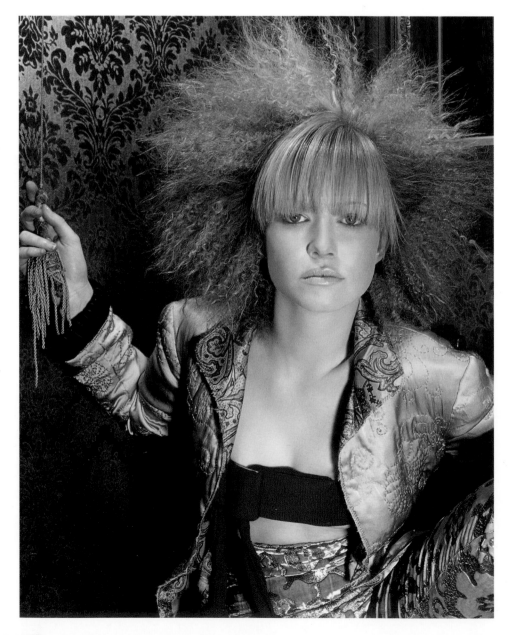

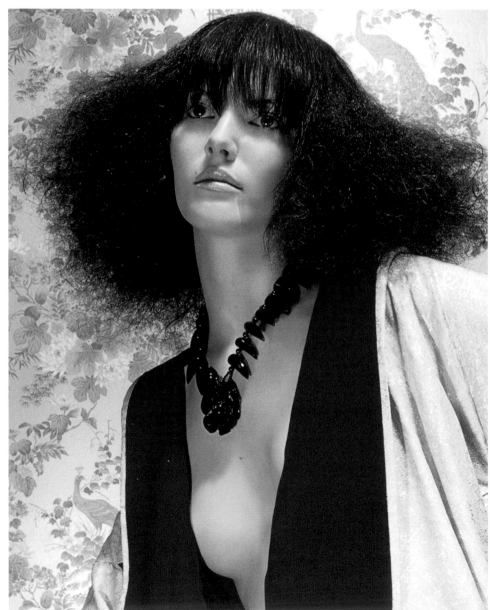

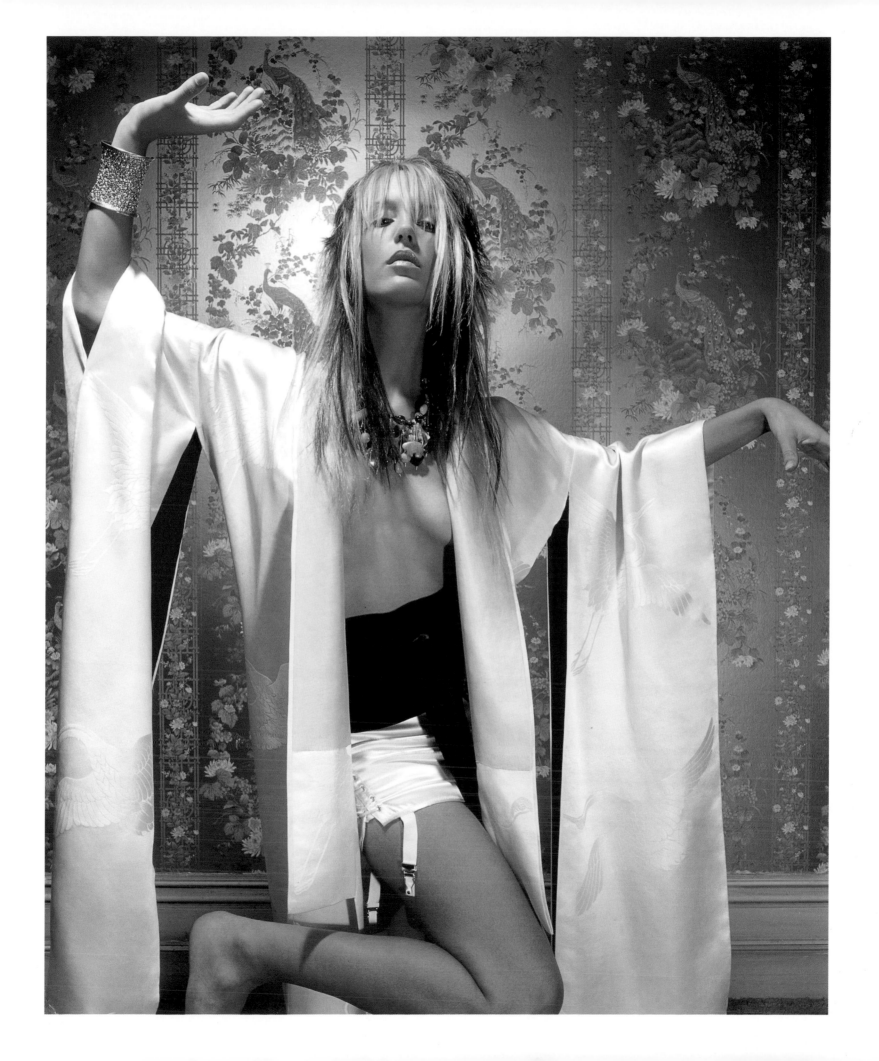

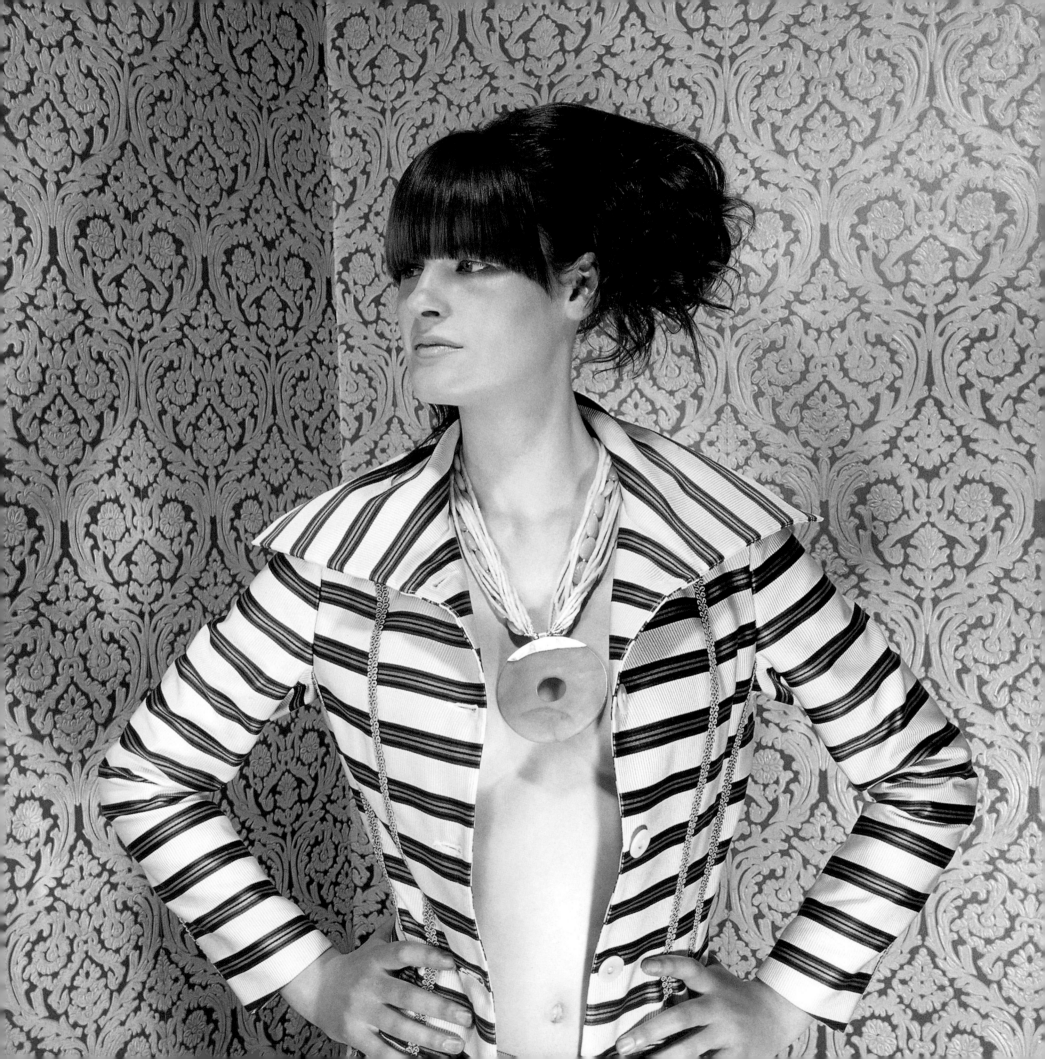

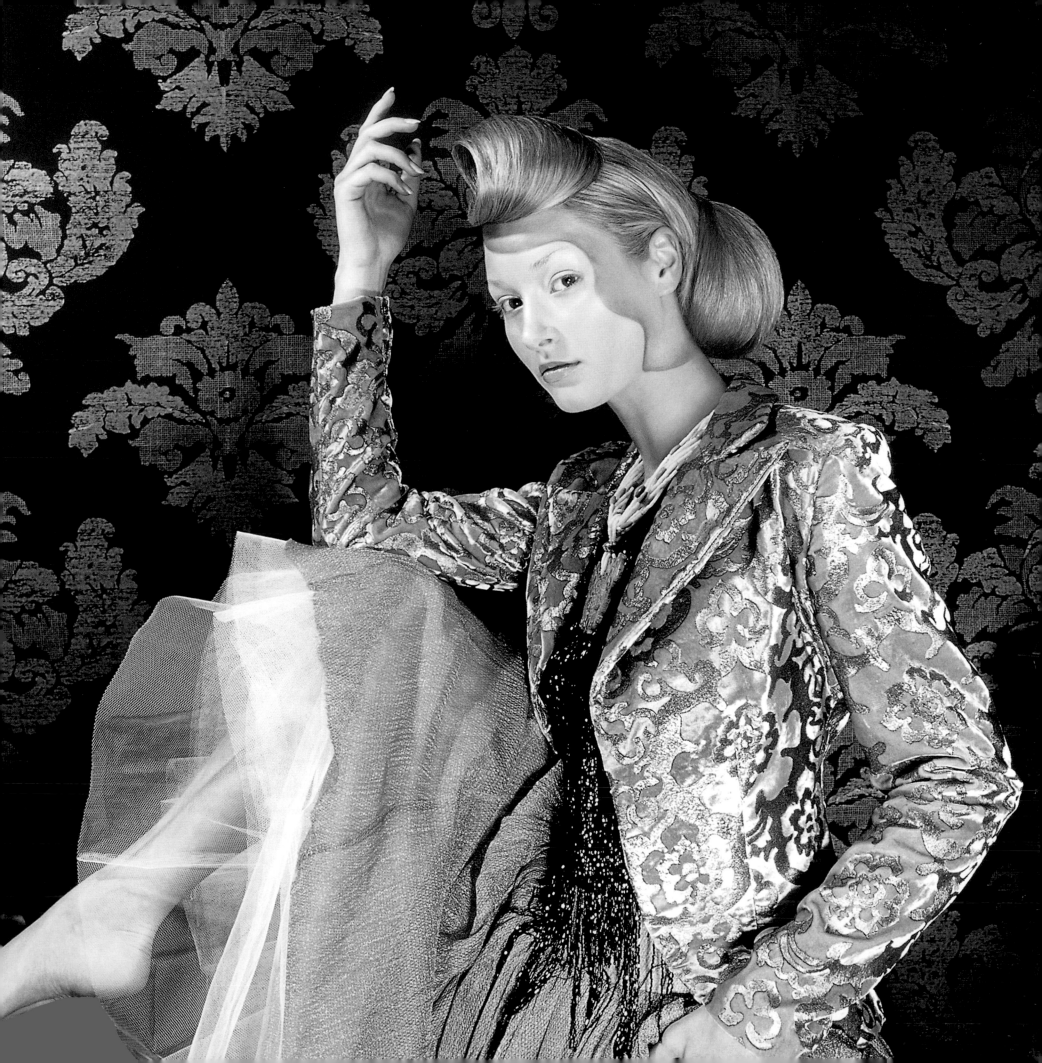

MARLIES MÖLLER pages 302–303

Marlies Möller Holding GmbH, Neuer Wall 61, 20354 Hamburg, Germany, www.marliesmoeller.com

Hair: Marlies Möller
Make-up: Astrid Michl
Photography: Bernd Böhm

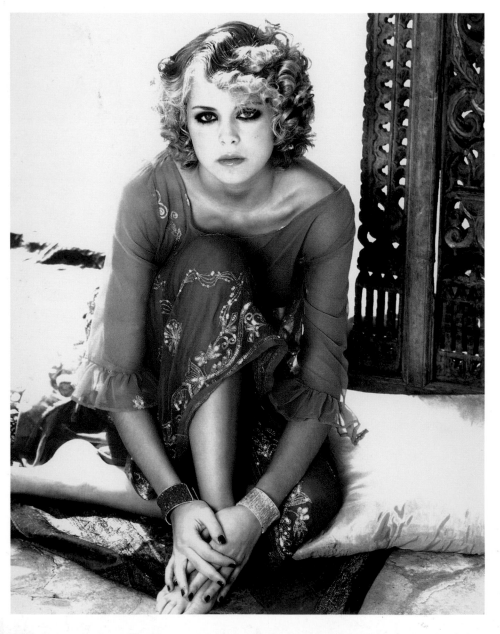
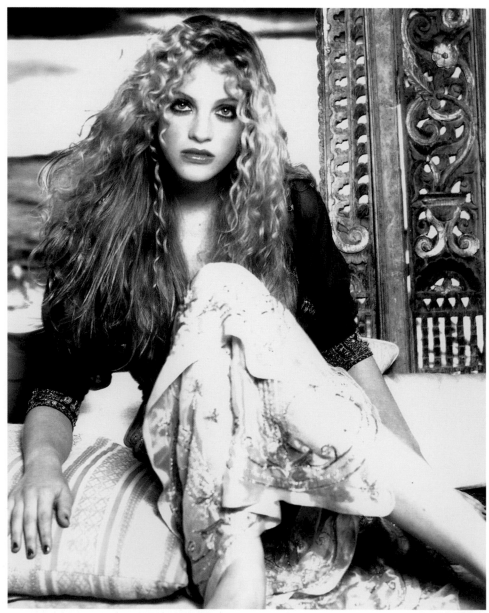

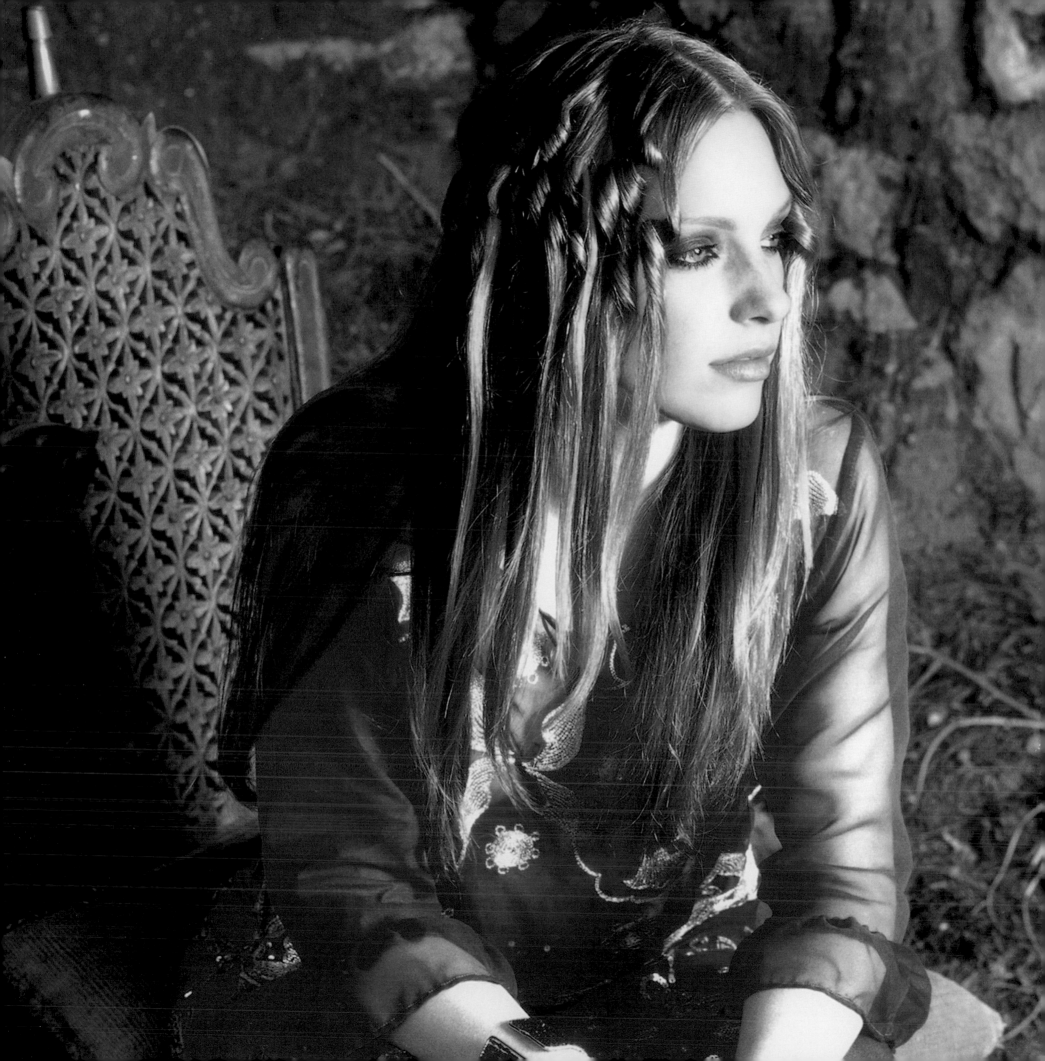

Hair: Carpy Coiffeur

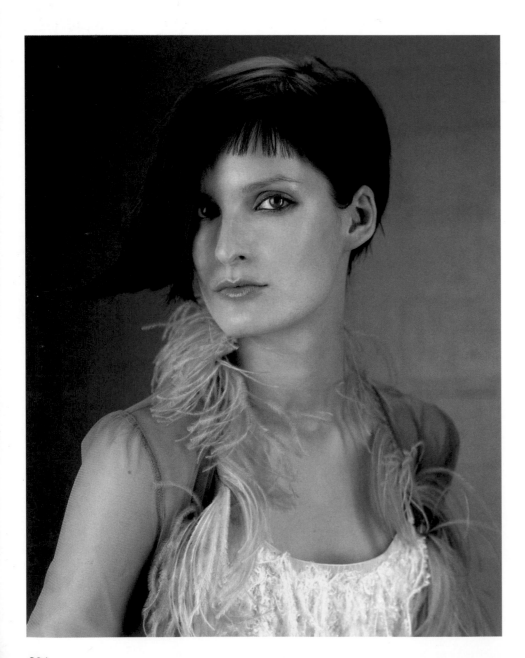

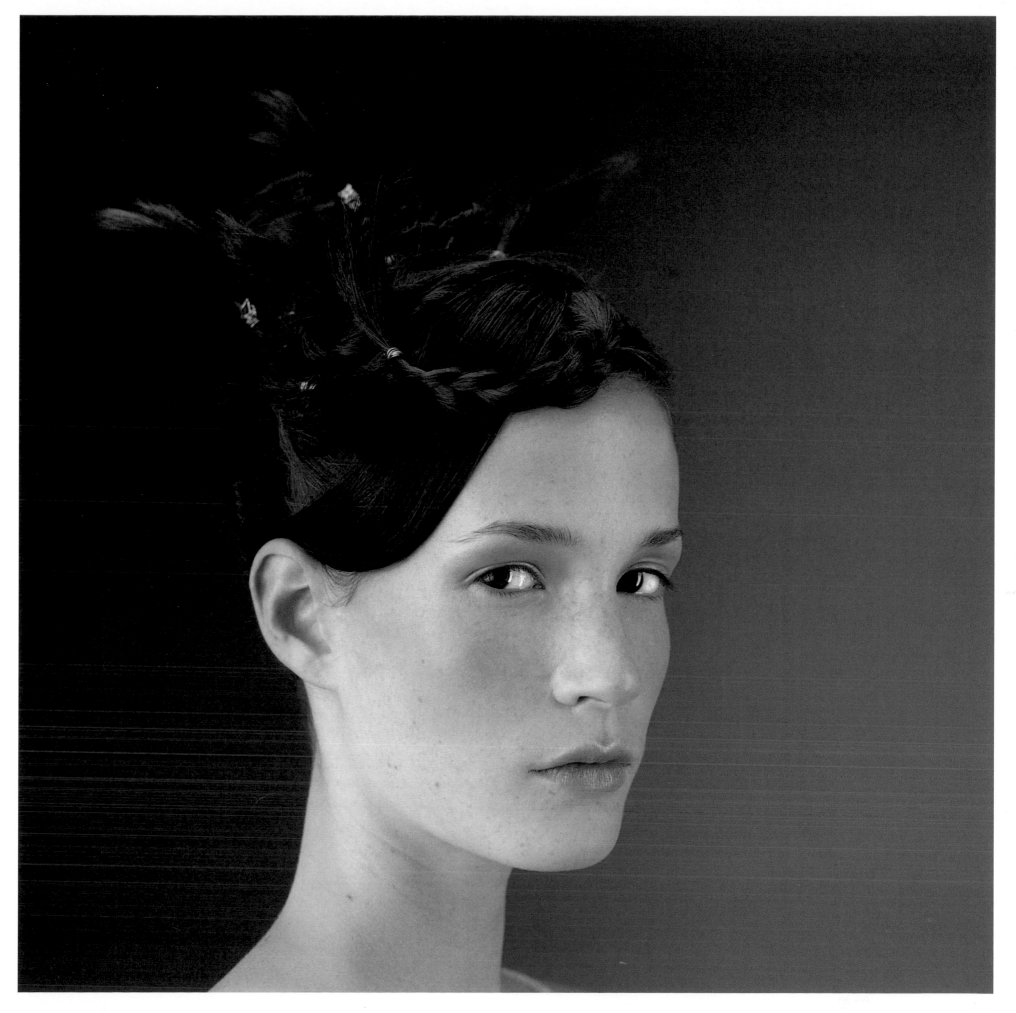

MARICARMEN MADRIGAL PELUQUERIAS pages 306–309

Sancho Dávila 31, 28028 Madrid, Spain, www.peluqueriasmadrigal.es

Hair: Madrigal Artistic Team
Make-up: Anita
Styling: Madrigal Artistic Team
Photography: Miguel Oriola
Model Agency: Colors

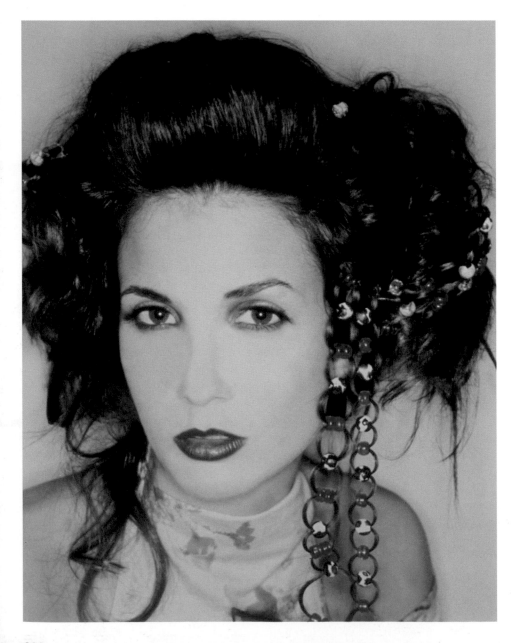

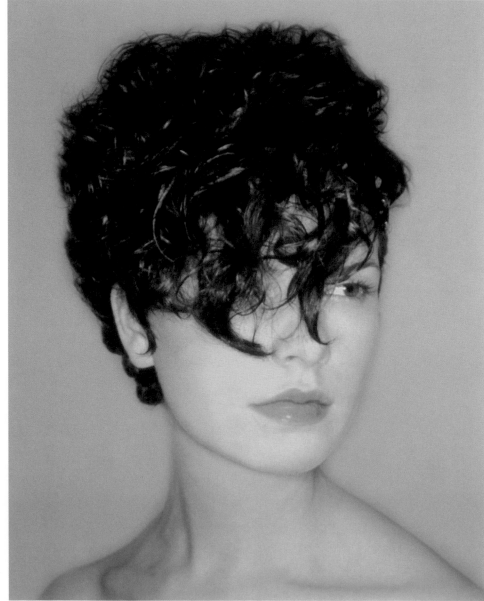

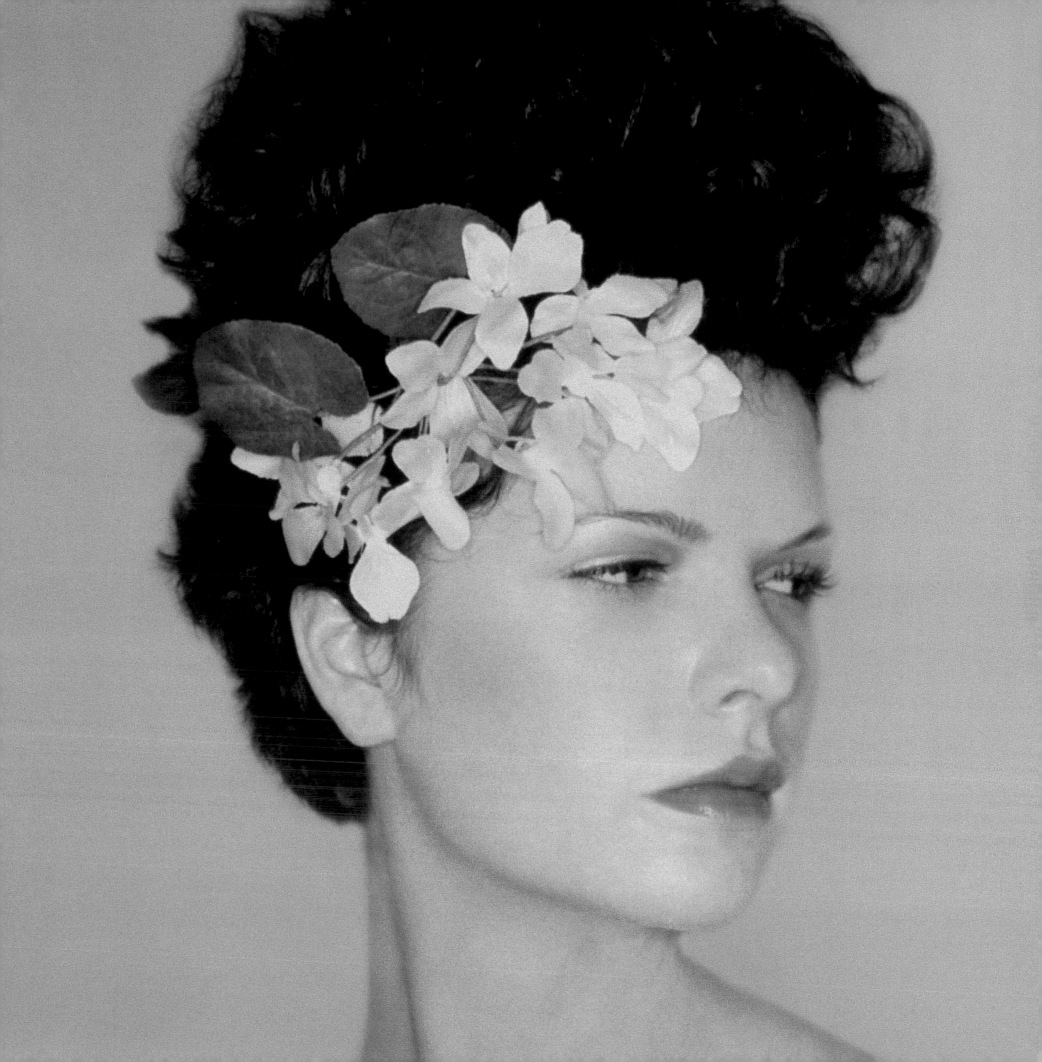

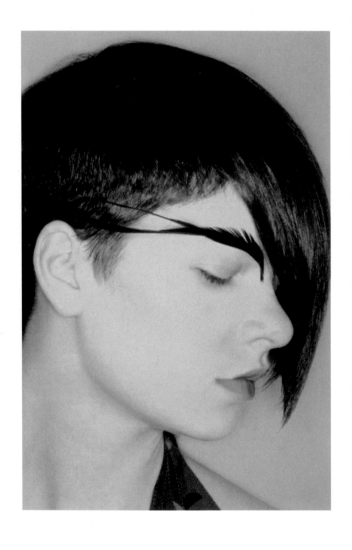
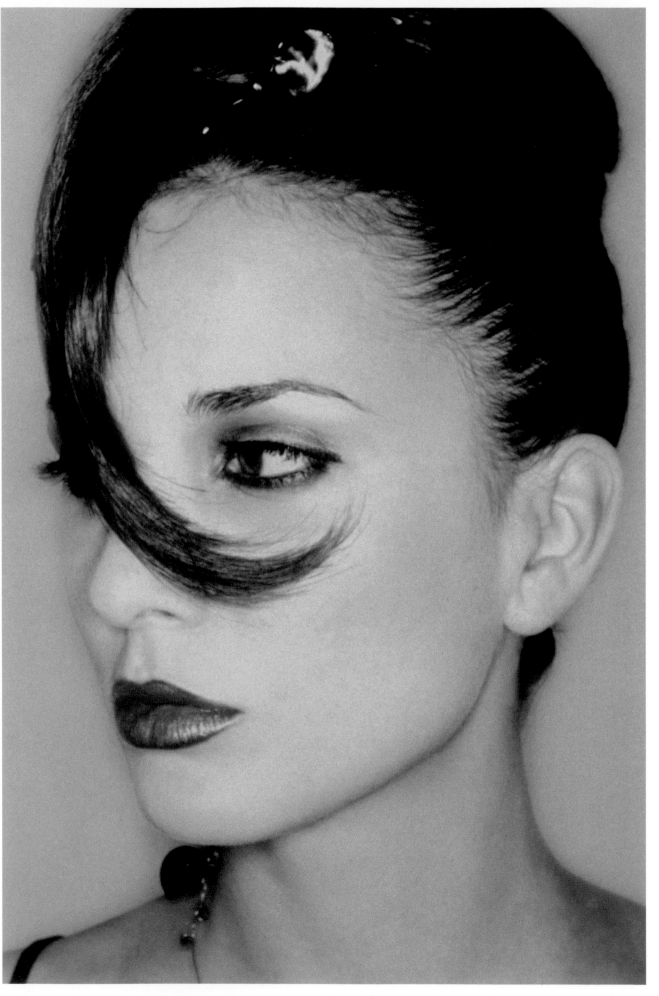

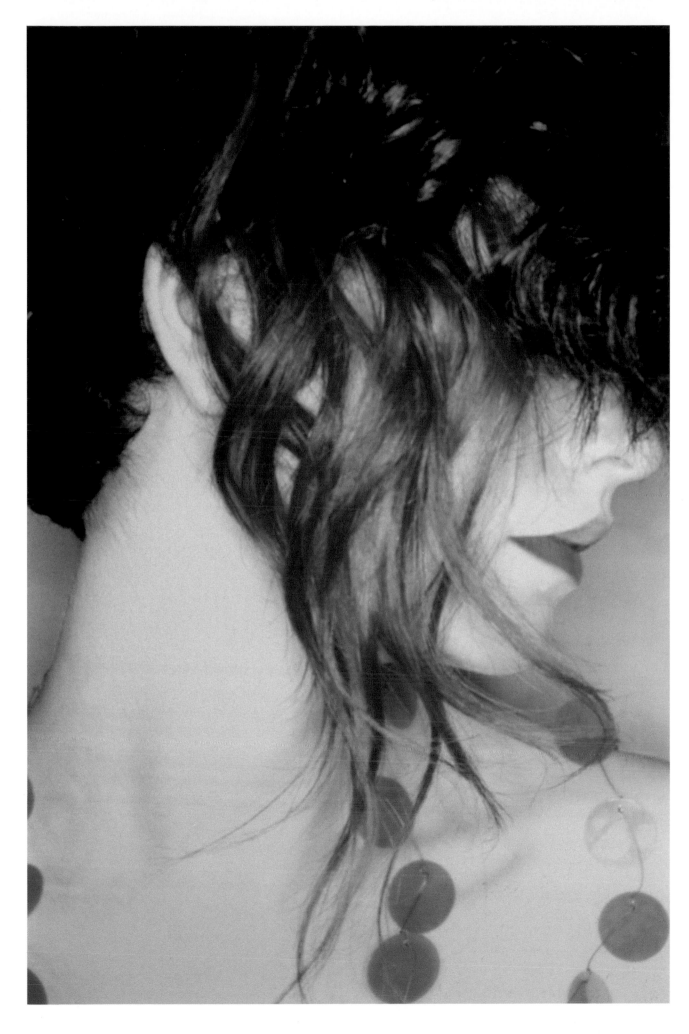

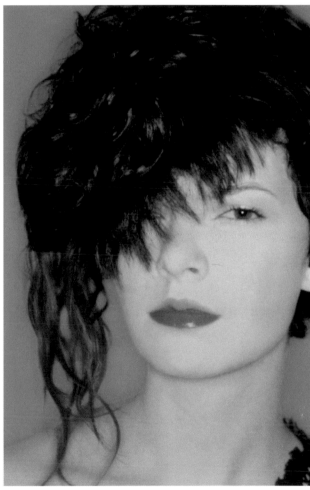

KRISAN pages 310–311

1 st Kikotö Boraross Ter, Budapest 1093, Hungary, www.kri-san.hu

Hair: Győző Krizsán
Salon: KriSan
Make-up: Viktória Bertalan
Styling: Zoltán Herczeg
Photography: Ádám Urbán
Models: Saci and Tissy

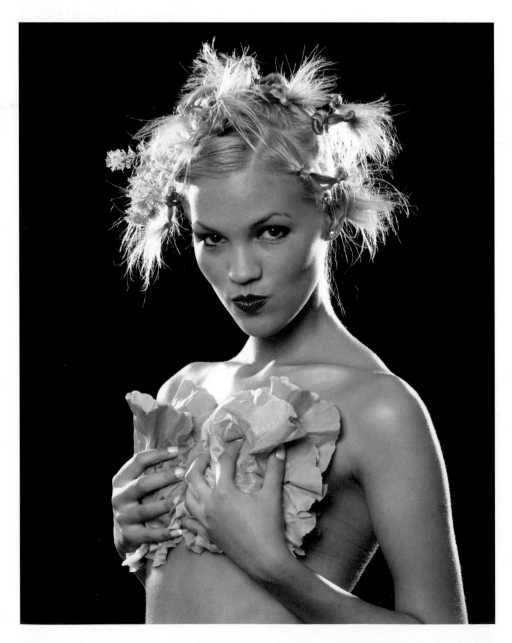

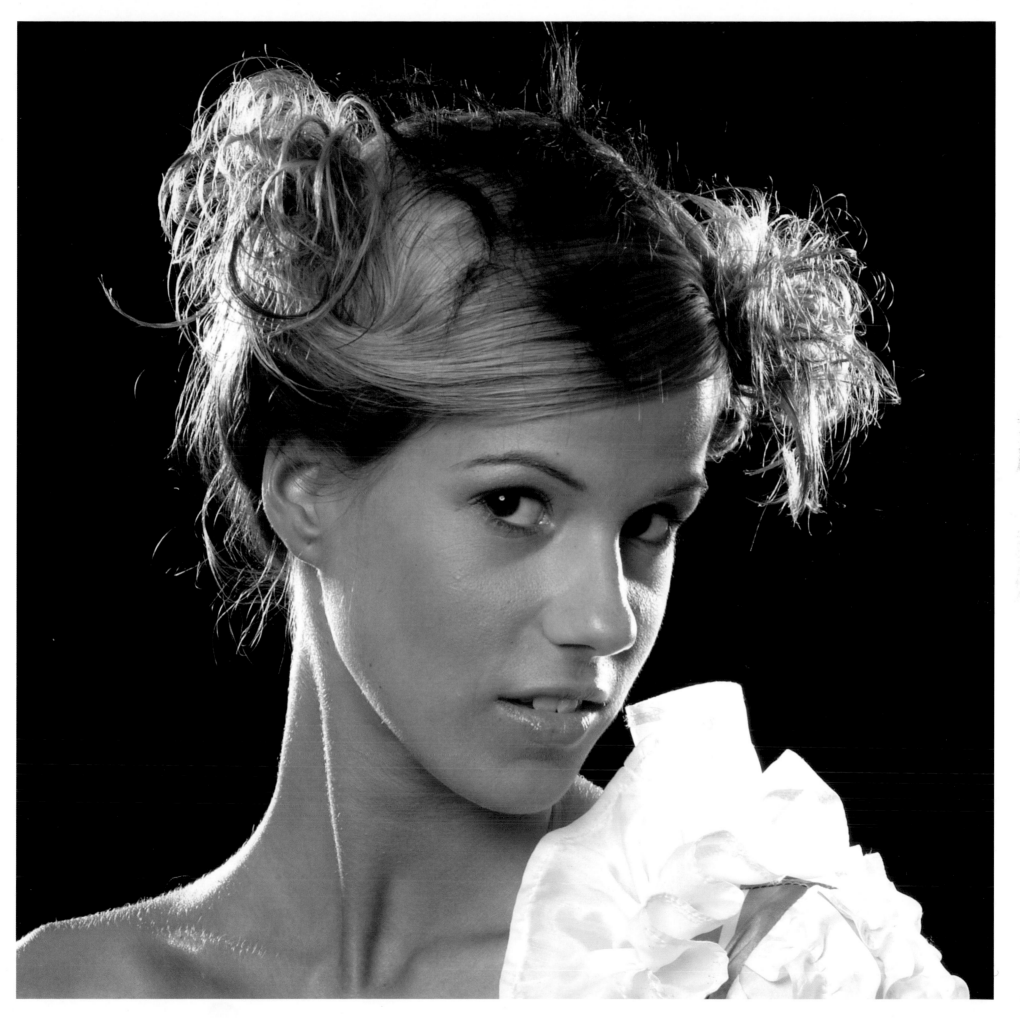

P.A.M. HAIR STYLE pages 312–313

Gontardplatz 10, 68163 Mannheim-Lindenhof, Germany, www.pam-hairstyle.de

Hair: Mandy van den Bosch-Macri
Salon: P.A.M. Hair Style
Photography: Rainer Zerback
Model: Olga Anselm

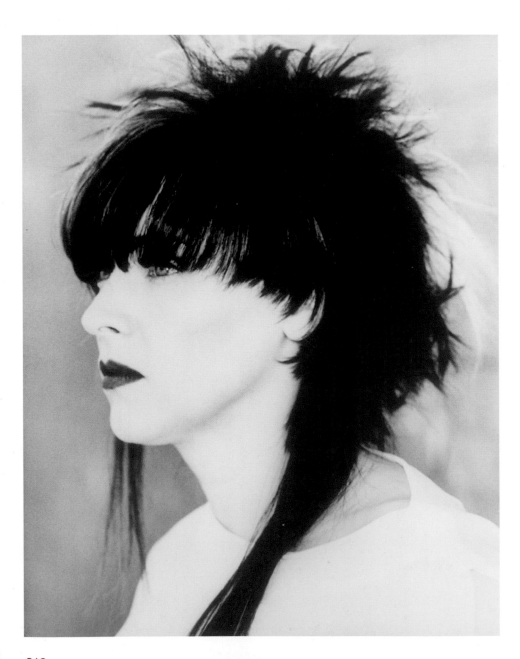

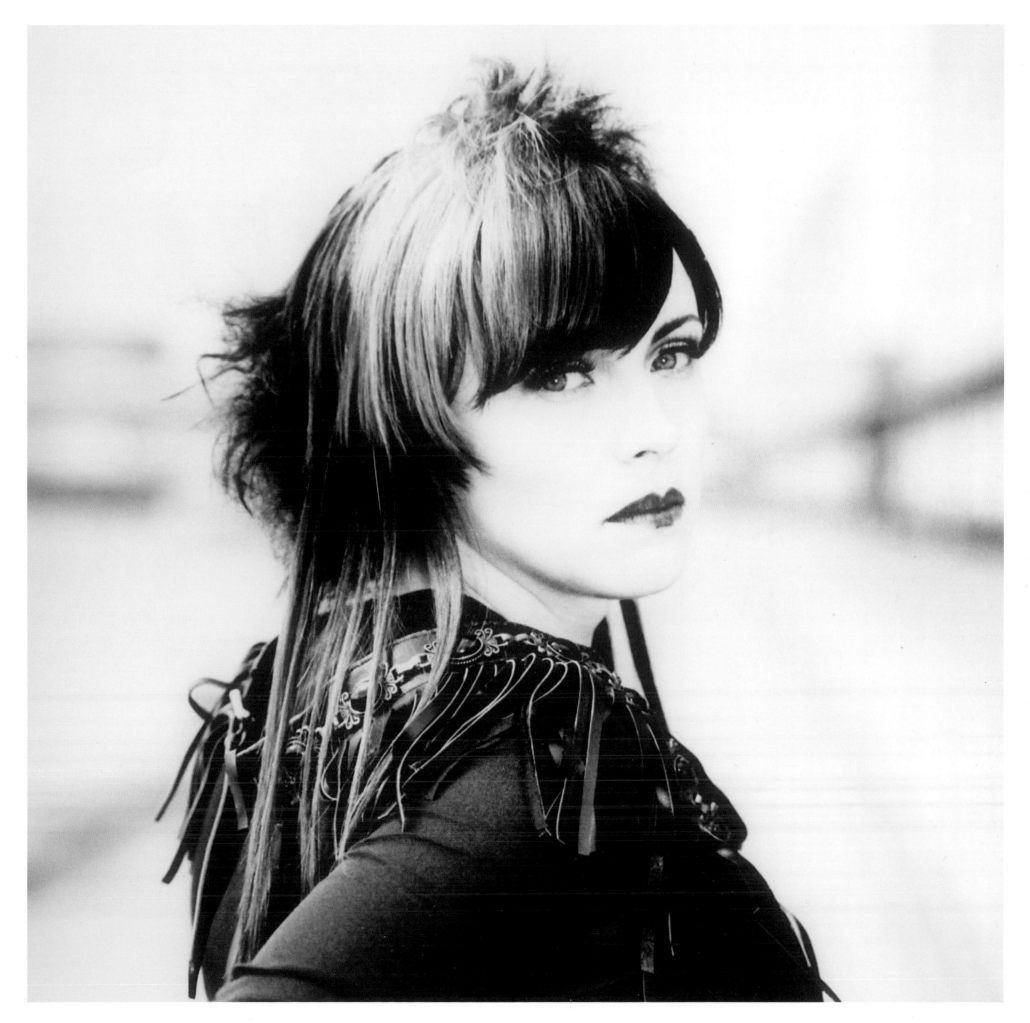

GO S GO pages 314–315

5-29-9 3F Jingmae, Shibya-ku, Tokyo 1500-0001, Japan, www.gosgo.jp

Hair: Shuij Kubota
Salon: Go s Go
Make-up: Yumi Iogi
Photography: Taro (Opuss)
Model: Maiko Akutagawa

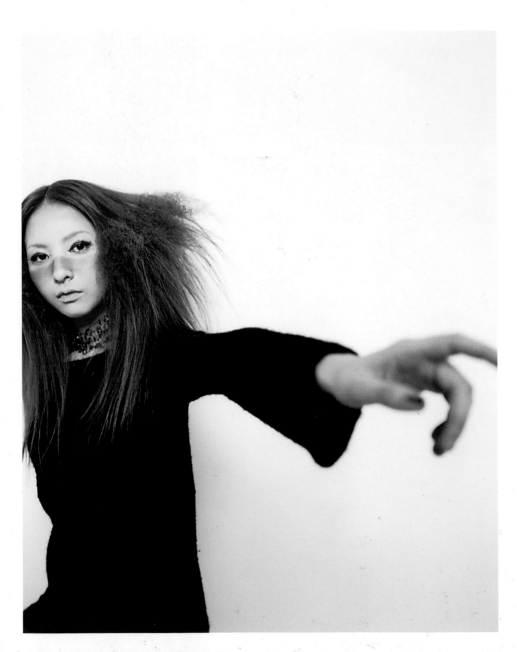

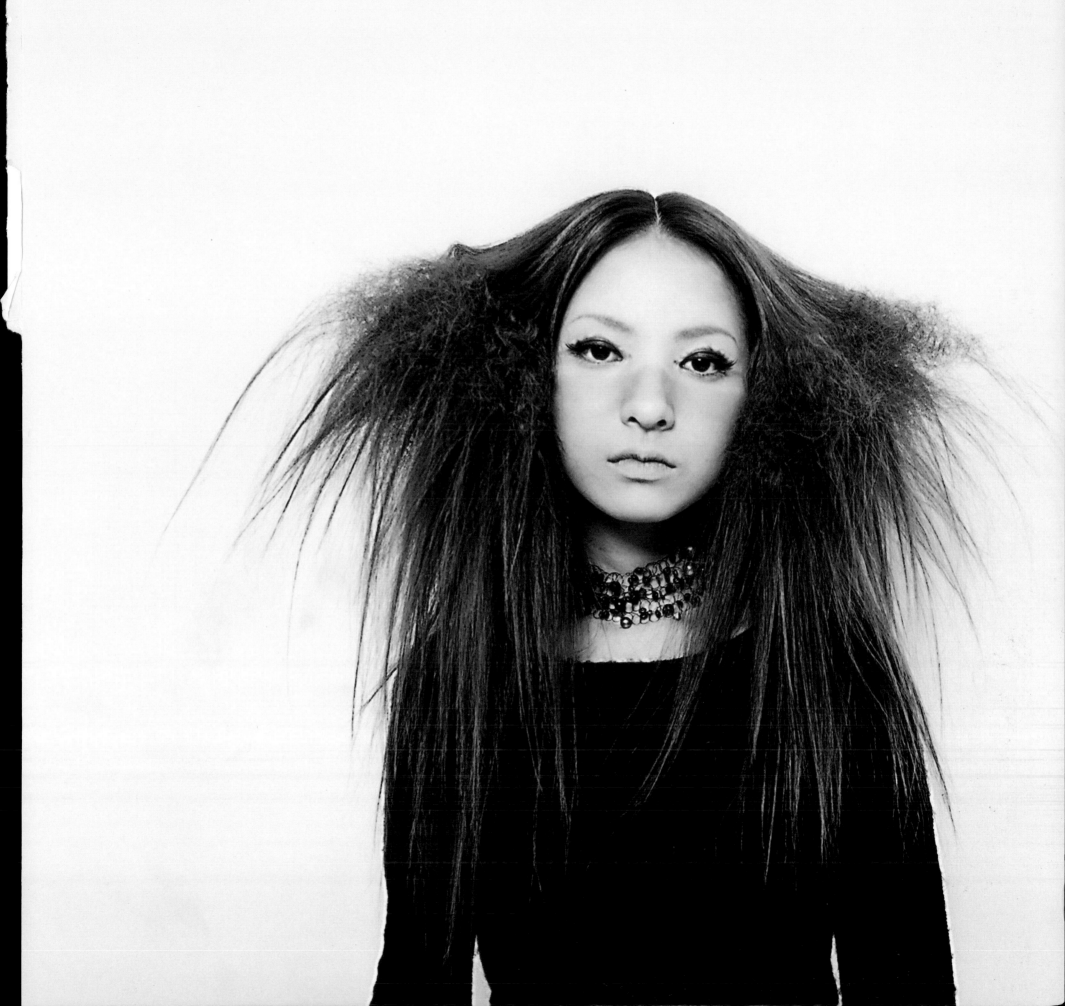

JEAN CLAUDE pages 316–317

Je sais Jean Claude, Via G. Paglia N. 19, I-24122 Bergamo, Italy,

Hair: Jean Claude
Photography: Gabriele Moleti

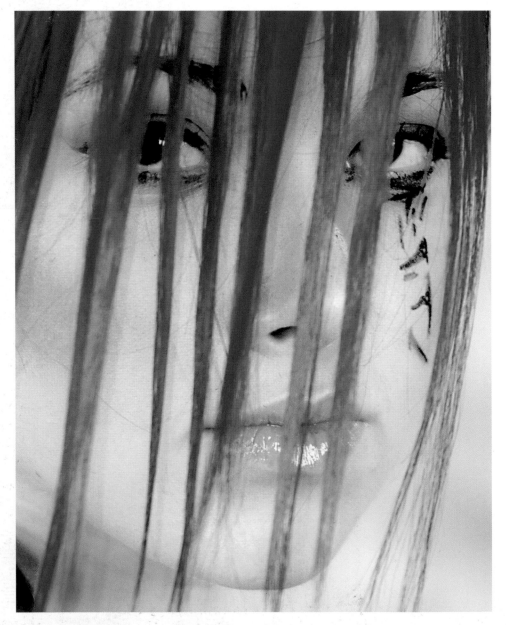

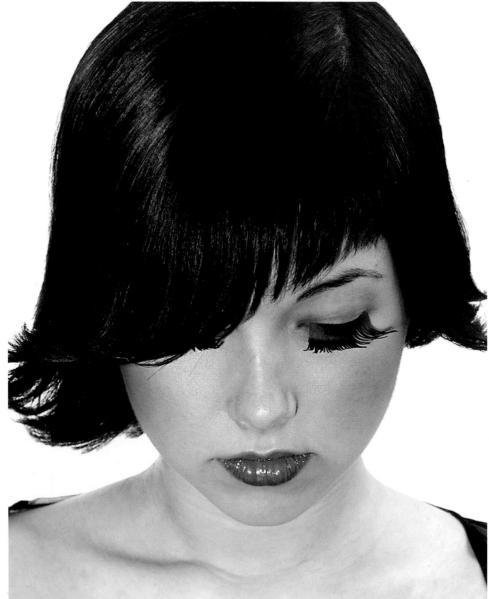

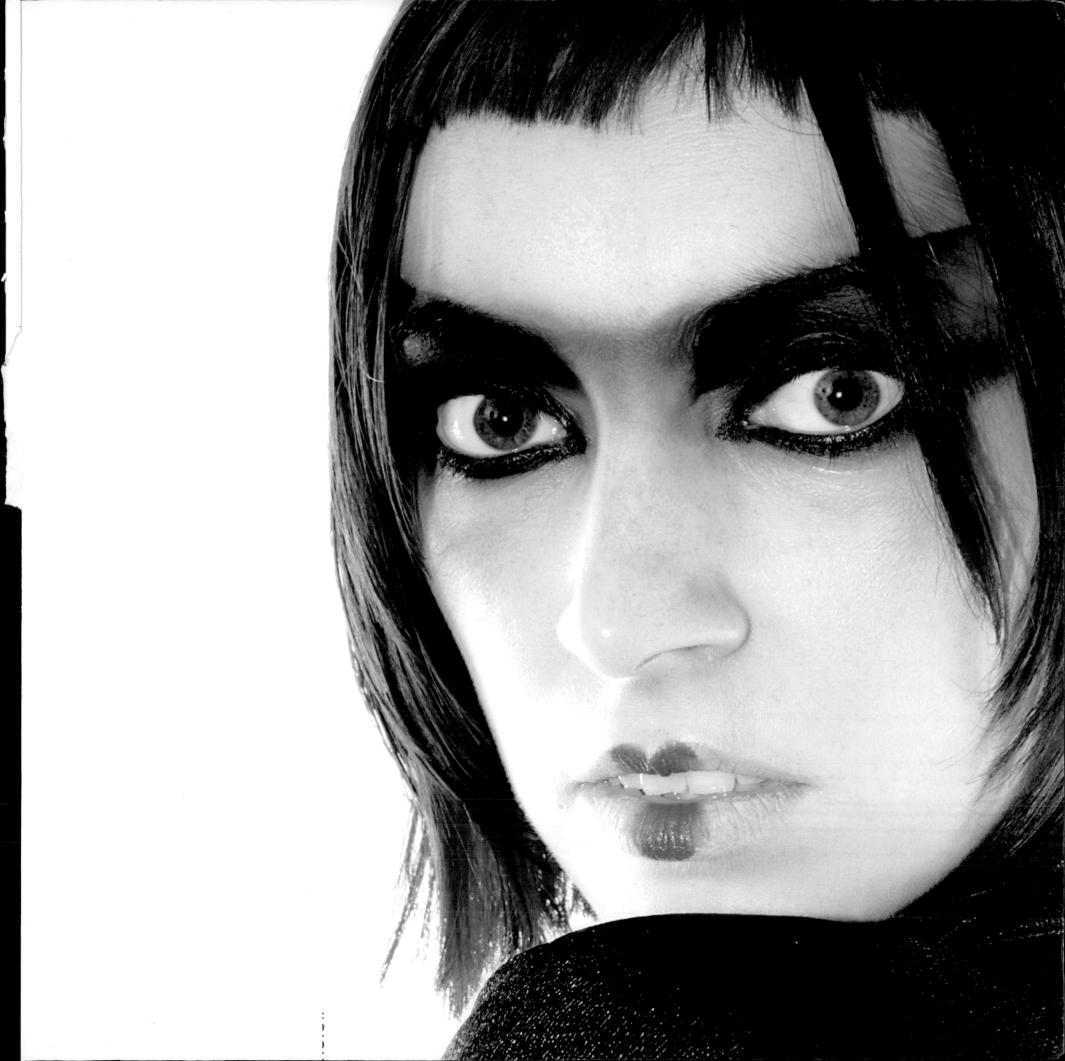

COUNTRY INDEX

Argentina

Silvia Aranza
Irigoyen 475
7300 Azul-Buenos Aires
Argentina

Austria

Concept Partizia Grecht
Operngasse 25
1040 Wien
Austria
www.concept-grecht.at

Australia

Cataldo's Salon
55 Northbourne Avenue
Canberra City ACT 2601
Australia
www.cataldos.com.au

Gritti Palace
66 Gawler Place
Adelaide SA 5000
Australia
www.grittypalace.com.au

Heading Out
225 Brunswick Street
Fitzroy VIC 3065
Australia

Mieka Hairdressing
308 Smith Street
Collingwood
Melbourne VIC 3306
Australia

Noddy's On King
88 King Street
Newton NWS 2042
Sydney
Australia

Raw Hair
95 Oxford Street
Darlinghurst NSW 2010
Australia

Tony & Guy St. Kilda
151 Fitzroy Street
St. Kilda VIC 3182
Australia

Tsiknaris Hair
169-171 Elizabeth Street
Brisbane QLD 4000
Australia
www.tsiknarishair.com

Bulgaria

Stylist Kapanov
14 Hristo Botev Blvd.
1000 Sofia
Bulgaria
www.kapanov.hit.bg

Canada

Entrenous
579 Richmond Street
London Ontario N6A 3G2
Canada
www.salonentrenous.com

Lounge Hair Studio
#100 - 1039 Richard Street
Vancouver BC V6B 3E4
Canada
www.loungehaistudio.com

Chile

Sebastián Ferrer
Av. Vitacura 5656
Vitacura
Santiago
Chile
www.sebastianferrer.cl

Czech Republic

Petra Mechurova Hair Design
Králodvorská 12
110 00 Praha 1
Czech Republic
www.petra.mechurova.cz

Denmark

Barikisu Larsen
Fælledvej 14C, 4th
DK 2200 København N
Denmark
www.barikisu.com

France

Sergio Bossi
38, rue Baron Le Roy
75012 Paris
France
www.sergiobossi.fr

Carpy Coiffeur
Ferme de la Liodère
37300 Joué-Lès-Tours
France
www.carpy.com

Claude Tarantino
Résidence de Villandry
4, rue Francois Lapierre
57120 Rombas
France

Eric Stipa
72, rue Nationale
37000 Tours
France
www.ericstipa.com

Jean Vallon
28, blvd. du Jeu de Paume
34000 Montpellier
France
www.jeanvallon.com

Germany

Beyer Friseur GmbH
Friedrich-Ebert-Straße 66
45468 Mülheim an der Ruhr
Germany
www.bybeyer.de

Capelli Group
Ziegeleistrasse 24 Tor 3
75417 Mühlacker
Germany
www.capelli-group.de

Michael Jung
Gärtnerstrasse 30
20253 Hamburg
Germany

Keller The School
Sindelfinger Straße 28
71032 Böblingen
Germany
www.keller-company.de

Marlies Möller GmbH
Neuer Wall 61
20354 Hamburg
Germany
www.marliesmoeller.com

Klaus Peter Ochs
KPOchs
Orber Straße 30
60386 Frankfurt am Main
Germany
www.kp-ochs.com

P.A.M. Hair Style
Gontardplatz 10
68163 Mannheim-Lindenhof
Germany
www.pam-hairstyle.de

Hungary

KriSan
1 st Kikotö Boraross Ter
Budapest 1093
Hungary
www.kri-san.hu

Indonesia

Rudy Hadisuwarno
Puri Pesanggrahan IV/NR 7
Bukit Cinere Indah
Jakarta 16514
Indonesia

Italy

Carlo Bay Hair Diffusion
Via Marsuppini 18 rosso
Firenze
Italy
www.carlobay.it

Jean Claude
Via G. Paglia n. 19
24122 Bergamo
Italy

Massimo Corsi
Via Roma 123
San Benedetto del Tronto
Italy

Gandini Club
Località Foroni 12
37067 Valeggio S/M (VR)
Italy
www.gandiniteam.com

James Hair Fashion Club
Via M. Curie 1/A
42100 Reggio Emilia
Italy
www.jameshairdiffusion.it

I Sargassi Training Centre
Via Ottaviano 6
(San Pietro)
00192 Roma (RM)
Italy

Studio Creativity
for Davines SPA
Via Ravasini 9/A
43100 Parma
Italy

Japan

Atelier KAZU
1-48-19-404
Sasazuka
Shibuya-ku
Tokyo
Japan
www.atelier-kazu.co.jp

Go s Go
5-29-9 3F
Jingumae
Shibuya-ku
Tokyo 150-0001
Japan
www.gosgo.jp

Kind Inc
351bld blf 3-5-1
Jingumae
Shibuya-ku
Tokyo 150-0001
Japan
www.hair-kind.co.jp

Malaysia

A Cut Above
Bangsar Shopping Center 285
Jalan Maarof 59000
Kuala Lumpur
Malaysia

Mexico

Antonio Bellver
Av. Coyoacán No. 425
Col del valle Entre Division
del Norte y Torres Adalid
C.P. 03100 México D.F.
Benito Juárez
Mexico
www.antoniobellver.com

New Zealand

Buoy
Skye Garden
Majestic Tower
100 Willis Street
Wellington
New Zealand
www.buoy.co.nz

Grace Hairdressing
64 Ghuznee
St. Wellington
New Zealand

Ginger Megg's & Associates
No. 7 St. Albans Street
Merival
Christchurch
New Zealand
www.gingermeggs.co.nz

Twistar Ltd.
189 Ridell Road
Glendowie
Auckland
New Zealand

Carl Watkins and Associates
74 Victoria Street
Christchurch
New Zealand

Norway

H2 Scandinavia AS
Thomas Angellsgt 5
7011 Trondheim
Norway
www.h2.no

The Philippines

Emphasis Salon
Rockwell Information Center
Estrella Cor. Amapola Sts.
Makati City 1200
Philippines

Poland

Jaga Hupalo & Thomas Wolff
Hair Studio
Ul. Burakowska 5/7
01-066 Warszawa
Poland
www.jagahairdesign.com

Russia

Academy of Hairdressing Art
Bolshoy Afanasjevsky
Pereulok 12
Stroenie 1
121019 Moscow
Russia
www.akd.ru

May Ltd.
Zanevskiy pr. 37
195112 St. Petersburg
Russia
www.may.spb.ru

Slovenia

Mic Styling
Sojer d.o.o. Trzaska 116
1000 Ljubljana
Slovenia
www.micstyling.com

Spain

Carité International
65 Tomas Montañana
46021 Valencia
Spain
www.newcarite.com

Cebado
Villarroel 40
08011 Barcelona
Spain
www.cebado.es

Carlos Gálico
P° Eduardo Dato N 2
28010 Madrid
Spain
www.carlosgalico.com

Llongueras
Berlin 39
08014 Barcelona
Spain
www.llongueras.com

Maricarmen Madrigal
Peluquerias
Sancho Dávila 31
28028 Madrid
Spain
www.peluquerias
madrigal.es

South Africa

Intercoiffure South Africa
ISJON
P.O. Box 4921
Halfway House 1685
Johannesburg
South Africa

Switzerland

Kuhn Intercoiffure
Tramstrasse 15
8050 Zürich
Switzerland
www.team-kuhn.ch

Taiwan

A-Square
61 Lane
233 TunHua S. Rd. Sec. 1
Taipei 106
Taiwan
www.a-square.com.tw

The Netherlands

Richard Koffijberg Hairdressers
Scheldestraat 8
1078 GK Amsterdam
The Netherlands
www.koffijberg.nl

Ad Peters
The Haircompany
P.O. Box 603
7400 AP Deventer
The Netherlands
www.adpeters.nl

United Kingdom

Antoinette Beenders
The Urban Retreat
174 High Holborn
London WC1 7AA
United Kingdom

Patrick Cameron
The Paddocks
Woodbank Lane
Chester CH1 6JD
United Kingdom
www.patrick-cameron.com

Damien Carney
London
United Kingdom
damienPcarney@aol.com

Clipso
57 Queens Road
Watford
Herts WD17 2QN
United Kingdom
www.clipso.demon.co.uk

Beverly Cobella
Cobella House
5 Kensington High Street
London W8 5NP
United Kingdom

Contemporary Hair
2 The Wynd
Marske-by-the-Sea
Saltburn TS11 7LA
United Kingdom

Anita Cox
62 Britton Street
Clerkwell
London EC1M 5UY
United Kingdom

Errol Douglas
18 Motcomb Street
The Halkins
Knightsbridge
London SW1X 8LB
United Kingdom
www.erroldouglas.com

Essensuals Hairdressing
19 Doughty Street
London WC1N 2PL
United Kingdom
www.essensuals.co.uk

Umberto Glannini
Warick House
159 Lower High Street
Stourbridge DY8 1TT
United Kingdom

Sean Hanna
26 The Broadway
Wimbledon
London SW19 1RE
United Kingdom

Haringtons
31 Green Lane
Nortwood Middlesex HA6 2PX
United Kingdom
www.haringtons.com

Headmasters
145-155 Ewell Road
Surbiton Surrey KT6 6AW
United Kingdom
www.hmhair.co.uk

Mark Hill Salon
Hogg Lane Kirkella
Hull North Humberside
HU10 7NU
United Kingdom
www.markhill.co.uk

Hype Coiffure
17 Tulse Hill
London SW2 2TH
United Kingdom

Ishoka Hairdressing & Beauty
11 Albyn Terrace
Aberdeen AB10 1YP
United Kingdom

Guy Kremer
Stonemasons Court
67 Parchment Street
Winchester SO23 8AT
United Kingdom

Jason Lea
Hairdressing Group
11 Lower Bridge Street
Chester
United Kingdom

McIntyre Hairdressing
50 Union Street
Dundee DD1 4BE
United Kingdom
www.mcintyres.co.uk

Medusa Hairdressing
6-7 Teviot Place
Edinburgh
United Kingdom
www.modusahair.co uk

Charlie Miller
13 Stafford Street
Edinburgh EH3 7BR
United Kingdom
www.charliemiller.co.uk

Hair & Beauty Partnership
60 Baker Street
London
United Kingdom

Stage Door
45 Horseferry Road
Westminster
London SW1
United Kingdom
www.stagedoor.co.uk

Trevor Sorbie International
27 Floral Street
Covent Garden
London WC2E 9DP
United Kingdom
www.trevorsorbie.com

Charlie Taylor
20-28 South Methven Street
Perth
United Kingdom

Richard Ward
162b Sloane Street
London SW1X 9BS
United Kingdom

USA

Teri Dougherty
1227 Muirkirk Court
Folsom California CA 95630
USA
www.teridougherty.com

Khamit Kinks
4 Leonard Street
New York N.Y. 10013
USA
www.khamitkinks.com

Stan Milton Salon
721 Miami Circle
Suite 102
Atlanta Georgia 30324
USA
www.stanmiltonsalon.com

Nedjetti
+973.923.4817
+646.236.6726 cell
USA
www.nedjetti.com
nedjetti@nedjettishhouseof
peace.com

ALPHABETICAL INDEX

A-Square 34
Academy of Hairdressing Art 66
A Cut Above 28
Silvia Aranza 126
Atelier KAZU 14
Carlo Bay Hair Diffusion 26
Antoinette Beenders 270
Antonio Bellver 102
Sergio Bossi 156
Buoy 160
By Beyer the Hair 274
Patrick Cameron 84
Capelli Group 286
Carité International 50
Damien Carney 196
Carpy Coiffeur 304
Cataldo's Salon 38
Cebado 180
Jean Claude 316
Clipso 290
Beverly Cobella 42
Contemporary Hair 130
Massimo Corsi 264
Anita Cox 8
Teri Dougherty 266
Errol Douglas 224
Entrenous 18
Emphasis Salon 214
Essensuals Hairdressing 148
Sebastián Ferrer 296
Carlos Gálico 178
Gandini Club 88
Umberto Giannini 280
Go s Go 314
Grace Hairdressing 198
Patrizia Grecht 140
Gritti Palace 114
Rudy Hadisuwarno 174
Hair Lounge 90
Sean Hanna 258
Haringtons 282
Heading Out 298
Headmasters 232
Mark Hill 260
Hype Coiffure 92
H2 Scandinavia AS 192
Intercoiffure South Africa ISJON 144
I Sargassi 46

Ishoka Hairdressing & Beauty 132
Jaga Hupalo & Thomas Wolff 52
James Hair Fashion Club 56
Michael Jung 48
Stylist Kapanov 182
Keller The School 284
Khamit Kinks 62
Kind Inc 158
Richard Koffijberg 118
Guy Kremer 24
KriSan 310
Kuhn Intercoiffure 122
Barikisu Larsen 60
Jason Lea 116
Llongueras 16
Lounge Hair Studio 3
Maricarmen Madrigal 306
May Ltd. 98
McIntyre Hairdressing 276
Petra Mechurova 70
Medusa Hairdressing 120
Ginger Megg's 72
Mic Styling 136
Mieka Hairdressing 124
Charlie Miller 238
Marlies Möller 302
Desmond Murray 74
Nedjetti 194
Noddy's On King 94
Klaus Peter Ochs 186
P.A.M. Hair Style 312
Roberto Perozzi 252
Ad Peters 82
Raw Hair 218
Trevor Sorbie International 248
Stage Door 228
Stan Milton Salon 68
Eric Stipa 128
Studio Creativity 202
Claude Tarantino 208
Charlie Taylor 204
Tony & Guy St. Kilda 262
Tsiknaris Hair 268
Twistar Ltd. 170
Jean Vallon 272
Richard Ward 246
Carl Watkins 112

151080